ASK YOUR GYNECOLOGIST

ASK YOUR GYNECOLOGIST

Answers to Over 200 (Sometimes Embarrassing) Questions Women Ask through Every Age and Stage of Their Lives

By
**R. Scott Thornton, MD, and
Kathleen Schramm, MD**

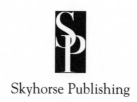

Skyhorse Publishing

10 9 8 7 6 5 4 3 2 1

Library of Congress Cataloging-in-Publication Data
Thornton, R. Scott.
Ask your gynecologist : answers to over 200 (sometimes embarrassing) questions women ask through every age and stage of their lives/ by R. Scott Thornton, MD and Kathleen Schramm, MD.
pages cm

Includes bibliographical references and index.

ISBN 978-1-62636-419-6 (alk. paper)

1. Gynecology—Miscellanea. 2. Generative organs, Female—Miscellanea. 3. Women—Health and hygiene—Miscellanea. I. Schramm, Kathleen. II. Title.
RG121.T486 2013
618—dc23
2013031956

ISBN: 978-1-62636-419-6

Printed in the United Sates of America.

Disclaimer

This book is intended as a reference volume only, not a definitive medical manual. The information is provided to help you make decisions regarding your health, but it is not intended to replace your medical doctors. This book should help you engage your doctors in meaningful discussion, but not replace their advice. If you suspect that you have a medical problem, you are encouraged to seek a professional healthcare provider. Prescribed medications and treatments should not be changed or discontinued without consulting the prescribing doctor and no new medication or treatment should be started without consulting a qualified healthcare provider.

Mention of specific brand name products, authorities, companies, and organizations does not imply endorsement of these by the authors or publisher. In addition, mention of specific companies, organizations, and authorities does not imply that these entities endorse the authors or the publisher. The brand names for drugs mentioned in this book are registered trademarks of their respective companies. The Internet addresses provided in this book are accurate as of the time this book went to press.

Acknowledgments

The authors would like to thank the following colleagues who have reviewed our book to ensure that its content is accurate and up-to-date:

Martin F. Freedman, MD
Co-Director
Division of Reproductive Endocrinology and Infertility
Temple University School of Medicine

Enrique Hernandez, MD, FACOG, FACS
The Abraham Roth Professor and Chair
Department of Obstetrics, Gynecology, and Reproductive Sciences
Section Chief, Gynecologic Oncology
Temple University School of Medicine

Beth Baughman DuPree, MD, FACS
Medical Director of the Holy Redeemer Breast Health Program
Adjunct Assistant Professor of Surgery at the University of Pennsylvania

Dr. Charles Lockwood, MD, MHCM
Dean, College of Medicine
Vice President for Health Sciences
Professor, Obstetrics and Gynecology
Ohio State University, Wexner Medical Center

The authors would also like to thank our agent Rita Rosenkranz (www.ritarosenkranzliteraryagency.com) for her encouragement and support in finding a home for our book and Emily Houlihan, our editor at Skyhorse Publishing, for polishing our text as needed.

Contents

Foreword • xxiii
Authors' Note • xxv
Introduction • xxvii

**Chapter 1: THE BIG PICTURE: WHEN TO SEE
A GYNECOLOGIST**

Why should I go to a gynecologist? • 1
How should I choose a gynecologist? • 3
What can I do if I'm too anxious and embarrassed to
    see a gynecologist? • 4
Why do I have such a hard time getting an
    appointment? • 5
When is the best time to schedule an
    appointment? • 6
Why do I have to wait so long in the doctor's waiting
    room? • 6
How often do I need to see a gynecologist? • 7
When should my daughter first see a
    gynecologist? • 8
My daughter has a problem and refuses to see a
    gynecologist. What should I do? • 8
Can my family doctor do the pelvic exam? • 9
Is douching a good idea? • 10
What do all those fancy words mean? • 11
What is the doctor doing during the
    examination? • 12
What is a Pap smear? • 15

How reliable are Pap smears? • 16

What is a mammogram? • 17

Are mammograms painful? • 18

Aren't mammograms dangerous? • 19

How reliable are mammograms? • 19

Why do I have to get a breast ultrasound? • 21

If breast MRI is more sensitive than mammography, should I get that instead of a mammogram? • 22

How can I lose this weight? • 23

What medications help you lose weight? • 28

When is surgery indicated for obesity? • 30

What can I do if I have pain? • 31

Chapter 2: THE MENSTRUAL CYCLE: WHAT'S NORMAL, WHAT'S NOT?

What's a normal cycle? • 37

I'm late for my period. Am I pregnant? • 38

I get my period only two or three times during the year. Is that okay? • 39

When my period comes, I flood. Is that normal? • 42

What does it mean when I get clots during my period? • 43

Is bleeding between my periods normal? • 43

Why do I get pain in the middle of my cycle? • 44

I get terrible cramps with my period. What's wrong? • 45

What can I do if I have PMS? • 46

I always get a headache at the beginning of my period. Why? • 51

My daughter is fifteen and still hasn't gotten her period. Should I be worried? • 53

Are tampons safe? • 54

Chapter 3: CONTRACEPTION: WEIGHING THE ALTERNATIVES

Is it possible to get pregnant the first time I have sex? • 56

What is natural family planning? • 56

What is barrier contraception? • 57

Is withdrawal a good method of contraception? • 60

How good are over-the-counter spermicides? • 61

Why should I use the birth control pill? • 61

Aren't birth control pills dangerous? • 62

What are all the side effects from the pill? • 64

Are there any medications I can't take with the pill? • 65

What should I do if I miss a pill? • 66

Will I have trouble getting pregnant when I stop taking the pill? • 67

Some birth control pills let you skip periods. Is there any reason not to use these? • 67

What is the minipill? • 68

What is the "morning-after" pill? • 69

What is the birth control device that is placed in the arm? • 71

I hear that there are shots that prevent pregnancy. Is that true? • 72

Are IUDs safe? • 73

How can I tell if my IUD is in place? • 75

How do I know which method of contraception is best for me? • 76

How are abortions done? • 77

Can I have a normal pregnancy after having an abortion? • 80

How is a tubal ligation done? Is it safe? • 80

Can my tubes be put back together? • 82

Why have my periods been irregular since my tubal
   sterilization? • 82
Is it better for my husband to have a
   vasectomy than for me to undergo a tubal
   sterilization? • 83
If I'm in menopause, can I still get
   pregnant? • 84

Chapter 4: SEXUAL RELATIONS

Why does it hurt when I have sex? • 85
Why don't I have orgasms? • 90
Where is the "G-spot"? • 95
Why don't I have any sex drive? • 95
Will my sexual pleasure decrease after a
   hysterectomy? • 98
Is oral sex dangerous? • 99
Is anal sex safe? • 100

Chapter 5: PELVIC INFECTIONS

Why does my vagina itch? • 102
Why do I keep getting yeast infections? • 104
Are yeast infections dangerous? • 106
How are yeast infections treated? • 107
Will yogurt or other natural products keep me from
   getting yeast infections? • 108
I have discharge but no itching or burning. Is that
   normal? • 111
What is PID? • 113
How can I tell the difference between a bladder
   infection and other pelvic infections? • 116
Do people still get syphilis? • 117
I have bumps that feel like warts. What are
   they? • 118

What is that painful sore down there? • 122

Can women get AIDS? • 126

Can you get hepatitis through sex? • 128

If I get a sexually transmitted infection, should I be
    tested for others? • 130

Why can't the gynecologist cure my
    infection? • 130

What can I do to avoid getting a sexually transmitted
    infection? • 131

How do I cope emotionally when I discover that I
    have a sexually transmitted infection? • 132

Chapter 6: WHY CAN'T I GET PREGNANT?

I've been trying to get pregnant for six months. Does
    this mean I have a problem? • 135

When is the best time in my cycle for
    conception? • 136

Do I need to see an infertility specialist? • 136

What is a BBT chart? • 137

How can the gynecologist tell if I have a
    problem? • 137

What about my husband? Should he be
    checked? • 144

Why does the doctor want to perform a
    laparoscopy? • 146

What is artificial insemination? • 146

When am I too old to get pregnant? • 147

Are there natural approaches that increase
    fertility? • 149

I hear that infertility drugs cause ovarian cancer. Is
    that true? • 151

Why do I feel as if I'm riding an emotional roller
    coaster? • 152

Chapter 7: **WHEN SOMETHING GOES WRONG: COMPLICATIONS OF EARLY PREGNANCY**

I missed my period and have a positive pregnancy test. Now I'm bleeding. Am I having a miscarriage? • 155

What needs to be done if I'm having a miscarriage? • 156

Why did I have a miscarriage? • 157

How long should I wait after a miscarriage before trying again? • 158

I had two miscarriages. Is there something wrong with me? • 158

What is a tubal pregnancy? • 161

I am pregnant and have pain. Do I have a tubal pregnancy? • 163

Is surgery always necessary to treat a tubal pregnancy? • 164

Can I get pregnant again after a tubal pregnancy? • 165

Chapter 8: **ENDOMETRIOSIS: THE GREAT MASQUERADER**

I was told I have endometriosis. What is that? • 166

If I have painful periods, does it mean that I have endometriosis? • 168

What other symptoms characterize endometriosis? • 168

How is endometriosis diagnosed and treated? • 169

If I have endometriosis, does that mean I can't get pregnant? • 173

Will endometriosis come back? • 174

My doctor said I'll eventually need a hysterectomy
because of my endometriosis. Is that
necessary? • 175

What happens to my endometriosis after
menopause? • 175

Chapter 9: DISORDERS OF THE UTERUS

What are fibroids? • 176

Will my fibroids turn into cancer? • 177

What problems do fibroids cause? • 177

When do fibroids need treatment? • 178

Can fibroids be treated with medications? • 180

What type of surgery is used to remove
fibroids? • 181

Are there any other nonsurgical treatments for
fibroids? • 185

Can fibroids grow back? • 186

Where do polyps come from? • 187

Can polyps turn into cancer? • 187

How are polyps removed? • 187

My doctor said my heavy bleeding is from
adenomyosis. Is that the same as
endometriosis? • 188

How can the gynecologist tell if I have
adenomyosis? • 189

How is adenomyosis treated? • 189

I'm sixty years old, and now I'm bleeding. Does that
mean I have cancer? • 190

What is endometrial cancer? • 191

How did I get endometrial cancer? • 192

How is endometrial cancer diagnosed? • 193

Why didn't this show up on my
Pap smear? • 194

Do I need a hysterectomy to treat endometrial
    cancer? • 194
I'm scared. What will happen if I don't do
    anything? • 194
I had a hysterectomy for endometrial cancer, and
    now my doctor says I need radiation therapy.
    Is that really necessary? • 195
Can I use hormone replacement after treatment for
    endometrial cancer? • 202
How often should I see the doctor after my treatment
    for endometrial cancer? • 202
My Pap smear is abnormal. Does that mean I have
    cancer? • 203
If my Pap smear is abnormal, why isn't the doctor
    doing something about it? • 203
What cervical conditions are
    precancerous? • 204
How do you diagnose LSIL and HSIL? • 205
How do you treat LSIL and HSIL? • 206
Why is my doctor treating my SIL differently
    than someone I know who has the same
    thing? • 207
Will SIL come back again after
    treatment? • 208
If the SIL can recur, why don't you just do a
    hysterectomy? • 208
What's the difference between cervical SIL and
    cervical cancer? • 209
How will I know if I have cervical
    cancer? • 209
How do you diagnose and treat cervical
    cancer? • 210
What are my chances of surviving cervical
    cancer? • 212

Chapter 10: DISORDERS OF THE OVARY

I was told I have a cyst. What is that? • 213

Why do I have pain from my ovarian
cyst? • 215

Do I need surgery if I have a cyst? • 217

What type of surgery is done for ovarian
cysts? • 218

How does the doctor know that my cyst is not
cancerous? • 218

The doctor says I have an ovarian tumor. Does
that mean I have cancer? • 219

Does ovarian cancer run in families? • 220

Are there screening tests for ovarian cancer? • 221

What symptoms will I have if I develop ovarian
cancer? • 222

If the tumor is on my ovary, why does the doctor
want to perform a hysterectomy? • 223

The doctor says all of the cancer was removed. Why
do I need chemotherapy? • 224

I know people who had chemotherapy
and died anyway, so why should I take
chemotherapy? • 224

Will I get sick from chemotherapy? • 227

How long will I get chemotherapy? • 228

Can I be cured, or will my cancer come
back? • 229

Chapter 11: PROBLEMS OF THE VAGINA AND VULVA

What is that lump by my vagina? • 231

Why do I keep getting boils? • 232

I constantly have burning in my vulva.
What can I do? • 234

The doctor wants to do a biopsy of the skin on my
   vulva. Does that mean I have
   cancer? • 236
How is vulvar cancer treated? • 237
Can you get vaginal cancer? • 238

Chapter 12: PROBLEMS OF THE BREAST

Why do my breasts hurt? • 240
Are breast implants dangerous? • 243
Can anything be done if my breasts are too
   large? • 244
I have a tender area in my breast. Does that mean I
   have cancer? • 245
Why does the doctor want to aspirate my breast
   lump? • 245
What does discharge from the nipple
   indicate? • 247
Is there anything I can do to prevent breast
   cancer? • 249
Is my risk of breast cancer increased if my mother
   had breast cancer? When should I get genetic
   testing? • 250
How can I tell if I have breast
   cancer? • 254
When is a breast biopsy necessary? • 256
Do I need to have my entire breast removed
   if there is cancer? • 257
I hear they can reconstruct your breast.
   Is that true? • 259
Why do I need radiation therapy after a
   lumpectomy? • 260
When is chemotherapy necessary? • 262
What is hormonal therapy? • 263

I was told I have CIS. Is that the same as breast
  cancer? • 266
How do you treat breast cancer that has spread to
  other parts of the body? • 267

Chapter 13: MENOPAUSE AND HORMONE REPLACEMENT: THE GREAT DEBATE

When will I reach menopause? • 270
Why do I have trouble sleeping? • 270
What is a hot flash? • 273
Why is sex painful since I stopped getting
  periods? • 274
I don't seem to have any sex drive. Is that because
  of menopause? • 275
I feel depressed. Does menopause
  cause that? • 277
What is the latest update on hormone
  replacement therapy? • 279
What type of hormones should I take? How are they
  given? • 282
What about bioidentical hormones? • 284
Do I have to wait until I stop getting periods to
  begin hormone replacement therapy? • 286
Is there an age at which it is too late to start
  hormone replacement therapy? • 287
Should I avoid hormones because they cause
  cancer? • 287
What side effects will I get from hormone
  replacement? • 289
Are there women who can't take
  hormones? • 291
What else can I take for my symptoms other than
  hormones? • 292

What are those new drugs that are supposed to
   replace estrogen, and are they safer? • 298
How can I tell if I have osteoporosis and what can
   be done to prevent it? • 300
What medications are used to treat
   osteoporosis? • 304

**Chapter 14: WHERE'S THE NEAREST
BATHROOM?**

Why do I always have to run to the
   bathroom? • 309
Is it normal to get up at night to go to the
   bathroom? • 312
Why do I lose urine when I cough or
   sneeze? • 313
Why do I keep getting bladder infections? • 317
What are those tests the doctor wants me to
   do? • 319
My doctor says I have interstitial cystitis. What's
   that? • 322

**Chapter 15: PELVIC PROLAPSE: THE "DROPPED
BLADDER"**

What is that bulge down there? • 327
How did this happen? • 328
What symptoms will I have from prolapse? • 328
I lose my urine. Is that because of my dropped
   bladder? • 329
Is pelvic prolapse dangerous? • 329
What can I do to keep my prolapse from getting
   worse? • 330
How is prolapse corrected? • 331
I hear that surgery doesn't always work.
   Why? • 334

Chapter 16: WHEN YOU NEED SURGERY

What are the complications of surgery? • 338

How long will I be in the hospital? • 345

Will I be "knocked out" during surgery, or can I have a local anesthetic? • 346

Why do I need a catheter in my bladder? • 348

What can I get to relieve pain after surgery? • 348

Will I feel nauseous after surgery? • 349

When can I return to work? • 350

What restrictions will I have after surgery? • 352

What is robotic surgery? • 353

What is the difference between a complete hysterectomy and a partial hysterectomy? • 354

When I have a hysterectomy, should my ovaries also be removed? • 355

How will the doctor perform my hysterectomy? • 356

Will a hysterectomy put me into menopause? • 357

Why do I have to be examined if I had a hysterectomy? • 358

If I have an ovarian tumor, does the whole ovary need to be removed? • 359

Will I need to take hormones after the surgery? • 359

Why do I need a catheter for so long after bladder surgery? • 360

Why am I losing urine after my bladder surgery? • 360

Why do I have pain in my shoulder after laparoscopic surgery? • 362

Why do I have so many incisions on my
   abdomen? • 362
Is laparoscopic surgery safer than regular
   surgery? • 362
Can I have laparoscopic surgery as an
   outpatient? • 363
How much pain will I have after laparoscopic
   surgery? • 364
Can hysteroscopy be done in the office? • 364
How much pain and bleeding will I have after a
   hysteroscopy? • 364

Epilogue • 365
Glossary • 366
Index • 383

Foreword

Having practiced obstetrics and gynecology for decades, I can tell you that our world can be a frightful place for any woman who doesn't know what to expect. Having come from a large extended family, I answer questions weekly from third cousins once removed about every aspect of their obstetrical and gynecologic concerns from pregnancies to ovarian cysts. However, not every woman has such a resource! One alternative to having a gynecologist for a relative is the Internet. But I have found that the explosion of data pouring out from the Internet can be paralyzing. Whom do you trust? Are you looking in the right place? Why are there so many different answers? These are only a few of the obstacles that women face before gathering the courage to make an appointment with their gynecologist.

I have known Dr. Scott Thornton since my medical student days. He was my chief resident and a terrific mentor: wise, well informed, and unflappable. Dr. Kathleen Ann Schramm adds her unique perspective as a psychiatrist. Together, they make a perfect team to render obstetrics and gynecology understandable to the lay audience, to serve as every woman's family doctor.

Over the years, I have dedicated much of my time to writing, reviewing, and editing numerous journals and textbooks to educate current and future physicians and I do it now on a daily basis as a dean. I have also spent countless long and sleepless nights caring for women with complicated and high-risk pregnancies. Needless to say, I have a little bit of experience in this field. Despite being an OB/GYN veteran, I never appreciated how critical the information in this book will be to women until I read it.

Throughout this book, Scott and Kathleen review the very basic to the very complex while keeping it easily digestible for those who do not have an RN, PA, CNM, MD, or DO behind their names. They give you honest and accurate information and advice on a variety of problems from yeast infections to breast cancer. Even more importantly, they keep you well apprised of some of the controversies in our field that could be important to you as you seek advice from your physician. Ultimately, you are getting an insider's view of the field of gynecology from a great physician team. Forget trying to find a doctor to join your family, as you now have a trusted gynecologist at your beck and call.

Dr. Charles Lockwood, MD, MHCM
Dean, College of Medicine
Vice President for Health Sciences
Professor, Obstetrics and Gynecology
Ohio State University, Wexner Medical Center

Authors' Note

Throughout *Ask Your Gynecologist*, we often include complementary and alternative medical (CAM) treatments for various gynecologic disorders. Complementary and alternative options are gradually gaining acceptance, not just with the public, but also with traditional medical practitioners. In some cases, their use is long overdue, but in other cases we seem to be putting the cart before the horse. In other words, herbs and supplements are often utilized without well-designed studies demonstrating their efficacy and safety. Keep in mind that the FDA (Food and Drug Administration) does not approve or regulate the manufacturing or sale of herbs and supplements.

The United States Pharmacopeia does enforce some standards in the manufacturing process. Companies that produce herbs meeting their requirements have the "USP Dietary Supplement Verified" seal of approval on their label. Looking for herbs with this stamp can help reassure you that you are buying a product with some quality.

You can join www.ConsumerLab.com, which conducts independent research on herbs and supplements. Also, if a label or advertisement says that a product has been scientifically tested, consider contacting the company for a copy of the study. Your doctor can review the study and help you determine the value of the research, the potential benefits of the herb or supplement for your condition, and the likelihood of adverse reactions based upon the study. Many doctors remain open to CAM treatments, even those that do not appear in traditional medical journals, but they will usually demand reasonable evidence of efficacy and safety based upon well-designed research. Just like traditional FDA-approved medications, herbs and supplements can have the potential for side effects and adverse reactions; you can't assume that a product is effective or safe just because it says so on the label or is available over the counter.

Many traditional gynecologists and general practitioners have little or no experience with using herbal supplements. Before using herbal products, consult a health professional with a background in complementary and alternative medicine, or at least consult a reputable online practitioner such as Dr. Andrew Weil (www.drweil.com) or Cathy Wong (www.altmedicine.about.com). You can also see if the Mayo Clinic (www.mayoclinic.com) or the National Center for Complementary and Alternative Medicine at the National Institute of Health (www.nccam.nih.gov) has reviewed the herb or supplement.

Introduction

You have a question to ask a gynecologist. Maybe it's about premenstrual syndrome, menopause, or that annoying pain that appears below your belly button. It isn't an emergency. Being considerate, you don't bother the doctor with a phone call. It only seems fair that you make an appointment to discuss this properly.

You nearly hit a car trying to decipher the multitude of signs outside the office building. There must be two hundred names on the directory at the entrance, but eventually you find the correct office. Terrific, you're right on time.

You spend another twenty minutes completing the questionnaire handed to you by the receptionist. Who dreams up these information sheets anyway? Even Uncle Sam doesn't get this personal.

Finally, the nurse calls you back to an examining room. Apparently, the staff forgot to pay the heating bill. The temperature is more conducive to chilling a Chardonnay than examining a naked woman. The nurse asks you to empty your bladder. She instructs you to totally disrobe. (Is it too late to back out now?) You put on a disposable gown made of tissue paper. You've been instructed to leave it open in the front. Well, you didn't really expect to maintain modesty, did you?

After an eternity, the doctor finally arrives. "Hello, I'm Doctor Stewart. What brings you in today?" Now is your chance. You ask your question, and the doctor magically transforms into one of the following:

- *The Great Evader:* He or she starts to give a reasonable reply, only to deftly switch in mid-response to a topic of no significance—one that is easier to discuss, such as the weather.

- *The Humorist*: He or she makes light of the situation. This relieves some of the tension that naturally occurs in a sensitive discussion, but still doesn't answer your question.

- *The Great Escape Artist*: He or she defers the question until the end of the examination and then mumbles a perfunctory response while backing out of the door, wishing you a pleasant day.

- *The Well-Intentioned but Desperately Short-of-Time Physician*: We hope most doctors fall into this category. They are well informed on a variety of topics pertinent to their specialty, but because of a large volume of patients, their schedule allows only ten to fifteen minutes per patient. They will do their best to give you informative answers, but often lack time to adequately address the issue.

As physicians, we empathize with both the patient and her doctor in this predicament. Periodically, we present seminars within our community. A worthy overview of almost any topic generally consumes one hour. Your doctor can't possibly spend that much time with a patient in the office on a regular basis and survive in today's medical climate—it is uncommon to schedule more than twenty minutes per patient. Brochures or videos can help educate patients, but they often don't provide enough information and tend to be impersonal.

We also realize that many women have questions that they never ask. Anxiety (let's be honest—going to the gynecologist is not the easiest task in the world) may cause anyone to forget to ask important questions. Some topics just seem too embarrassing to bring up. Many women deem their questions too "stupid" to ask.

With this in mind, *Ask Your Gynecologist* was conceived. It is dedicated to all of the women who have walked into a gynecologist's office with a question and left with an unsatisfactory answer (or left without asking the question). We will examine the most commonly asked questions and give valuable insight and advice.

Before starting, we want to tell you a little about ourselves. After all, you should know the background of the authors who are giving you advice. Dr. Thornton is an expert in the field of gynecology. He graduated from the University of Pennsylvania School of Medicine and completed a residency in obstetrics and gynecology at Pennsylvania Hospital, one of the premier training programs in Philadelphia. Since that time, he has maintained an extremely successful private practice at Holy Redeemer Hospital and Medical Center, just outside Philadelphia. Dr. Thornton currently serves as Director of New Horizons Menopause Center and Chairman of the Cancer Committee at Holy Redeemer Hospital and Medical Center. He maintains a fellowship at the American College of Obstetrics and Gynecology. Dr. Thornton is the founder and director of Women's Health Seminars, an organization dedicated to the education of women.

Dr. Schramm graduated from the Medical College of Pennsylvania, where she earned her medical degree, completed a residency in psychiatry, served as Chief Resident, and was awarded multiple honors. She then completed a fellowship in Child and Adolescent Psychiatry and subsequently served as Director of the Child and Adolescent Residency Program. She thrives in a private practice in child, adolescent, and adult psychiatry at Southampton Psychiatric Associates in Ivyland, Pennsylvania. Her multiple roles of female physician, psychiatrist, and wife of a gynecologist (she is married to Dr. Thornton) provide Dr. Schramm with a unique perspective on the physical and emotional difficulties women face in gynecology.

Although we are providing you with valuable information on a variety of gynecologic conditions, never forget that your best resource is still a personal gynecologist. Keep in mind the following pointers when you consult a gynecologist:

1. *Don't make assumptions!* When you develop a symptom such as unusual bleeding, pelvic pain, or vaginal discharge, don't assume that a disaster is brewing. Your symptom may not indicate a problem. Keep in mind that most gynecologic disorders are not life-threatening and can be remedied. On the other hand, don't assume that your symptom is normal. Most delays

in treatment occur because patients fail to seek appropriate attention.

2. *Avoid self-treatment.* It's been said, "He who treats himself has a fool for a patient." Always see a professional for evaluation and treatment. The people you hear plugging various cures over television, radio, and the Internet aren't paid to solve your problem. They're paid to sell a product. Using over-the-counter products without the advice of a medical professional is playing Russian roulette with your health. Likewise, this book is not intended to replace your gynecologist. It should supplement the information he or she provides and give you a basis for meaningful discussion.

3. *Educate yourself.* Educate yourself, but choose your resources carefully. We have tried to provide unbiased information in this book. Books, pamphlets, and audiovisual resources produced by the American College of Obstetricians and Gynecologists or other reputable medical institutions are reliable sources of information. Your doctor may have these or other resources available in the office. Be leery of information transmitted through television news shows, magazines, and Internet blogs and forums, which is often oversimplified or distorted.

4. *Don't be afraid to ask "dumb" questions.* The odds are pretty good that your doctor has heard the same question from many other women. Make a note of your questions when you think of them. There is a good chance that you'll forget a question when you get to the office if it is not written down.

5. *Communicate clearly with your doctor's office.* When you call the office, state whether your problem is urgent. Your doctor will find time to see you promptly if the problem is really an emergency. But don't cry wolf. If you portray everything as an emergency, your doctor may eventually learn to ignore your complaints. If you anticipate a lengthy visit because you have a complex problem or an extensive medical history, inform the receptionist and ask for more time. If the

receptionist cannot accommodate you, ask to speak with the physician or find a new doctor.

6. *Don't compare yourself to other people.* Doctors cringe when they hear "My Aunt Ginny had this same problem and her doctor said . . ." Every patient and problem presents a unique set of circumstances. Recommendations applicable to one patient may not be appropriate for another. We have also seen patients ignore recommendations because their mother (or uncle, or neighbor . . . the list goes on) didn't "think it was a good idea." If you feel uncomfortable with your doctor's recommendation, ask more questions or seek a second opinion. Don't be influenced by people—no matter how much they love you—who do not have medical credentials.

7. *Trust your doctor, but don't blindly follow the advice.* When your doctor recommends a specific treatment, he or she should explain the rationale behind it. If further clarification is necessary, ask more questions. If you still feel uncomfortable, seek a second opinion. But avoid the tendency to run around obtaining multiple second opinions. If your doctor meets the following criteria, you are probably in good hands. He or she should:

   • Have a good reputation among other healthcare professionals.
   • Offer rational, concise explanations for his or her recommendations.
   • Provide you with alternatives and options when they exist.
   • Have extensive experience in dealing with the disorder in question.

Without further delay, let's embark on our exploration of the world of gynecology.

1

THE BIG PICTURE: WHEN TO SEE A GYNECOLOGIST

Why should I go to a gynecologist?

Carol doesn't see the sense in going to a gynecologist. She doesn't plan on having any babies and isn't in a relationship. Her Aunt Martha never went to the doctor and lived into her nineties. She doesn't have a family history of breast cancer and let's face it, if she gets any other kind of cancer, she'll probably die from it anyway. Having someone examine you while you are nearly naked is at best embarrassing and at worst mortifying. Why should she subject herself to it?

There are many women like Carol who talk themselves out of a gynecologic exam, rationalizing their negligence with flawed logic. It's amazing how many people like Carol don't even want to talk about cancer, never mind be screened for it. They have "ostrich syndrome": They believe that if they bury their heads in the sand and don't look for it, then it won't happen.

If you are destined to develop cancer, it will occur whether or not you're screened. Screening, however, helps the doctor discover cancer early, increasing the chances of successful treatment. A glance at the history of cervical cancer treatment clearly shows the importance of early detection. The incidence of cervical cancer in the 1950s was thirty to thirty-five cases per one hundred thousand per year in women over the age of twenty. With the advent of the Pap smear (a test that detects this cancer), the incidence of cancer dropped to only ten cases per one hundred thousand women—and this despite an epidemic rise in the sexual transmission of HPV viruses that predispose women to cervical cancer. Although the media seem to be fond of locating women who develop cervical cancer in spite of screening, such problems are rare. Without a doubt, the institution of regular screening with Pap smears was tremendously successful. With the recent addition of HPV screening, it is even more successful. At various points in your life, you will also be screened for breast, colon, vaginal, vulvar, and ovarian cancer. We'll delve into the specifics of these conditions later.

Family planning is another important reason for consulting a gynecologist. A large number of pregnancies are accidental. Reasons given by younger women include these:

- "I didn't think I could get pregnant the first time."
- "We did it only once."
- "He said he loved me." (The "he" in question has long since left.)
- "I don't know how this happened." (This is our personal favorite.)

Unintended pregnancies also occur in the later reproductive years. Older women can be taken by surprise just like younger women:

- "But I was told I couldn't get pregnant at my age."
- "Well, we were meaning to get around to doing something more permanent."
- "I didn't think a woman could get pregnant this late in life."

Your best chance of having the right size family at the right time in your life is to practice family planning. Your gynecologist is the best person to help you in this endeavor. There are a wide variety of contraceptive options and other techniques to help you plan for the best time to have your baby.

Finally, regular appointments with your gynecologist can provide you with a greater understanding of your body and health. Throughout your life, you will face a wide range of normal and possibly abnormal developments. During your reproductive years, you may confront premenstrual syndrome, menstrual irregularities, fibroids, endometriosis, infertility, and concerns related to pregnancy. In the post-reproductive years, you will go through menopause. You may also have concerns regarding bladder dysfunction or other problems related to changes in the pelvic area as you get older. As the years advance, the risk of developing cancer increases. Visiting your gynecologist on a regular basis ensures that these issues can be addressed promptly.

How should I choose a gynecologist?

Locating a competent and caring gynecologist can be a challenge. Many women find a doctor based on the recommendation of a friend or neighbor. However, such recommendations can be misleading. Doctor "X" may be very congenial, but incompetent. A general practitioner whom you trust is more qualified to suggest someone to you. If your doctor is a man, ask whom his wife visits for her exams. If your general practitioner is a woman, ask her whom she sees.

If you are new to the area, first determine which of the nearby hospitals has the best reputation. Then call the hospital and ask to speak with the nurse in charge of the labor and delivery suite. He or she works with the physicians on a daily basis and should be able to make a reasonable assessment of the doctor's capabilities and bedside manner. Also contact the nurse in charge of the operating room for an assessment of the doctor's surgical skills. Communicating with these people is more valuable than contacting the hospital's referral service. The referral service can provide you with the names of gynecologists in your vicinity but cannot comment on their level of competence. You will want to make sure that the physician is Board Certified in Obstetrics and Gynecology and that he or she participates in your insurance plan. You can search the name of the physician via Internet sites such as Administrators in Medicine (www.docboard.org) to make sure that they are in good standing with your state's licensing bureau and see if the physician is reviewed on consumer sites such as Angie's List (www.Angieslist.com). Once you identify a physician it is reasonable to call their office and ask the office manager the following questions:

- How long is the usual wait for an appointment? What if it is an emergency?

- What is the average waiting time once you have reached the office?
- How long does it take for a doctor or nurse to call you back when you call with a question?
- Does the practice cross cover with another group?

Should you try to locate a female gynecologist? You may assume that a female gynecologist will be more empathetic in treating your problems. That is not necessarily true. Most men who choose gynecology as a profession are very personable and enjoy treating women. Often older women seek a male gynecologist, presuming that he will be more competent than a female simply because few women of their generation became physicians. Try to choose a doctor on the basis of ability and disposition, not gender. If you are particularly anxious about visiting a gynecologist and feel that you will be more comfortable seeing a female doctor, then try to find one. Otherwise, concentrate on locating the best physician, regardless of gender.

What can I do if I'm too anxious and embarrassed to see a gynecologist?

Cindy can't help herself. She knows that it's crazy. She must be the only twenty-five-year-old woman in the entire world who has not seen a gynecologist. Most of her friends didn't have much of a choice. They needed contraception or had a problem that required them to see a doctor. Cindy, however, was a bit of a late bloomer and only now feels like she is in a relationship that could lead to sexual intimacy. She knows she should see a gynecologist, but just can't get herself to do it.

Cindy is not alone. Many women never, or rarely, visit a gynecologist for this very reason. The embarrassment of having a gynecologist examine you can be overwhelming. The fact that he or she examines thousands of women every year doesn't provide much consolation. You may also fear that the doctor will discover a serious problem.

Understanding the purpose of your visit may help you overcome your reservations. It will be especially important for you to choose a gynecologist who can make you feel comfortable.

To help overcome your anxiety, consider accompanying a friend on her visit to a gynecologist. The gynecologist's office will not seem as ominous if you know you are not there for an exam. Then consider making an appointment just to talk. Conversing with the doctor while you are fully clothed eases some of the tension and enables you to feel more at ease. The doctor can take your history and explain the procedures involved in an examination.

If you feel comfortable with the doctor, schedule an examination. For emotional support, consider bringing a friend who can either stay in the waiting room or come in with you during the exam. A nurse from the office can also serve in this capacity (many doctors routinely have a nurse in the room during exams; if not, you may request one).

Why do I have such a hard time getting an appointment?

You finally get through to the doctor's office after hearing busy signals all day. Well, at least you're close to getting an appointment, right? *Not!* The receptionist gives you an appointment just this side of eternity. Why?

Most good physicians have a backlog of routine appointments. They have developed a large base of patients, and other doctors refer additional patients to them as well. Therefore the appointment schedule may extend well into the future. It is critically important to communicate clearly to the receptionist if your problem is urgent. He or she usually will add you to the next office session. For a true emergency, be prepared to visit the emergency room. If you think your problem demands prompt attention and the receptionist seems to be putting you off, leave your name and phone number. Ask for the physician to call you back at his or her earliest convenience. You can then discuss the situation. If it is necessary, the doctor will find a way to see you. If you prefer a specific date or time for a routine appointment, call the office well in advance. Usually your request can be honored.

When is the best time to schedule an appointment?

It depends on what type of visit is necessary. When an extensive discussion of a topic is required, inform the receptionist while scheduling your appointment. Extra time can be allotted. Inquire as to the best point in the schedule for a lengthy discussion. This may be the last appointment of the day. You will possibly have to wait longer if the doctor is behind schedule, but at least you will have more time to talk. This applies only if the doctor does not have surgery or an important meeting scheduled after hours, so check with the staff. When you come, bring a written list of your concerns and questions. Time is valuable, so stay on the subject of your healthcare and avoid small talk.

Ideally, you should not schedule an appointment on the day that the doctor covers deliveries. If a woman in labor needs attention, the doctor will be eager to finish the office session. You also run the risk that the doctor will leave for a delivery in the middle of office hours, which really fouls up the works. Your best chance for getting in and out quickly is to get an appointment at the beginning of the office session.

> ### Communicate!
> *If you have:*
>
> • *A complicated problem*
> • *Many questions*
> • *More than one problem*
>
> *Ask the receptionist for more time.*

Try not to schedule your appointment on a day that is near your next menstrual period, presuming your periods are reasonably predictable. The exam will be messier and more embarrassing. If your menstrual flow comes on the day of your visit, call the office. If your flow is light or your problem urgent, you may be asked to come in for your visit anyway.

Why do I have to wait so long in the doctor's waiting room?

Julie rushes out of work, runs down the stairs to the parking garage, hops in her car, and heads to the doctor's office. She knows there may be traffic at this time of day but doesn't want to be late for her appointment. She cuts through the back streets to avoid traffic lights and turns into the office complex. She quickly parks and races up to the office. Glancing at her watch, she is relieved to see that she is right on time. She opens the door to find that the doctor's waiting room appears only slightly less crowded than a bus terminal.

Sound familiar? You arrive on time, only to find a waiting room full of patients. It is frustrating to discover an office running far behind schedule when you had the courtesy to arrive on time. This problem isn't easily rectified. It is partly caused by the amount of time allotted for each patient, which is determined by how much time the average visit is expected to consume. However, the doctor cannot predict what types of problems will appear on a given day. If a series of complex problems arises, it will be very easy to fall behind schedule. Some patients arrive late for their appointments. This sets the schedule further behind. Certainly, many doctors underestimate the amount of time needed for the average patient and should allow more time for each appointment. If waiting is a problem, schedule your appointment early in the day. You can also call ahead on the day of your visit to see if the office is running on schedule. If the doctor is far behind, see if you can arrive later or reschedule your visit.

How often do I need to see a gynecologist?

Many people will only see a doctor when they think they have a problem. However, that is not a good way to stay healthy and live longer. After initial visits, women should be examined annually. If a problem warrants closer observation, the doctor will recommend more frequent visits. A family history of a gynecologic cancer may also indicate a need for more than one exam per year. There are many problems that are easier to treat when they are found early. Others can be prevented from getting worse with early intervention. Finally, cancer rarely presents with symptoms when it is early, so regular examinations by your doctor, along with appropriate screening tests such as Pap smears and mammography, are essential.

When should my daughter first see a gynecologist?

The standard recommendation is to consult a gynecologist at age eighteen or at the onset of sexual activity, whichever comes first. We see you parents cringing. It's amazing how many parents say, "There is no way that my daughter could be sexually active!" Unless your daughter is locked in the attic, make no assumptions. Certainly if an adolescent is having a physical problem or has concerns, she should be evaluated earlier. Usually, initial discussions of menstruation, normal female development, and sexuality are addressed at home and at school. If parents feel uncomfortable discussing gynecologic topics, they should bring their teen (or preteen) to the doctor for education. This also gives your daughter an opportunity to discuss concerns she may not be willing to share at home. Assure her that she will have complete confidentiality. Let her know that she can talk to the gynecologist without being examined. Do not attempt to pry information from the doctor. If your daughter wants to, she can ask the doctor to speak with you.

My daughter has a problem and refuses to see a gynecologist. What should I do?

Talk to your gynecologist. It may be that your daughter has a problem that doesn't require an office visit. Ask her if she would be more comfortable seeing a female gynecologist, or a doctor other than your own. She may think that information shared with your doctor will be transmitted back to you. Or she may feel more at ease with the family doctor or pediatrician rather than a stranger. If the problem is beyond his or her scope, a gynecologist can be consulted.

Depending on the problem, a pelvic ultrasound scan may provide the physician with the information required to manage a problem. An ultrasound can be performed without having a patient remove her clothes (thereby diminishing the embarrassment) and is painless.

Can my family doctor do the pelvic exam?

Many physicians trained in family practice and internal medicine are able to practice basic gynecology. If comfortable with their skills, they can perform routine gynecologic exams and obtain Pap smears. They also may handle common gynecologic problems. This is reasonable as long as they are aware of their limitations. It is logical to assume, however, that a gynecologist will be more skilled in this area. For that reason, many women would rather see a gynecologist for their examinations.

Maggie and Tina's Story

Maggie's daughter Tina has a steady boyfriend, or at least what counts as steady in this day and age. Tina has been seeing Robbie for three months now. She's only sixteen and has never asked any questions about sex. In fact, Maggie tried to get her to use a thin tampon during swim season, but Tina refused, saying it hurt too much. Maggie wonders what she should do next. If Tina won't use a tampon, she can't be having sex, right? Should she take Tina to see a gynecologist? Maggie's gynecologist has a younger female partner, Dr. Jaffe, who would be perfect for Tina, but Maggie doesn't think Tina will allow an exam. When she raises the possibility with her daughter, Tina reacts. "No way, Mom! You've got to be kidding."

Several weeks later, Tina finally opens up to her mother. Was it the threat of seeing a gynecologist or the Rocky Road ice cream? Probably the Rocky Road. Their best mother-daughter moments were always shared over ice cream. Tina reassures her mother that she and Robbie are just friends. She is not engaging in any sexual activities. Maggie lets her know that she can talk about these things openly. She tells Tina that she hopes her daughter will wait until she is in a long, committed relationship before considering sex. However, she wants Tina to know that the most important thing is for her to be protected against pregnancy and sexually transmitted infections if and when Tina becomes sexually active.

Six months later, Tina misses three periods in a row. Maggie gives her a pregnancy test even though Tina swears that she has not been sexually active. The test is negative. Maggie is relieved but at the same time understands that this is not normal and that she should take her daughter to the gynecologist. Tina refuses. Maggie asks herself, "What should I do now?"

Maggie calls her gynecologist, Dr. Johnson, who suggests that Tina will feel comfortable with Dr. Jaffe and informs Maggie that she can first bring Tina to the office just to talk with Dr. Jaffe. Maggie then asks if it would be okay for Tina to see Dr. Winwood, their family doctor. Tina already trusts Dr. Winwood, who has managed her asthma for many years. Dr. Johnson concurs and recommends that Dr. Winwood call them after he has seen Tina if he needs any advice on treating Tina's gynecologic problem.

Tina agrees to see Dr. Winwood. After her visit, Dr. Winwood calls Dr. Jaffe and together they resolve Tina's problem.

Is douching a good idea?

No! For the most part, douching does more harm than good. The manufacturers of feminine hygiene products would like to convince you that these products are necessary for cleanliness. Wrong! Except when certain problems occur, the vagina maintains a normal bacterial population on its own. Douching temporarily reduces the normal bacteria, thereby giving less desirable bacteria or yeast an opportunity to dominate. If you have excess discharge or an odor, there might be a vaginal condition requiring treatment. Don't douche or use other over-the-counter products. Make an appointment with the gynecologist. Women may also develop an allergic or irritant reaction to one or more substances in the douche. Your doctor may instruct you to douche under certain circumstances, but avoid douching on a regular basis.

What do all those fancy words mean?

Sandy and Scott have been trying to conceive for an eternity. Sandy's gynecologist tried to help them without success, so he sends them to an infertility specialist, Dr. Kennedy. Sandy and Scott aren't there for more than five minutes when Dr. Kennedy goes into his spiel on the ten thousand causes of infertility. Unfortunately, he might as well be speaking Greek. It doesn't take long before Sandy and Scott are confused.

We often accuse lawyers of creating their own vocabulary so we will need them to interpret it for us. This is somewhat hypocritical of us, since doctors have done the same thing. After all, what is an endometrium, anyway? Here we'll explain terms used in describing the pelvic anatomy (see the illustrations below). Throughout the book, other terminology will be clarified. You will also find a glossary at the end of the book.

- *Uterus*: The uterus is the reproductive organ located in a woman's pelvis that serves as an incubator for the developing fetus. It is primarily composed of muscular tissue called the myometrium. You can thank the myometrium for those wonderful labor pains and menstrual cramps. The inside of the uterus is lined with a layer of tissue referred to as the endometrium. It is predominately composed of glandular tissue. Each month, it is modified by hormones in preparation for pregnancy. If pregnancy does not occur, the endometrium is shed, creating the menstrual period.
- *Cervix*: The cervix is the portion of the uterus that protrudes into the vagina, commonly referred to as the opening of the uterus.
- *Ovary*: The ovaries are the female glands containing the eggs necessary for reproduction. The eggs reside in structures called follicles, which also produce the female hormones estrogen and progesterone.
- *Fallopian tubes*: These tubular structures transmit the egg to the uterus from the ovaries. An ovary and a fallopian tube are on each side of the pelvis.

- *Vagina*: The vagina is a tubular canal connecting the outside of the body and the uterus. It allows for penetration by the penis so that sperm can be deposited and sent on their journey toward the egg. Most people are familiar with the term *vagina*, but we never make assumptions about this. We still recall a teenager who decided to name her newborn daughter *Vagina* (not Virginia). On her way out of the delivery suite she overheard the term and liked the sound of it. We can only hope she changed her mind once enlightened about its meaning.
- *Vulva*: The region immediately external to the vagina, the vulva includes smaller inner folds referred to as the labia minora and larger outer folds referred to as the labia majora, which are covered with pubic hair. These are also called the inner and outer "lips" of the vagina.
- *Bladder*: Similar to a water balloon, the bladder is a structure that serves as a holding station for urine until you're ready to void. (At least you hope it waits until you're ready.) It is located immediately in front of the uterus. The ureters are the tubes that bring urine to the bladder from the kidneys. The urethra is the tube that carries urine outside the body from the bladder. Its opening is located directly above the vagina.
- *Clitoris*: This small, protuberant structure is located between the uppermost reaches of the labia minora. It is directly above the urethral and vaginal openings. In most women, this is the genital structure most associated with generating sexual pleasure (sure, now we have your attention).

What is the doctor doing during the examination?

Many women don't have a clear understanding of what goes on during the pelvic exam. However, one thing is crystal clear. When someone is examining that part of your body, any amount of time is too long. What takes so long?

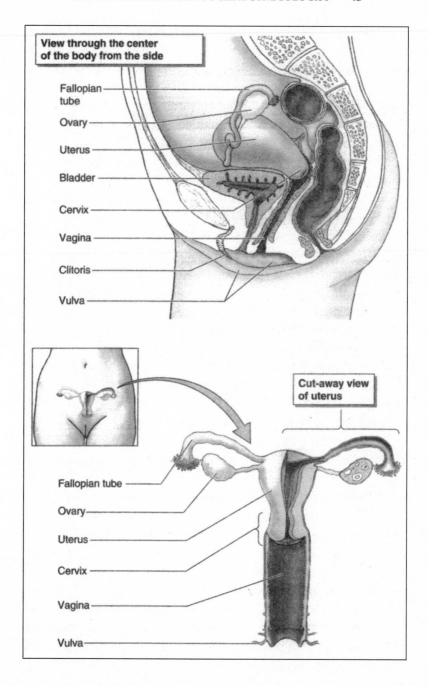

View through the center of the body from the side

Fallopian tube
Ovary
Uterus
Bladder
Cervix
Vagina
Clitoris
Vulva

Cut-away view of uterus

Fallopian tube
Ovary
Uterus
Cervix
Vagina
Vulva

First, the doctor will inspect the external genitalia. This includes the vulvar lips, clitoris, and the opening of the vagina (referred to medically as the vestibule). The opening of the urethra (referred to as the urethral meatus) and the perianal region are also examined. Any unusual change in color, thickness, or texture of the skin in these areas is noted. The doctor also searches for skin lesions such as warts, cysts, and ulcerations.

A speculum is then inserted into the vagina. Opinions concerning this instrument range from "uncomfortable" to "instrument of torture." The speculum is a long, narrow device inserted into the vagina in a closed position and then opened to allow the doctor to see the vagina and cervix. Speculums are available in a variety of sizes. Your doctor should be able to find one that allows a clear view without making the procedure too uncomfortable. The amount of discomfort you feel depends on how tightly your pelvic muscles contract around the speculum. Your natural reflex is to tighten your muscles. However, you can learn to relax them. These muscles are related to those that control voiding. Relax them as if you are ready to void (don't worry; you won't actually have an accident). Also think about relaxing your buttock muscles. When you tighten your pelvic muscles, your bottom will actually start to rise. Concentrate on relaxing your bottom, and the exam will be easier. Take slow, deep breaths, exhaling completely, to relax yourself. The typical speculum feels as if it just emerged from a refrigerator. You can suggest that warming it might be in order. At this point, the doctor may obtain a Pap smear (see the next question). Finally, as the speculum is removed, the vagina is evaluated for abnormalities.

Looking through the speculum, the doctor can see only the vagina and cervix, but cannot gain information regarding the uterus, fallopian tubes, or ovaries. Therefore, he or she will perform a bimanual examination, placing one or two fingers into the vagina while placing the other hand on your lower abdomen. Using mild to moderate pressure, the doctor can feel the size, shape, and mobility of the internal organs. If you momentarily feel pain during the exam, do not misinterpret that as representing a problem. The ovaries do not like being pushed around. Once again, relaxation is of the utmost importance. Without it, the exam is more uncomfortable, and the doctor cannot get the necessary information. The doctor may also perform a rectal or rectovaginal (one finger in the rectum and one in the vagina) exam. Structures in the posterior part of the pelvis are often assessed better through the rectum. A rectal exam should be performed on women over age fifty as a screening for rectal cancer.

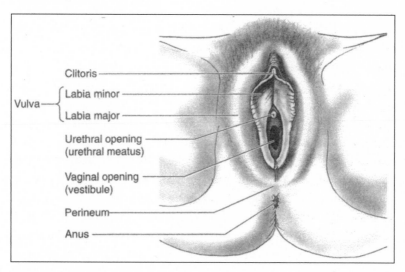

What is a Pap smear?

The Papanicolaou (named after the man who introduced the technique), or "Pap" smear, is a procedure whereby the gynecologist gathers cervical cells for microscopic examination. He or she takes the specimen while the speculum is open inside the vagina. A brush or small spatula is used to obtain the cells. In most cases the procedure is not painful, although it may feel unusual. If it is painful or uncomfortable, take solace in knowing that it doesn't take long to acquire the specimen. A specially trained technician (referred to as a cytologist) or physician (referred to as a pathologist) analyzes the cells on a slide. They use a microscope to find precancerous or cancerous changes of the cervix.

The Pap smear screens women for cervical cancer only. Often women harbor the incorrect notion that the Pap smear is used to detect all types of malignancies. It does not reveal endometrial, ovarian, or vulvar cancer. If an abnormality is seen on the vaginal wall, a separate smear can be performed to screen that area.

Since we now know that high-risk strains of HPV (human papillomavirus) are the actual cause of cervical cancer, your physician may also have the Pap smear specimen tested for HPV. We will learn more about this virus in our chapter on sexually transmitted infections. If a woman has had a total hysterectomy (removal of the entire uterus, including the cervix) for benign disease (noncancerous conditions), Pap smears are no longer required. In the past, post-hysterectomy Pap smears of the vagina were performed, but this is no longer recommended since primary vaginal cancer is very uncommon.

In the past, Pap smears were routinely acquired on an annual basis. With the addition of high-risk HPV testing, it is now recommended that low-risk women can be screened less frequently (ask your doctor if you qualify as low risk). Current recommendations are for women to start getting Pap smears at age twenty-one (regardless of when they become sexually active). Pap smears (without HPV) are recommended every three years between ages twenty-one and twenty-nine. Routine HPV testing is not recommended between twenty-one and twenty-nine. Prevalence of HPV is high in this age group and most women who acquire HPV in their twenties will clear the virus. It is recommended that women ages thirty through sixty-five get a Pap smear with high-risk HPV testing every five years or just a Pap smear every three years. Recent recommendations suggest that Pap smears can be discontinued after age sixty-five because cervical cancer is rarely seen after this age. Having said that, most physicians will continue Pap smears beyond sixty-five.

How reliable are Pap smears?

Periodically, network television airs news segments depicting the inaccuracies of various diagnostic medical techniques. However, the stories create a devastating misimpression by focusing on the relatively small percentage of failures. The Pap smear has been a very valuable tool in the screening of cervical cancer and has been immensely success- ful in reducing mortality from this cancer. False negative rates do run as high as 20 percent, meaning that there is a one in five chance that an abnormality may be missed on a single Pap smear. That sounds scary, but that statistic is misleading. First, assuming you are examined regularly, if an abnormality is not detected on an initial Pap smear, it is extremely likely that it will be dis- covered on a subsequent smear while it is still in the precancerous stage (cervical cancer usually develops slowly). At this stage, the condition is still readily treatable with a variety of conservative techniques. Second, current methods have improved the accuracy of Pap smears tremen- dously. New technologies that use a computer to screen Pap smears and new methods of collecting cells for the Pap test have improved its accuracy. Finally, the addition of HPV screening has immensely helped doctors focus on women who may be at higher risk for cervical cancer.

> *Even if your Pap smears are done less frequently, you still need to be seen on an annual basis. Cervical screening is only one of the many reasons for your annual visit.*

What is a mammogram?

You walk into the office shortly after turning forty. Your gynecologist enters the room. "I hear congratulations are in order. You recently had a birthday. Of course you know what that means."

"No, what?" you ask.

"We now recommend that you get an annual mammogram," the doctor says with a slightly sadistic grin.

Great! *you think.* Could this day get any better?

As you're being examined, it dawns on you that you don't really know much about mammography. You're not stupid. You know that it takes pic- tures of the breasts. But what are they really looking for? How can they tell when something is abnormal?

A mammogram is an X-ray of the breasts. A technician places each breast between two plates and takes pictures. The radiologist interprets the images, looking for calcifications and subtle densities within the breast tissue that could represent cancer. The majority of screening mammograms have no abnormalities. If a nodule is found, the size and shape of the nodule is evaluated to determine whether it might be cancerous. Other factors taken into consideration include the sharpness of the margins (the edges or borders of the nodules) and any associated small calcium deposits. A small nodule with a regular shape and smooth margins suggests a benign (noncancerous) density, such as a cyst. Scattered, large calcifications are fairly common and are usually benign. An enlarging nodule that is irregular and has indistinct margins suggests cancer. Small, clustered calcium deposits are also suspicious. In these situations, the radiologist recommends a breast biopsy (a tissue sample) because early detection is important in the treatment of breast cancer.

Are mammograms painful?

Yes and no; the answer definitely depends on whom you ask. Most women find mammography somewhat uncomfortable, but tolerable. A small number of women find mammography painful. Often these women have fibrocystic breasts (see page 240). However, regular mammograms are particularly important for women with fibrocystic breasts because they are "lumpier" and more difficult to examine, making the detection of cancer more difficult.

Mammograms will also be more uncomfortable when performed shortly before your menstrual period. Cystic areas in the breasts are more prominent at this time, which can make the interpretation of the mammogram more difficult. Schedule your mammogram early in your menstrual cycle (right after your period), and both you and your radiologist will be happier.

If you are menopausal, mammograms will be more uncomfortable if you are using hormone replacement therapy. Don't misinterpret the discomfort as a sign of a problem. If the pain is intolerable, discuss the situation with your gynecologist. He or she may be able to adjust your hormone regimen to remedy the problem.

The amount of discomfort associated with the mammogram previously varied according to the technician. Their task was difficult: If they squeezed the plates too hard they would cause pain, but if they didn't squeeze hard enough the quality of the study was compromised. This subjective factor has since been eliminated by modern equipment that automatically adjusts for the right amount of pressure.

Aren't mammograms dangerous?

Sooner or later you will run into someone who never gets a mammogram because they are convinced it is dangerous. After all, a mammogram uses radiation. Isn't that dangerous? Can't that cause cancer itself?

Although mammograms involve a small exposure to radiation, it is a low dose. You are actually exposed to a similar dose of radiation from the environment each year. Any small increase in risk from this low dose of radiation must be compared with the benefit of diagnosing breast cancer earlier. While acknowledging that there may be a small risk from mammography itself, most reputable organizations, like the National Cancer Institute, feel that the benefits from mammography far outweigh the risks. Mammograms do not prevent breast cancer, but they do reduce the death rate from breast cancer through early detection.

How reliable are mammograms?

If you live long enough, you will eventually encounter someone who develops advanced breast cancer even though they were conscientious in obtaining their mammogram every year. This begs the question of how effective mammograms are at picking up early cancers. If mammography is not really effective at picking up early cancers, there's no point in getting them.

The quality of radiologic equipment used for mammography varies. Studies have also shown that different radiologists can interpret the same breast images differently. Because of these variables, it is important to go to a facility with state-of-the-art equipment (such as digital mammography machines) and physicians who specialize in breast imaging and acquiring breast biopsies when indicated. Your gynecologist, who is the doctor primarily responsible for breast cancer screening, can recommend a facility that provides reliable results. Make sure the facility is accredited by the American College of Radiology.

The value of mammography for women over age fifty is not questioned. In this age group, approximately 90 percent of breast cancers are detected through this procedure. Early detection results in a 30 percent decrease in mortality (deaths from the cancer). Women over fifty should undergo mammograms annually.

The benefits of mammography for women under age fifty are somewhat more controversial. Because breast tissue in younger women is denser, it is more difficult to spot a cancer on the images and more cancers are missed. Another concern is that breast cancer in young women often behaves aggressively. Therefore, detecting it at an earlier stage may not improve survival rates as much. Recent studies suggest, however, that regular screening with high-quality equipment does reduce the number of deaths due to breast cancer in this age group. Current recommendations for this age group vary, with most reputable organizations recommending mammography every one to two years beginning at age forty. Since 75–85 percent of all breast cancer is diagnosed in women who have no family history for breast cancer, it is important that all women are screened after age forty on a regular basis.

Interpretation of mammographic abnormalities is not an exact science. The radiologist cannot always be certain whether a finding is benign or cancerous. A breast ultrasound (see the next question) may help determine the nature of an abnormality. MRI (magnetic resonance imaging) is also used, particularly in high-risk women, to distinguish between normal and abnormal breast tissue. Thermography (detecting temperature differences between normal and abnormal tissue) and scintimammography (using a radioactive tracer to provide tumor-specific imaging) are additional imaging methods used to supplement, not take the place of, mammography in women who have particularly difficult breasts to image, such as women with dense breasts, fibrocystic breasts, and breast implants. Tomosynthesis, a new form of mammography, utilizes 3-D imaging that may also improve detection in women who have dense breasts that are difficult to image.

There will be "interval cancers" that grow fast between screenings and subtypes of cancer, such as lobular, that are difficult to detect with screening mammography, but the vast majority of cancers will be detected early using screening mammography.

Why do I have to get a breast ultrasound?

Sue was a little hesitant, but finally talked herself into getting a mammogram. No sooner is she home than she finds a message on her answering machine asking her to call the radiology department. She quickly calls the designated number and speaks with Nancy from radiology, who explains, "Something showed up on your mammogram. This doesn't necessarily mean that it is anything bad, but the radiologist wants you to come back to take extra pictures of that area and get a breast ultrasound." Sue tries not to get overanxious, but it is difficult. Her sister Heidi developed breast cancer at fifty-five and Sue can't help but think that she must have cancer too.

She calls her gynecologist, Dr. Jones, to see what he thinks. Dr. Jones reassures Sue that 10 percent of the time the radiology department calls patients back for additional pictures and the vast majority of the time everything turns out to be fine. He explains, "Although mammography effectively reveals a breast nodule or mass, it cannot tell whether it is solid or cystic (fluid filled). A breast ultrasound provides this information. A fluid-filled structure is considered a cyst, and therefore benign. The risk of cancer is greater with a solid mass. It is usually biopsied."

A breast ultrasound does not replace the mammogram, but rather gives additional information. If your mammogram is normal, a breast ultrasound is usually not necessary. However, this may change with the development of automated 3-D breast ultrasounds, which recently received FDA approval for screening women with dense breasts and a normal mammogram. Moving forward, facilities may begin to implement this technology in their screening protocols.

If breast MRI is more sensitive than mammography, should I get that instead of a mammogram?

Sue returns to the radiology facility. They take additional pictures of her breast and indeed there is something there, but the ultrasound shows it to be a simple cyst. She is reassured by the radiologist and her gynecologist that this is quite common and benign. Since the cyst is not bothering her, she doesn't need to do anything about it.

She calls her sister Heidi and shares this information with her. Heidi is relieved. "That's so good. I was worried for you. I wonder if you should get a breast MRI instead of mammography. Ever since I had my cancer, the breast surgeon orders an annual MRI."

Sue considers this suggestion. "I'll have to ask Dr. Jones about that when I see him next year." She is left pondering, Who gets a breast MRI and who doesn't?

Mammography is still the standard of care for screening for breast cancer. Breast MRI can be more sensitive at detecting breast problems, but it is extremely expensive (which means your insurance won't pay for it), prone to a higher incidence of false positives (saying there is a problem when there really isn't), and requires more sophistication in its interpretation. Because of its high sensitivity, it should be considered in the following circumstances:

- High-risk patients who are determined to have a greater than 20 percent lifetime risk of breast cancer, using one of the accepted breast cancer risk calculators, such as the Gail risk assessment model

- Patients with a history of atypical hyperplasia on biopsy

- Patients with a personal history of breast cancer or DCIS or LCIS (discussed in chapter 12)

- Patients with a breast implant when there is a suspicion of rupture

- Patients with a known BRCA1 or BRCA2 genetic mutation. These mutations significantly increase the risk of breast and ovarian cancer. Most insurance companies will cover a breast MRI under these circumstances, as well as for patients who have a first degree relative with a BRCA mutation and have not had testing themselves or patients with other genetic syndromes associated with an excess risk for breast cancer.
- Patients with a history of radiation therapy to the chest between the ages of ten and thirty. The Children's Oncology Group's guidelines recommend that patients treated with this type of radiation (as a child, teen, or young adult) start screening five to eight years after finishing their treatment or at age twenty-five, whichever is later.

How can I lose this weight?

Jamie, Helen, Linda, and Betty decide to form a weight loss support group at their church. They were always talking about doing this but never committed to the idea until today. Pastor Rachel preached on how your body is a temple and you have to take care of it. They now gather for the first time and begin to share their stories.

Jamie, the youngest, speaks first. "I can't believe how much weight I've gained since having my baby. I used to be the person who could eat anything in college without gaining weight. Pregnancy really killed me. I put on fifty pounds and I know that's too much, but I thought most of it was water weight and would leave me after the pregnancy. Now I'm left with trying to get rid of an extra thirty pounds."

Helen responds, "You think you have problems now, just wait until menopause. I was doing fine until I stopped getting periods. Ever since then I gain weight just by looking at food and it all goes right to my middle. I'm convinced that losing my hormones has slowed down my metabolism or something."

Linda laughs. "I'm sorry, I didn't mean to laugh, but I went through menopause three years ago. I had terrible hot flashes so my doctor put me on hormone replacement therapy and I've done nothing but gain weight since that time. I was going to blame my weight gain on getting hormones, not losing them."

Betty, the matriarch of the group, joins the discussion. "Well I don't know about hormones, but it seems like I put on weight every year. Looking at me now at 250 pounds, you wouldn't know that thirty years ago I was only 130. I never thought that three to four pounds a year could add up to much, but it sure does."

Many women can relate to the frustration shared above. The nurse has the gall to weigh you immediately upon entering the exam room. How could you possibly have gained another five pounds? You haven't been eating any differently. This isn't fair!

Excess weight gain is something that can develop at any age and is especially common in the menopausal years, often settling in one's midsection and creating that unsightly "midriff bulge." Some studies suggest that menopause is related to a modest increase in weight gain with an accelerated accumulation of central body fat that exceeds changes normally attributed to the aging process. Estrogen replacement may curb some of this tendency. However, hormonal changes alone don't cause the amount of weight gain commonly seen in postmenopausal women. Weight gain in midlife occurs irrespective of the timing of menopause and also occurs in men. In midlife we tend to be less active in our everyday life and exercise less than we did earlier. In addition, muscle mass naturally decreases with age. If you don't do anything to replace this muscle, your body will burn fewer calories. If you continue to eat as usual, you will gain weight. Whether your weight gain is linked to menopause itself or aging and lifestyle is less important than understanding that it can be prevented with proper exercise, diet, and lifestyle modifications.

Currently, more Americans are overweight than normal weight. What is overweight? As a rule, a woman who is five feet tall should weigh one hundred pounds. You can then add five pounds for every inch above five feet, plus or minus 10 percent. If you're not sure, your doctor can refer to a chart that indicates a normal range of weight. If you are more than 20 percent overweight, he may even use that hideous term *obese*. Weight gain occurs when you consume more energy (as food) than you burn. Weight problems can result from certain medical conditions such as hypothyroidism or medications. However, heredity, eating habits, and lifestyle usually dictate your weight.

Tackling your weight problem is a difficult endeavor. There are no shortcuts or instant cures for the problem. The most sensible approach is a gradual change to a healthy diet and increased exercise. Fad diets that severely restrict calories are not the answer. When these diets are discontinued, weight rebounds, often shooting higher than before. Modest reduction in calories (three hundred to five hundred) is reasonable and usually occurs when changing to a lower-carbohydrate diet rich in fruits and vegetables. Excess carbohydrates and unhealthy fat, especially saturated fat and trans fat, should be severely reduced. Help can also be obtained by consulting a nutritionist (check with your local hospital). Your change in habits should consider the following:

- Avoid alcohol—it is "empty calories" with no nutritional value.
- Eliminate sweets (soda, candy, cake, cookies, pie, et cetera).
- When eating a carbohydrate product such as bread, pasta, or rice, switch to a whole-grain product and limit your quantities.
- Don't try to eliminate fat altogether from your diet. To remain healthy, approximately 30 percent of your diet should come from the consumption of healthy fat. In addition, fat is more satiating, so you are less likely to eat between meals. Most of your fat consumption should come from monounsaturated or polyunsaturated fat (fish or plant-based oils such as olive oil). Saturated fats (animal fat such as red meat and full-fat dairy products), with the exception of virgin coconut oil, should be limited. Trans fat products should be eliminated altogether. Trans fat usually occurs in processed foods like margarine, commercial baked goods, and fast food.
- Never eat fast food!
- Cook your own food. This allows you to use healthy ingredients, enables you to see exactly what you are putting into the recipe, and allows for better portion control. It also tends to make you eat slower since you want to appreciate the work you put into your meal.
- Eat slowly. When you eat slowly, your brain can catch up to your stomach in realizing that you are getting full. You can

also trick your brain into thinking that it needs less by eating something bulky, such as a salad, or drinking a glass of water before your meal. You can also eat a small portion of something high in protein and fat, such as a handful of nuts, twenty or thirty minutes before your meal.

- Incorporate a source of protein into each meal.
- Drink plenty of water—up to six glasses of water every day (unless you must restrict fluids for other health reasons).
- Avoid second helpings.
- Use a salad plate instead of a dinner plate to reduce your portion sizes.
- If hungry between meals, choose a healthy snack (fruit) over an unhealthy snack (ice cream, potato chips).
- Eat at regular intervals throughout the day. Eating next to nothing for breakfast and lunch and then inhaling everything in sight at the end of the day is not healthy, and you won't burn up many of those calories while you're sleeping.
- Don't associate eating with other activities (reading, watching television).
- Try not to eat for the wrong reasons (boredom, stress, depression).
- Eat out less often—when you do eat out, be selective in your choices.

Tracking your food intake is a great way to lose weight. The simple act of recording your food intake in a journal, computer program (ex. www.myfooddiary.com), or phone app prevents you from overeating. Simple smartphone apps like "Lose It!" enable you to track what you're eating no matter where you are located.

Adding a regular exercise routine to your daily regimen is essential for continued health. Not only does exercise burn up calories, but it improves your general conditioning, health, strength, and mobility. However, don't be fooled into thinking that exercise gives you a license to eat whatever you want. Most people overestimate the amount of calories burned during exercise. Exercise is employed as an adjunct to proper eating, not in its place. Exercise does not have to be tedious and boring. Choose an activity that you enjoy, such as tennis, golf, swimming, or dancing. Even thirty minutes of brisk walking every day will make a difference. For a more disciplined approach, look into your local YMCA or fitness center. Incorporate strength training (weights or resistance machines) into your exercise schedule. This will help maintain your muscle mass, which in turn helps you burn calories more efficiently. Also consider adding yoga or Pilates. Both of these help maintain strength and flexibility and will help with conditioning the core part of your body (midsection), which is often problematic in menopause. Of course let's not ignore all of those excuses we have for not exercising:

- "I don't have the time to exercise." Do you have time to read or watch television? If so, you have the time to exercise. Both of these can be done while exercising. Buy a treadmill or exercise bike and put it in front of the television to make it harder to ignore.
- "I'm too tired to exercise. By the end of the day, I'm exhausted!" It seems paradoxical, but exercise is more likely to energize you than cause fatigue.
- "I have arthritis (or bursitis, or tendinitis—insert your own *itis*) so I can't exercise." Nice try, but we're not buying it. There is usually some form of exercise that can be adapted to suit your medical condition. In the case of arthritis, you will probably do well in a swimming pool (pool aerobics are great), which takes the weight off your joints.

We are talking about a serious commitment. You have to dedicate yourself to changing years of poor eating habits. In some cases, we're talking about a major overhaul in lifestyle. However, if you have the resolve to make this commitment, you will not only lose the pounds, but keep them off.

For more information and help with healthy eating, go to www. choosemyplate.gov.

What medications help you lose weight?

As the group discusses various strategies for weight control, Helen thinks she has a solution. "Can't you just take medications that help you burn up calories? When I was growing up, the doctor gave my mother something to help boost her metabolism."

Linda responds, "I don't think they do that anymore. I think it's dangerous. I once asked my doctor about that and she said it was too risky, so she doesn't prescribe those medicines. She told me to go to Weight Watchers."

"Did that work for you?" asks Helen.

"Yeah, it worked while I was doing it, but as soon as I stopped going to the meetings, I fell back into my old habits."

So what's the deal? Are you like Helen? Taking a pill to lose weight sounds good to many people. Medications can help you lose weight, especially when coupled with a diet and exercise regimen. However, the additional weight loss is often modest (usually about ten pounds), tends to level off after six months, and rebounds when the medications are discontinued. You must change to a healthier diet and exercise to maintain weight loss over the long run. Prescription medications are only indicated in severely obese patients with a BMI (Body Mass Index, calculated from your height and weight) of thirty or above (or twenty-seven and above if there are additional obesity-related conditions such as diabetes). You can go to www.nhlbi.nih.gov/guidelines/obesity/BMI/bmicalc.html to calculate your BMI.

The first class of medications used for weight loss is appetite-suppressant medications, which promote weight loss by decreasing appetite or increasing the feeling of being full. Medications in this class include phentermine, phendimetrazine, diethylpropion, and lorcaserin (Belviq), a newcomer that received approval by the FDA in June of 2012. Historically, phentermine has been the most commonly prescribed. There are a myriad of side effects that may appear with the use of appetite-suppressant medications. Most of the side effects are mild and usually improve with continued use. They cannot be used in people with certain medical conditions and serious, even fatal, outcomes have been reported. It is important that these medications be prescribed only by physicians with a thorough understanding of their potential adverse effects. Medications in this class should generally be used for several weeks, or several months at most. They are not intended for long-term use.

The second class of medications approved for weight loss is lipase inhibitors, or fat blockers. Xenical (orlistat) was approved for weight loss and is now available over the counter under the trade name Alli. Lipase inhibitors work by blocking 30 percent of dietary fat absorption. Side effects include abdominal cramping, gas passage, leakage of oily stool, increased number of bowel movements, and the inability to control bowel movements. The side effects may be worsened by eating foods that are high in fat, so patients should combine the medication with a low-fat diet. They reduce the absorption of some vitamins, so patients taking Xenical or Alli should take a multivitamin at least two hours before or after taking the medication.

There are additional medications normally used to treat other conditions that are used off-label, in other words without FDA approval for weight loss, including buproprion (antidepressant), topiramate and zonisamide (anti-seizure), and metformin (diabetes). Recently the FDA approved a drug called Qsymia, a combination of topiramate with phentermine (see above). Combining the two drugs increases the amount of weight loss, but also potentially increases the number of side effects and risks. Women taking Qsymia must use reliable contraception because topiramate can cause birth defects. People with recent or unstable heart disease or stroke should also not take Qsymia because of potential heart risks. Once again, they should only be used in situations where their benefit clearly outweighs the risk. No medication prescribed for weight loss should be used in a patient who is only mildly or moderately overweight.

Alpha-lipoic acid (800–1800 mg/day) is an antioxidant supplement used for weight loss in the complementary and alternative community. Alpha-lipoic acid helps your body process sugar into energy. It is also used by some in the treatment of diabetes. Diabetics and patients with thyroid disorders require special monitoring when using this supplement.

When is surgery indicated for obesity?

Betty shocks the group by telling them that she's going to have a stomach banding procedure. "I've tried all of the diets. Weight Watchers worked while I was going to meetings, but I couldn't stick with it at home. I've also done Nutrisystem and Jenny Craig. They worked as long as I ate their meals, but once I started cooking for myself, I gained back all my weight. I tried Trevose Behavior Modification, but they kicked me out for cheating. I'm ashamed to admit it, but I just don't have the self-control to stick with one of those programs."

Jamie interjects, "I thought that surgery was dangerous. My mother's best friend had that surgery and she says that she gets reflux every time she eats."

Undeterred, Betty continues, "I was told there are risks, but most people do well. The surgery is easier now because they can do it laparoscopically. I already have diabetes and high blood pressure, and my doctor says I'll need to get all of my joints replaced if I don't do something to get this weight off me now."

Yes, surgery may seem rather drastic, but it can be a lifesaver for people like Betty who have failed other methods and face multiple medical complications from their weight. Roughly one in twenty-five Americans are morbidly obese. Bariatric (obesity) surgery, which includes gastric banding and gastric bypass techniques, is indicated for anyone with a BMI of forty or above (roughly one hundred pounds overweight for men and eighty pounds for women) or for someone with a BMI of thirty-five or above if they have obesity-associated conditions such as hypertension, diabetes, heart disease, sleep apnea, or high cholesterol. In these situations, the risk of getting sick or dying from obesity-related conditions outweighs the risk and potential complications of surgery. Improved surgical techniques and the availability of laparoscopic surgery have greatly improved outcomes from bariatric surgery. In the vast majority of cases, surgery successfully helps men and women dramatically reduce their weight, improving the quality of their life tremendously. Of course, surgery should still be combined with dietary changes and exercise in order to optimize benefits. Most bariatric surgery programs hold periodic information sessions that can help you decide whether this option is right for you.

What can I do if I have pain?

Jody doesn't know what to do. She's had pain in her lower abdomen for two years now. It seems to be getting worse as time goes by. She has seen her internist and gynecologist multiple times and they keep insisting that everything is normal. It almost seems like they think that it's all in her head. Well, it's not! There's something wrong. She just knows it. It doesn't seem to be associated with any other symptoms, so no one has been able to figure it out. What can she do at this point? How many more tests are available? Her gynecologist mentioned laparoscopy to look inside, but implied that it was unlikely to show anything. She doesn't want to go through surgery for no reason, but she can't continue living with this pain. Maybe she should see one of those pain specialist doctors.

Anyone who has had chronic pain can sympathize with Jody. There is nothing worse than pain! Even patients who avoid the doctor's office like the plague relent when pain occurs. It's one of the more common reasons for a woman to see a gynecologist. Any pain in the lower abdomen or pelvic region is assumed to be related to the female organs. Although this may indeed be the case, there are multiple causes of pain.

You should see a doctor if your pain is severe, worsening, recurring, or disruptive to your daily life. Changes in your bowel function, bladder function, or menstrual cycle or a rise in your temperature to above one hundred degrees should also prompt you to seek help. Initial evaluation can be made by your primary care doctor or your gynecologist. It is probably most appropriate to see your primary care doctor if the pain is in the middle or upper abdomen or associated with gastrointestinal symptoms (nausea, vomiting, diarrhea, constipation). Your gynecologist can evaluate unexplained pain in the lower abdomen. Before seeing the doctor, try to characterize your pain. How long does it last? Is it constant or intermittent? How frequently does it occur? Is it sharp or dull? Does it occur at a particular time of your menstrual cycle? Is it worse with specific types of movement? This information will help your doctor evaluate your condition.

Pain accompanied by nausea and vomiting or change in bowel function is usually gastrointestinal in origin. Upper abdominal pain can result from problems involving the stomach (gastritis, ulcers, and reflux esophagitis), pancreas, liver, and gallbladder. Lower abdominal pain can be caused by colitis, irritable bowel disease, diverticulitis, or appendicitis. Cancer within the abdomen can cause pain, so do not ignore persistent discomfort. If one of these conditions is suspected, your doctor may consult with either a surgeon (in the case of appendicitis or other surgical conditions) or a gastroenterologist (for conditions that do not require surgery).

Pain associated with bladder symptoms, such as frequency and urgency of urination, painful urination, or bloody urine, is usually urologic in origin. Possible causes include infection of the bladder or kidneys, kidney stones, cancer, and interstitial cystitis. These are explored in our chapter on bladder disorders.

Muscle strain or spasm can also produce pain in the lower abdomen or pelvis. This may occur because of strain or injury to the abdominal, back, or pelvic floor muscles. Muscle spasm may also result from disc disease or arthritis in the spine. Damage to nerves emerging from the lower back or coursing through the pelvis may also cause pelvic pain.

Pelvic pain can also arise from many gynecologic conditions. We'll only briefly describe them here because most are explored in other chapters.

1. *Infections*: Pelvic inflammatory disease is an infection of the uterus, fallopian tubes, and ovaries. It is often associated with sexually transmitted organisms. Common symptoms include lower abdominal or pelvic pain, fever, and discharge. Pain limited to the vagina or vulva may be caused by herpes or vaginitis. Pelvic infections are addressed in chapter 5.

2. *Complications of pregnancy*: Miscarriage and ectopic pregnancy (a pregnancy located outside the uterus, usually in the fallopian tube) may cause pain. If you have missed your usual menstrual period and develop pain, you should be evaluated promptly. Refer to chapter 7 for more information about these conditions. Your doctor can easily exclude complications of pregnancy by obtaining a blood pregnancy test (referred to as an HCG or B-HCG test).

3. *Ovarian cysts and tumors*: When the ovary develops a cyst or growth, it enlarges. You may sense fullness or a dull ache in the pelvic region. If a cyst ruptures, you may experience a sharp pain that goes away within a day or two. An enlarged ovary may also twist and turn, causing intermittent pain. Ovarian cysts are common, and most disappear spontaneously. However, large or persistent cysts may require surgery. Benign tumors and ovarian cancer may also cause pelvic pain. Ovarian cysts and tumors are reviewed in chapter 10.

4. *Uterine conditions*: Uterine fibroids are benign smooth muscle tumors that develop within the wall of the uterus. It is uncommon for fibroids to cause pain, although they may do so if they enlarge markedly and press on other organs or outgrow their blood supply and undergo a process called degeneration. Adenomyosis is a condition in which the inside lining of the uterus (endometrium) "grows" into the muscular wall of the uterus (myometrium). Adenomyosis causes menstrual cramps and heavy menstrual flow, worsening in a woman's late thirties or forties. Uterine cancer may cause pelvic pain, although this is often a late symptom; abnormal bleeding would usually signal the cancer's presence much earlier. We discuss fibroids and adenomyosis in chapter 9.

5. *Endometriosis*: Endometriosis is a condition in which endometrial tissue (normally found lining the inside of the uterus) is located outside the uterus. It may cause painful menstrual cramps, chronic pelvic pain, or painful intercourse. We will discuss endometriosis and its related problems in chapter 8.

6. *Adhesions*: Adhesions (scar tissue) can form as a result of anything that causes inflammation in the pelvic region, including pelvic infections, endometriosis, and prior surgical procedures. Pain from adhesions is usually chronic in nature and often unassociated with other symptoms.

7. *Functional pain*: You can have "functional" pain that does not come from disease. This seems counterintuitive. If everything

is normal, why is there pain? Painful menstrual cramps (dys-menorrhea) may occur without other disease. This is par-ticularly true if you have always had painful periods. Some women will get recurrent mid-cycle pain associated with ovulation. These and other menstrual disorders are discussed in chapter 2.

You can see from this list (if you're not totally confused by now) that there are myriad potential causes for pain in the lower abdomen. Sometimes the source of the pain is obvious. It can, however, be very perplexing. Your doctor may have to approach the problem one step at a time, gradually eliminating causes until he or she correctly diagnoses the condition. The evaluation begins by taking a careful history and performing an examination. If the source of your pain is not obvious, the doctor will order laboratory tests such as blood work, urine studies, or imaging studies to gain more information. These might include any of the following:

- *Pelvic ultrasound*: This imaging scan uses sound waves (no radiation) to generate a picture of the pelvic organs. Ovarian cysts and tumors, fibroids, pregnancy (normal and abnormal), pelvic abscesses, and large kidney stones can all be revealed by ultrasound.

- *Computed tomography (CT or CAT scan)*: This type of X-ray produces images of the internal organs. This information can help the doctor diagnose benign or malignant tumors as well as certain types of inflammatory conditions (appendicitis, diverticulitis).

- *Magnetic resonance imaging (MRI)*: This method of viewing the internal organs uses a magnetic field. Certain types of abnormalities can be seen more easily or clearly with MRI.

- *Barium enema*: Barium is placed into the colon through the rectum. The contrast material helps a radiologist detect lower bowel problems on X-rays. If there is a need to evaluate the upper intestinal tract, barium can be swallowed before an X-ray is taken.

- *Intravenous pyelogram (IVP)*: In this procedure, dye is injected into a vein, the kidneys excrete the dye into the urinary tract, and X-rays are taken, providing good images of the kidneys, ureters, and bladder.

Telescopic instruments may be used for further examination if the source of pain is still unclear. The gastrointestinal tract can be evaluated by either endoscopy (placing a flexible telescopic instrument down the throat) or colonoscopy (you guessed it—through the rectum). Cystoscopy enables a urologist to look into the bladder. Gynecologists use either a hysteroscope to look into the uterus without making an incision or a laparoscope to look into the abdomen through a tiny incision near your navel. Sometimes these procedures are done in an office setting, and other times they're performed as outpatient surgery. A local anesthetic, intravenous sedation, or general anesthesia may be used for these procedures.

Treatment of pain varies according to its source, but is likely to include medications called analgesics. You are already familiar with the more common ones, such as acetaminophen (Tylenol) and NSAIDs (nonsteroidal anti-inflammatory drugs including Advil, Motrin, and Aleve). More intense pain is treated with drugs containing narcotics. These will be more effective at relieving pain but generally have more side effects, such as nausea, constipation, and drowsiness. They should not be taken if you must be alert for any reason, especially if you will need to drive a car or operate machinery. (Then again, if you're in that much pain, you probably should be at home resting.)

Chronic pain is particularly distressing. Not all pain can be eradicated. At other times, chronic pain ensues even when the immediate source of pain has been treated successfully, which is difficult to cope with physically and emotionally. Other medications may be added to analgesics to treat chronic pain. Antidepressants have been used successfully for patients with chronic pain. They act on pain impulses at a different location than analgesics do, and the two can be used together. Anticonvulsants (anti-seizure medications) may also play a role in treating chronic pain. Two additional medications, gabapentin (Neurontin) and pregabalin (Lyrica), are also commonly used for chronic pain, although their mechanism of action is not clearly understood.

Complementary modalities such as biofeedback, relaxation techniques, physical therapy, nerve stimulators (such as TENS, which creates tiny electrical nerve impulses at the affected site to block pain impulses), hypnosis, and acupuncture may also be effective in treating chronic pain. Healthcare providers in the alternative community have used proteolytic enzyme supplements (ex. Wobenzym) in the treatment of pain. They are primarily used for digestive disorders and by athletes to accelerate recovery from exercise, injury, and surgery. However, proteolytic enzymes may help reduce pain caused by inflammatory disorders such as rheumatoid arthritis. They are generally considered safe with the most common side effect being upper gastrointestinal distress, such as reflux. White willow bark (Salix Alba) is also used to treat inflammation. The active ingredient, salicin, is similar to aspirin. Like aspirin, white willow bark can lead to gastric ulcers if used at high doses for a prolonged time. Reasonable doses (standardized to 120–240 milligrams of salicin) for a limited period of time appear to be safe. Both proteolytic enzymes and white willow bark have blood thinning properties and should not be combined with other drugs that have anticoagulant effects, including aspirin and NSAIDs like ibuprofen (Advil, Motrin) and naproxen sodium (Aleve). Boswellia, curcumin, ginger, and devil's claw are additional alternative products with anti-inflammatory properties. Glucosamine, capsaicin cream, and Arnica gel are common over-the-counter products used for back and joint pain, with variable degrees of success.

Often a multidisciplinary approach that involves several doctors and therapists is the best answer for patients with chronic pain syndrome. Emotional support is often required. A competent therapist may be a critical resource in coping with the psychological struggles associated with chronic pain. It is also reasonable to ask your primary care doctor to refer you to a doctor who specializes in the management of chronic pain.

2

THE MENSTRUAL CYCLE:
WHAT'S NORMAL, WHAT'S NOT?

What's a normal cycle?

Joni is confused. Sometimes she gets her period in three weeks, while other times it comes in six. Her girlfriends all seem to have regular periods, approximately every four weeks. Some of them are on the pill and Joni knows that birth control pills keep you regular, but even her friends who aren't on the pill seem to have regular periods. There must be something wrong with her. Right?

Many concerns about menstruation are based on a misunderstanding of the normal menstrual cycle. Any variation within the cycle may be interpreted as abnormal and worrisome. Explaining the menstrual cycle is only slightly easier than outlining Einstein's theory of relativity, but let's try.

The menstrual cycle is composed of two phases. It begins with the follicular phase. Located in the ovaries, follicles are small fluid-filled structures that contain an egg. The cycle begins when one of the follicles matures, generally over the course of two weeks, and produces estrogen. Estrogen stimulates the endometrium (the lining of the uterus), causing it to thicken. When follicular maturation is complete, the egg is released to embark on its journey down the fallopian tube. This is referred to as ovulation. After ovulation, the second phase of the menstrual cycle, called the luteal phase, begins. The follicular structure (now referred to as the corpus luteum) continues to produce estrogen.

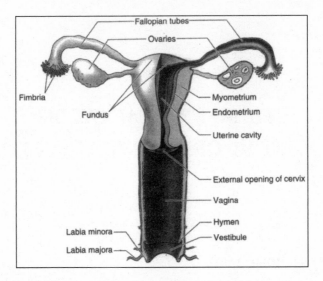

It also produces a second hormone called progesterone. Progesterone alters the endometrium, preparing it for implantation of a fertilized egg. If the egg is not fertilized, the ovary stops producing the female hormones. Without hormonal support, the endometrium is shed as a menstrual flow, commonly known as the period. The cycle begins again as another follicle matures.

The average length of a complete cycle is four weeks. It is, however, common for the cycle to vary in length from three to five weeks. It is most variable when menstrual periods first begin and then again as menopause approaches. Some women never achieve a regular cycle. If your cycle varies between three to eight weeks, and your menstrual flow lasts for less than one week, don't worry about it. If you are bleeding more frequently than every three weeks or have not had a menstrual period in eight weeks, you should contact your gynecologist. You are probably no longer having ovulatory cycles, and hormonal intervention may be necessary.

I'm late for my period. Am I pregnant?

Lucy calls her best friend Karen. "I can't believe I am pregnant!"

Karen is taken aback. "How can you be pregnant when you haven't even had sex?"

Lucy confesses, "I did last month after the prom. I didn't tell you because I didn't want you making a big deal out of it. Now I'm late for my period. I must be pregnant."

"Did you use any protection?" asks Karen.

"Of course," replies Karen. "I'm not that stupid. We used a condom."

"Did you get a pregnancy test?"

"Not yet," admits Lucy, "but why else would I miss my period?"

This question is associated with the most anxious moment in one's life. "I'm late for my period . . . help!" Often, though, a missed period does not indicate pregnancy. The menstrual cycle may simply be out of sync. In this situation, the body's normal signals that control ovarian function have become confused. Ovulation doesn't occur, and the ovary fails to produce progesterone. Without progesterone, the endometrium will not be shed, and thus no period occurs. If your pregnancy test is negative, your doctor can prescribe a short course of progesterone to induce the menstrual flow. It is not prudent to wait longer than two to three months before beginning progesterone. During the time you are not ovulating, the ovary continues to produce estrogen, stimulating the endometrium and causing it to thicken. Eventually, the endometrium will break down, causing heavy or erratic bleeding.

I get my period only two or three times during the year. Is that okay?

This may sound great. No bleeding, and think of all the savings on pads and tampons. Heck, while you're at it, why can't you get rid of periods altogether? Unfortunately, this is not in your best interest.

Infrequent menses (called oligomenorrhea) and totally absent menses (amenorrhea) usually mean that you are not ovulating on a regular basis. Both conditions can produce heavy or erratic bleeding and eventually increase your risk for developing endometrial cancer.

There are numerous reasons for skipping a menstrual period. Some are quite simple, such as stress or anxiety. Abrupt weight gain or loss and vigorous exercise are also culprits. Certain medications alter your cycle by interfering with the female hormones. Various medical disorders can upset your cycle. The most common is thyroid disease. Your doctor may order blood work to rule out endocrine (hormonal) disorders if the problem is recurrent.

If your menstrual periods are infrequent, talk to your gynecologist. Usually, no distressing problem is found. Your gynecologist will recommend either progesterone or oral contraceptives to improve your hormonal balance, decreasing the chance of experiencing erratic bleeding.

Donna and Lisa's Story

Donna and Lisa are coworkers, both in their late forties, approaching menopause. They have both started to skip periods and don't know what to make of it.

Donna is very conscientious when it comes to her healthcare. Friends and coworkers like Lisa have told Donna that she is overanxious, but Donna ignores them. Whenever someone makes a snide remark, she replies, "You only get to go through life once, so I'm going to make sure that I stay healthy."

Donna has allowed herself to skip one month as long as she gets her period the next month, but now it's been more than two months since her last period and she's getting concerned. She gives her gynecologist, Dr. Kerber, a call. "Dr. Kerber, I'm sorry to bother you, but I haven't had my period for two and a half months and I'm a little concerned. Is this normal? Am I just going through menopause?"

Dr. Kerber replies, "It's a good thing that you called me, Donna. It's not very common for the ovaries to turn off like a switch. Most women will miss periods before menopause because their hormones are out of sync. In that situation, you have an imbalance between the two hormones estrogen and progesterone. Your ovaries continue to make estrogen during the months that you're missing your period, so the lining in your uterus continues to thicken, but your ovaries fail to produce progesterone and you don't get your period. Eventually the thickened lining inside the uterus breaks down, often causing heavy, prolonged bleeding. Fortunately, we can prevent that from happening. I'm going to give you two weeks of progesterone, which is what your ovaries would have done if they were working properly. After you have finished the progesterone, you will get a period and probably get back on track. If not, you can call me whenever you go more than two months and we will repeat the progesterone. This will keep your hormones in balance and will prevent you from getting into trouble."

Lisa is more laissez-faire when it comes to her health. She sees Donna overreacting to the least little ailment and is determined that she will never be a hypochondriac like her. Skipping periods at this point is no big deal. After all, that's what is supposed to happen when you get near menopause.

Lisa ignores her skipped periods. In fact, she's thrilled. Here she is in menopause and doesn't even have any symptoms. She feels great. No hot flashes or night sweats. No mood swings. Life is good! Four months later, she begins to bleed. *Well how about that. A period after all this time,* she thinks. Only this doesn't seem to be any normal period. She's flooding, going through Maxi pads every hour! After several days of heavy bleeding, she's starting to feel lightheaded and calls her gynecologist, Dr. Drew. "I don't know what's going on," she begins. "I just missed a few periods and now it seems like the floodgates have opened."

Dr. Drew seems more than just a little annoyed. "Why didn't you call me before this? If you had called me earlier, we could have prevented this. I'll put you on some progesterone and hopefully the bleeding will stop, but if it doesn't we'll have to take you to the operating room for a D&C!"

Despite high doses of progesterone, Lisa continues to bleed. Dr. Drew performs a D&C and hysteroscopy to exclude other causes of Lisa's heavy bleeding and places her on high doses of birth control pills after surgery, which finally controls her bleeding.

Donna and Lisa were both experiencing the same alteration of their menstrual cycle. One thought to call her doctor and the other didn't. The lesson to be learned from hearing their stories is when you notice an alteration in your menstrual cycle, call your gynecologist. Let him or her decide if it is normal. Don't assume anything!

When my period comes, I flood. Is that normal?

Do Not Wait!

If you bleed:

- *Longer than one week*
- *Between your periods*
- *More often than every three weeks*
- *Less often than every eight weeks*
- *Progressively heavier over time*

Call your gynecologist now!

Assessing your bleeding can be surprisingly difficult. What one person considers heavy may be normal to another. If you are saturating Maxi pads every hour or two, your bleeding is unusually heavy. Occasionally, a woman has a history of heavy menstrual periods her entire life. This condition may be normal, but if you have it, you should be checked to make sure that you don't have a problem with blood clotting.

If your menstrual flow is becoming progressively heavier, it is abnormal. Don't let this persist without investigation. What seems to be a mere nuisance now could become a life-threatening hemorrhage in the future. If the timing of your period is erratic, your problem may relate to abnormal production of the female hormones. In this case, artificially regulating your cycle corrects the problem. However, if your cycle appears to be regular, the heavier flow is probably caused by an intrinsic disorder of the uterus, such as fibroids, polyps, or adenomyosis. Your doctor will probably want a pelvic ultrasound scan to give a clearer picture of your pelvic organs. An endometrial biopsy, D&C (dilation and curettage, in which the endometrium is scraped and the sample is evaluated under a microscope), or hysteroscopy may be needed. These are discussed extensively in chapter 9.

If your flow is heavy, drink more fluids than usual to ward off dizziness. Also take an iron supplement to prevent anemia. Iron often irritates the gastrointestinal tract, resulting in constipation or diarrhea. Your doctor can recommend a brand of iron that is less likely to produce these effects.

What does it mean when I get clots during my period?

Blood clots during menstrual flow can be startling. Because of their striking appearance, it can be easy to assume that they mean that something is wrong. Actually, blood clots do not reflect a specific problem. If blood remains inside the uterus long enough, it will clot. However, copious, large clots reflect heavy bleeding and should be brought to the attention of your doctor.

Is bleeding between my periods normal?

Bleeding between periods is referred to as intermenstrual bleeding. When you ovulate, you get a hormonal surge, and you may have light bleeding for a day or two. Mark on your calendar the day the bleeding occurred, and wait for your next menstrual period. If your menses follows the bleeding episode by two weeks, assume it is normal.

Intermenstrual bleeding that occurs at other times in the cycle is not acceptable. The abnormal bleeding may be caused by a hormonal variation. However, as you advance in age, other conditions such as fibroids, polyps, and even cancer become possibilities. Other less likely culprits include cervical or vaginal lesions, endometriosis, uterine infection, and ovarian disorders. Your doctor can readily eliminate vaginal or cervical causes for the bleeding if these structures appear normal on your speculum exam and your Pap smear is normal.

If you are younger than age thirty-five and your exam is normal, further evaluation may not be necessary. If the intermenstrual bleeding persists over several months, your cycle can be regulated artificially to correct the problem. If it does not respond to hormonal manipulation, additional studies should be undertaken. These may include pelvic ultrasound, endometrial biopsy, D&C, and hysteroscopy.

Over the age of thirty-five (some doctors may say forty), intermenstrual bleeding may indicate precancerous and cancerous uterine conditions. Although this is the least likely cause of your problem, it is the most critical to diagnose. Evaluation of the endometrium with an endometrial biopsy, D&C, or hysteroscopy is mandatory. A pelvic ultrasound is also helpful. If no underlying condition is discovered, the doctor will attempt hormonal regulation with either progestational agents or oral contraceptives.

Why do I get pain in the middle of my cycle?

You're in the supermarket. You're just about to reach for the frozen lasagna when suddenly a pain appears out of nowhere. After a few hours it subsides, but you're still wondering, "What was that?" If it occurred in the middle of your cycle, you just experienced mittel-schmerz. Discomfort is often felt in the pelvis during ovulation. Usually the pain is transient, but it can persist for a day or two. When severe, it is termed *mittelschmerz* (from the German words meaning "middle pain"). If you menstruate two weeks after the pain occurs, no special investigation is necessary. If the pain is severe, take acetaminophen (Tylenol or generic equivalent). If the pain is disabling and you do not wish to become pregnant, consider asking your gynecologist to prescribe oral contraceptives (the birth control pill). By inhibiting ovulation, they will solve your problem.

I get terrible cramps with my period. What's wrong?

You don't have to suffer!

If you have a long-standing history of painful periods, ask your doctor about reducing the frequency of your periods with continuous birth control pills like Seasonique and Lybrel.

Cramps are induced by the release of substances called prostaglandins from the endometrium (inner lining of the uterus), causing contractions in the muscular wall of the uterus. The wall of the intestines also has a muscular layer, which may also be affected by the prostaglandins. Therefore, nausea and loose bowel movements often accompany uterine cramps. Nonprescription medications that offer relief by combating prostaglandins include ibuprofen (Advil and Motrin), naproxen sodium (Aleve), and ketoprofen (Orudis). Oral contraceptives, which thin the endometrium, are also used. Menses then become lighter and less painful.

Dietary supplements that may help with dysmenorrhea (the medical word for menstrual cramps) include magnesium (200–400 mg daily), vitamin E (800 IU), vitamin B6 (100 mg daily), vitamin B1 (100 mg daily), and Omega-3 fatty acids (3 gm daily, divided with meals). Supplemental vitamin D may also be beneficial. In one study, women were given either 300,000 IU (international units) of Vitamin D or placebo (similar-looking product but without medicine). The treatment group had a 41 percent reduction in menstrual pain whereas the placebo group experienced no benefit. Most doctors would not recommend giving patients that much vitamin D, but you can certainly safely take 1,000 units of vitamin D (significantly more than 1,000 if you are deficient). Ask your doctor to check your vitamin D level (25-OH Vitamin D). There are studies that also show that a low-fat vegetarian diet reduces the duration and intensity of dysmenorrhea.

If your menses only recently became painful, you may have an underlying disorder. A common offender is endometriosis, a condition in which endometrial tissue is found outside the uterus. Endometriosis is particularly suspected if the pain starts during the days leading up to your menses. (See chapter 8 for more information.) Other causes for pain include adenomyosis, pelvic infection, uterine polyps, and fibroids. These are described extensively in other chapters.

Inform your gynecologist if your menstrual periods are unusually painful. He or she may want to obtain more information through pelvic ultrasound or cultures. If no obvious source for your pain is found, the doctor will recommend anti-prostaglandins or oral contraceptives. If your pain is severe, laparoscopy or hysteroscopy may be indicated. Laparoscopy is a surgical procedure that allows the doctor to view the internal pelvic organs through a telescopic instrument inserted into the abdomen. Hysteroscopy is a telescopic look at the inside of the uterus that is done by way of the vagina, without making an incision.

What can I do if I have PMS?

Premenstrual syndrome (PMS) encompasses a wide range of physical and emotional symptoms that repetitively occur during the week or two immediately preceding your menses. Common physical symptoms include breast tenderness, fluid retention, bloating, and fatigue. Appetite changes, food cravings, headaches, nausea, constipation, dizziness, clumsiness, and a host of other physical symptoms have also been linked to PMS. Common emotional symptoms include mood swings, irritability, anxiety, and depression. You don't have to experience all of these symptoms to have PMS, but the symptoms must occur only premenstrually. If you are not sure, keep a diary to establish the timing of your symptoms. PMDD, or Premenstrual Dysphoric Disorder, is a particularly severe form of PMS with similar symptoms but severe enough to interfere with work, social activities, and relationships. Before a doctor makes the diagnosis of PMDD, he or she will rule out other emotional disorders—such as major depression or panic disorder—as the cause of the symptoms. Women with a personal or family history of mood disorders—including major depression or postpartum depression—are at greater risk for developing PMDD.

Despite many claims, nobody really understands the cause of PMS and PMDD. Many assume that the symptoms are produced by alterations in the levels of the female hormones estrogen and progesterone. Since the disorder appears in women only between the onset of menstruation and menopause, this theory appears logical. Most scientific studies have established that hormone levels are normal in patients with PMS, although some studies point to more subtle variations that may have an impact. It appears that certain individuals are more sensitive to various hormonal effects in certain areas of their body. Premenstrual mood and anxiety disorders are likely created by alterations in chemicals produced in the brain referred to as neurotransmitters, such as serotonin.

The physical symptoms of PMS are easier to

Just a Bad Day?

Mary walks into the kitchen, where her ten-year-old son John has somehow managed to knock over the milk carton next to his cereal bowl. "Now look what you've done! I can't leave you alone for two seconds. You're supposed to be at the bus stop in five minutes and I'm supposed to be at work in twenty. What's wrong with you? Why are you so careless?"

Mary gets to work only to find her coworkers socializing around the coffee machine. "This is just great! Jim told us that our project has to be in by the end of the day, and you guys are just hanging out. Well, you can be lazy, but I'm getting to work. Someone has to do something around here."

It is the end of the day. Mary and her husband Jim are watching TV when he affectionately rubs her leg. "Not tonight, Jim. I'm not in the mood, my breasts are killing me, and I feel bloated."

Is Mary just having a bad day? Maybe, but more likely she has PMS. We all have bad days, but if you have emotional or physical changes that recur every month before your period, you probably have PMS.

control than the emotional ones. Swelling in the hands or feet is caused by fluid retention. Eliminating salt from your diet is an initial step to approaching this problem. A mild diuretic ("water pill"), a medication that helps your kidneys excrete excess fluid, can be prescribed. Bloating reflects increased intestinal gas. It may be associated with constipation. Often a change in diet will help reduce these symptoms. Avoid foods that increase gas production (beans, cabbage, broccoli, carbonated beverages) and increase your fiber intake. Beano, an over-the-counter medication, can be used prior to eating to reduce gas production. Additional over-the-counter preparations containing simethicone (MYLICON or Gas-X) dissipate gas in your bowel, thereby increasing comfort after eating.

Breast tenderness may decrease if fluid retention is eliminated. Diindolylmethane (100–300 mg per day) has been shown to be an effective treatment for breast pain. Decreasing caffeine consumption (coffee, tea, colas, and chocolate),

One Size Does Not Fit All

Rachel is the sort of patient who looks for an easy fix for any given problem. She's not about to change her lifestyle habits in order to solve a problem. "Just give me a pill, Doc" is her mantra. Appropriate treatment for Rachel might include a "water pill" for her fluid retention and an antidepressant like Prozac for her premenstrual depression and irritability.

Abby is a patient who always looks for natural solutions to her health issues. She has a holistic "mind, body, spirit" mentality. Abby is instructed to limit salt, sugar, alcohol, and caffeine. Her doctor suggests smaller, more frequent meals and dietary supplementation with B-6, calcium, magnesium, and Omega-3 fatty acids. She is advised to increase her yoga from once a week to twice, and meditation and exercise are recommended for stress reduction. If her mood does not improve with the above changes, she should consider a PMS product containing Chasteberry and St. John's wort.

supplemental vitamin E (400–800 IU per day), evening primrose oil (3 to 4 gm per day), and Ginkgo Biloba (60–240 mg) have also been tried and appear to help some women, although medical evidence demonstrating their benefit is scanty. Nonprescription pain relievers containing acetaminophen (Tylenol) or ibuprofen (Advil, Motrin) should also be considered. If your breast tenderness is particularly severe, special medications can be prescribed (discussed in chapter 12). However, they all have potential side effects that may be undesirable. Your doctor can review these with you if the preceding suggestions are not helpful. Eating five or six small meals daily, high in protein and complex carbohydrates (vegetables, whole grains, legumes) and low in simple carbohydrates (refined sugar, soft drinks), can help you keep food cravings in check.

The emotional symptoms associated with PMS are more difficult to manage. Many solutions have been touted as successful, only to fall short under closer scrutiny. Progesterone supplementation has been extensively utilized for PMS in the past, but most well-designed studies do not support progesterone having a greater benefit than a placebo (a pill that contains no medication). Dietary supplementation with vitamin B6 (100 mg per day—do not exceed this dose or it could be dangerous), calcium (600 mg twice daily), magnesium (200–400 mg per day), and Omega-3 fatty acids (3 gm per day, divided with meals) have been recommended and are supported in at least some studies. One has to be careful in attributing therapeutic value to a treatment for PMS because there is a very high placebo effect. If you are really convinced that something should help you, there is a good chance it will, but the positive effects won't last.

Complementary and alternative practitioners recommend Chasteberry (20 mg) and St. John's wort (300 mg per day), and there are at least some studies to support their use. It should be noted that St. John's wort decreases blood levels of oral contraceptives, theoretically making them less effective. If patients choose to take St. John's wort, they may want to use a backup method of contraception such as a condom or diaphragm, or at least use an oral contraceptive with higher doses of estrogen and progesterone. Femal and Serelys (two tablets daily), a pollen extract, has been shown in a small study to help with premenstrual sleep disorders but not other symptoms. Other alternative products that have been used for the emotional symptoms of PMS and PMDD include black cohosh, evening primrose oil, dong quai, kava kava, tryptophan, DHEA, and melatonin. None of these have consistently shown a benefit, and in some cases, they have proven dangerous. Homeopathy in the treatment of PMS and PMDD has not been well studied. In one small study it was not found to be better than placebo.

Lifestyle modifications can help with the emotional symptoms of PMS. We already mentioned dietary modification, which should include reduction of caffeine, salt, sugar, and alcohol. All of these in one way or another can affect your mood. Next, start a vigorous exercise program. Exercise not only strengthens the body but also relieves tension and elevates mood. Stress adversely affects mood so you should try to schedule stressful activities earlier in your cycle. Incorporate stress-reduction activities such as meditation, yoga, and massage during the second half of your menstrual cycle.

There are many over-the-counter medications for the treatment of PMS (Midol PMS, Premsyn PMS, Pamprin). Most of these contain acetaminophen (as does Tylenol), a mild diuretic, and an antihistamine that has sedative effects. You may gain some relief with these products, particularly if you *really* think they will help. However, they are mild and not likely to be successful with severe PMS or PMDD. Feminine hormone creams containing hormonal extracts from yams have also been recommended for PMS, but once again, there is inadequate evidence to confirm their effectiveness.

The mainstay for treating the emotional symptoms of severe PMS or PMDD in traditional medicine is the class of antidepressants called SSRIs (selective serotonin reuptake inhibitors). The most common SSRI used for this purpose is fluoxetine (Prozac). When this was found to be effective for PMS, the pharmaceutical industry introduced Sarafem, which is the same fluoxetine found in Prozac. Other SSRI medications can also be used for PMDD. These medications should be started at a low dose (paradoxically, starting at a higher dose may actually increase anxiety) and titrated upward until your depression or anxiety symptoms improve. Doctors may initially use these SSRI medications on a continuous, daily basis. If symptoms improve, it can be limited to the two weeks leading up to your menstrual period. Birth control pills are also sometimes tried in patients with PMS. The oral contraceptive Yaz received an indication for the treatment of PMDD from the FDA.

I always get a headache at the beginning of my period. Why?

We're talking big-time, throbbing headaches. They appear before or during the first few days of your menstrual period. You may be experiencing menstrual migraine headaches. Your hormone levels drop immediately before the onset of your flow. This can trigger a migraine headache. Typically, a migraine brings a severe pain limited to one side of your head. Sometimes it is preceded by visual effects, such as flashing lights or partial loss of vision. Nausea and vomiting may accompany the headache. Intolerance to loud noises and bright lights is common. Migraines are more common in women than men. Common triggers for migraines include changes in humidity, changes in altitude and barometric pressure, flashing lights, loud noises, changes in sleeping habits such as oversleeping, missed meals, hormone changes, and certain foods. If you're predisposed to migraines, the following foods may induce a headache:

- Bananas (more than half a banana daily)
- Beans (lima, fava, snow peas)
- Chicken liver, pâté
- Chocolate
- Citrus fruit (more than half a cup daily)
- Coffee, cola, tea (more than two cups daily)
- Figs, raisins, papayas, avocados, red plums (more than half a cup daily)
- Herring (or any food that is fermented, pickled, or marinated)
- MSG (monosodium glutamate—may be found in soy sauce, meat tenderizer, seasoned salt, Chinese food, salad bars)

- Nuts, peanut butter
- Pizza
- Processed meats (sausage, bologna, pepperoni, salami, hot dogs, bacon)
- Ripened cheeses (cheddar, Swiss, Stilton, Brie, Camembert)
- Sour cream (more than half a cup daily)
- Sourdough bread

Now that we've eliminated all your favorite foods, you may decide you'd rather have a headache. Actually, everyone is unique. The above list is only a guide. Keep track of your diet to see which foods trigger your migraines, and adjust your food choices accordingly.

There are a number of approaches to the treatment of migraine headaches. Some women gain adequate relief with over-the-counter or prescribed analgesics (painkillers).

For many people with migraine attacks, triptans are the drug of choice. Medications in this class include sumatriptan (Imitrex), rizatriptan (Maxalt), almotriptan (Axert), naratriptan (Amerge), zolmitriptan (Zomig), frovatriptan (Frova), and eletriptan (Relpax). Side effects of triptans include nausea, dizziness, and muscle weakness. They are not recommended for people at risk for strokes and heart attacks. One of the triptans, Imitrex, has been combined with naproxen sodium (the medicine in Aleve). The drug Treximet has proven more effective in relieving migraine symptoms than either medication on its own. Sometimes, doctors will recommend starting a triptan medication a day or two before you normally get your menstrual migraine, and continuing it through the menstrual period. This may stop a headache from developing at that time.

Another class of medications used to treat migraines is the ergots. Ergotamine and caffeine are combined in many drugs (Migergot, Cafergot). These drugs are cheaper than the triptans, but also usually less effective. Dihydroergotamine (Migranal) is an ergot derivative that is more effective and has fewer side effects than ergotamine. It is also available as a nasal spray and in injection form.

Doctors will sometimes prescribe medications that can reduce the frequency of migraines. Medications used for this purpose include certain types of antidepressants, beta-blockers, calcium channel blockers, anti-seizure medications, and Botox. A complete discussion of these is beyond the scope of this book, but ask your doctor about them if your headaches are frequent.

Menstrual migraines may be triggered by prostaglandins released at menstruation. Anti-prostaglandin medications such as ibuprofen (Motrin, Advil) or naproxen sodium (Anaprox, Aleve) may reduce the frequency of migraines. Estrogen fluctuations may also trigger migraines. This may be prevented by starting an estrogen supplement near the end of the cycle (for example, between days twenty-four and twenty-eight for cycles lasting twenty-eight days). For unpredictable cycles, estrogen can be started when premenstrual symptoms (breast tenderness, bloating) occur. The estrogen is continued during the first few days of the menstrual flow.

If you get migraines, you should make a concerted effort to eat balanced meals at regular intervals and avoid alcohol and caffeine. Dietary triggers should be reduced at times when you seem vulnerable to migraines. Stress reduction and regular exercise are also beneficial. Biofeedback and acupuncture have been found effective in reducing migraine headache pain. If skilled therapists offer these treatments in your area, you might try them.

Additional information can be obtained at the National Headache Foundation website (www.headaches.org).

My daughter is fifteen and still hasn't gotten her period. Should I be worried?

Angie's daughter Stephanie has been pouting all week. Angie is used to her daughter's moods fluctuating, but this funk is longer than usual. She catches up with her daughter after school and finally confronts her. "What's up with you, Steph? All week long you have been in a foul mood."

Stephanie tries to be dismissive. "It's nothing."

Her mother proceeds, undeterred. "Don't tell me it's nothing. I want to help you, but I can't if you won't tell me what's going on."

Stephanie is irritated by her mother's insistence but shares anyway. "If you must know, all the girls in school are making fun of me. They've all gotten their periods and I haven't. I must be a freak or something. What's wrong with me that I can't be like other girls?"

Just like Stephanie, your daughter will feel embarrassed if her friends are menstruating and she is not. It seems that they are progressing into womanhood, leaving her behind. Reassurance is all that is necessary. There is a wide variation in the onset of the first menstrual period, which is referred to as menarche. The average age of onset is twelve, but up to sixteen may be normal. The development of other sexual characteristics such as breast formation and pubic hair typically precedes menarche, as does the growth spurt. If these are not present by age fourteen, consultation with an endocrinologist or a gynecologist who specializes in endocrine disorders is recommended. If these sexual characteristics are developing and growth is on schedule, then it is reasonable to wait until age sixteen before seeing a specialist. Also, it is common for the menstrual period to be erratic in the year following menarche. If the cycle ranges anywhere from three to eight weeks apart and the duration of flow is less than a week, no action is necessary. Her cycle will likely become regular within one to two years, without treatment.

Are tampons safe?

In 1980, toxic shock syndrome was diagnosed in a number of menstruating women. Mass hysteria followed. We can understand the panic. A person could be placed in solitary confinement for a month and not come up with a name as ominous as toxic shock syndrome. What is this terrible disease? It causes fever, diffuse rash, and faintness during menstruation or shortly thereafter. Nausea, vomiting, diarrhea, cramping, disorientation, and loss of consciousness are also common. Toxic shock syndrome is caused by the release of toxins from a bacterium called Staphylococcus aureus. This bacterium is present in the vaginas of approximately 5 percent of all women. The disease can also be seen in men and non-menstruating women who develop other types of infections from the bacteria. Although toxic shock syndrome can be severe, it is rare. Even at its peak, the incidence did not exceed fifteen cases per one hundred thousand menstruating women per year. It was found to be associated with the use of superabsorbent tampons, particularly one called Rely. Women began to question the safety of tampons. After the Rely tampon was withdrawn from the market, the incidence decreased to one per one hundred thousand women each year. You should not avoid using tampons because of a concern about toxic shock syndrome. It does, however, make sense to avoid superabsorbent tampons (labeled as such on the package), unless your flow is very heavy and you expect to change tampons frequently. Tampons should not be left in place for a prolonged time greater than eight hours.

You may be concerned about injuring yourself when you insert a tampon. Don't worry: Genital injury caused by placing or removing tampons is extremely uncommon. Virginal women may have difficulty. Using slender models of tampons with lubrication such as K-Y Jelly may help in that situation. If you still have difficulty, schedule a gynecologic exam.

3

CONTRACEPTION: WEIGHING THE ALTERNATIVES

Is it possible to get pregnant the first time I have sex?

Dr. Stewart asks Beth, an eighteen-year-old patient, what she's using for contraception.

"Nothing," replies Beth, "I don't need anything."

"So you're not engaged in any sexual activity?" asks Dr. Stewart.

"Well, not much," replies Beth. "We don't have sex very often."

You'd be surprised how many women—particularly teens—think that multiple sexual encounters are required for conception to occur. Many times when we ask a woman who says she has missed her period whether she might be pregnant, she responds, "No, I only had sex once." Sometimes, once is enough. The time to think about contraception is before you achieve that level of intimacy.

What is natural family planning?

No, this doesn't refer to growing children organically, without antibiotics or pesticides, although that doesn't sound half bad. Natural family planning refers to the prevention of pregnancy without using "artificial" contraceptives. Instead, couples refrain from intercourse during the time in the woman's cycle when the chance of conception is the greatest—anywhere from five days before ovulation through two days after. The key to natural family planning's success is determining the day of ovulation. In most cases, ovulation will predictably occur fourteen days before the next menstrual period. For example, if a woman's cycle interval (the number of days from the first day of one period to the first day of the next period) is thirty-two days, she ovulates on day eighteen and would abstain from intercourse on days thirteen through twenty.

If you wish to proceed with natural family planning, you must pinpoint your day of ovulation by charting your basal body temperature with a digital basal thermometer. Your doctor can provide you with a chart and instructions. In this method, you check your temperature immediately upon awakening each morning. Your temperature usually dips slightly on the day of ovulation and rises approximately a half degree twenty-four hours after ovulation. By reviewing the chart, you can determine when ovulation has occurred. Ovulation predictor kits (First Response, Fertile-Focus) can be purchased for approximately twenty-five dollars and are fairly accurate. If you really want to splurge, you can purchase a fertility monitor (Clearblue Easy Fertility Monitor, OvaCue Fertility Monitor). These are quite accurate, but will run you two to three hundred dollars. Most women would only make this kind of investment if they were trying to determine their day of ovulation in hopes of enhancing their chance of conception. In this case, you are trying to avoid conception.

Checking your cervical mucus can also help determine the day of ovulation. Your cervix (the opening of the uterus) produces mucus that is secreted into the vagina. Before ovulation, the mucus is voluminous and has a watery texture, and when you observe this, you should refrain from intercourse. After ovulation, the mucus is reduced in amount and becomes thicker.

A high level of motivation is required to carry out successful natural family planning. Before deciding whether to use this method, you should be aware that surveys indicate a 25 percent failure rate over the course of one year.

What is barrier contraception?

You can't erect a barricade to hold off the millions of sperm attacking your egg, but you do have the benefit of barrier contraception.

The Right Fit

Donna is a twenty-eight-year-old woman who recently got married. She has been using oral contraceptives for ten years. She sees Dr. Jones for her annual checkup. "I think I want to stop using birth control pills."

"Any particular reason why?" asks Dr. Jones.

"It's just that I have been on them for such a long time that I think I should take a break."

Dr. Jones attempts to reassure her. "You know there is no reason why you have to stop birth control pills at this point, unless you want to get pregnant."

"Well, I don't really want to get pregnant for a couple of years, but I was thinking I could use something else," replies Donna. "It doesn't have to be as effective as the pill. It wouldn't be the end of the world if I got pregnant at this point."

"In that case, you may want to use a diaphragm," responds Dr. Jones. Donna

Barrier contraceptives include condoms, diaphragms, the vaginal sponge, and spermicides. They do just what their name implies: they form a barrier between his sperm and your egg. These contraceptives function as physical barriers (condoms and diaphragms), chemical barriers (spermicides), or both (the vaginal sponge or using a diaphragm with spermicide).

The diaphragm is a dome-shaped rubber device inserted into the vagina prior to intercourse. It is used with a spermicidal cream or jelly to enhance protection. Apply spermicide to the diaphragm, which must be inserted no more than two hours prior to intercourse. It must remain in place for at least six hours after intercourse. If you have intercourse again before six hours, place another application of spermicide into the vagina. Your doctor will fit you with a diaphragm of the correct size and will instruct you on proper placement. Be sure you can insert and remove the diaphragm properly before leaving the office. If the diaphragm fits properly, it shouldn't agrees and sets up an appointment.

Donna represents a good candidate for barrier contraception. Barrier contraceptives are good for women who want to postpone conception without using a hormonal product. Barrier contraceptives are not as effective as hormonal contraception, so they are best used in situations where pregnancy is acceptable if the contraceptive fails. The effectiveness of barrier contraception can be increased if both partners use a product (ex. diaphragm and condom together), but this obviously requires an extremely motivated couple.

feel uncomfortable. Replace it every two years or if it develops holes or tears. Have the size checked if you gain or lose more than twenty pounds. Also have it rechecked after pregnancy. When used properly, diaphragms are 85–90 percent effective at preventing pregnancy.

Cervical caps are smaller, dome-shaped devices that fit tightly on the cervix. Although more effective than the diaphragm, they are generally more difficult to use. Currently, they are not in widespread use in this country, although this may change. For more information about their availability, contact your doctor.

Condoms are available in male and female versions. They are readily available over the counter in most pharmacies. The male condom is a sheath, usually composed of latex, placed over the erect penis. Condoms should be removed before the penis is limp to prevent leakage of semen into the vagina. Female condoms are also available and are effective, although generally more cumbersome to use. The female condom is composed of a nitrile or polyurethane (types of plastic) pouch with a ring at both ends. The inner ring is placed deep in the vagina while the external ring remains outside. One advantage of the female condom is that it may be less disruptive than the male condom because it may be inserted up to eight hours prior to intercourse. Do not use a male and female condom at the same time.

One of the biggest advantages of condoms is protection against sexually transmitted infections (see chapter 5). However, some male condoms, such as Naturalamb, are made of animal membranes that do not afford this protection. For the best defense against pregnancy and disease, use latex condoms. Condoms are approximately 90 percent effective at preventing pregnancy. Their success is increased with the addition of a spermicide.

If you are allergic to latex (as evidenced by the fact that your vagina becomes inflamed whenever you use a condom), consider trying either the female condom or a male condom made with polyisoprene (Durex Avanti, Lifestyles SKYN).

Is withdrawal a good method of contraception?

Prom night, Saturday, May 4, 2012:

All the kids go to Atlantic City for the after-party. Ricky and Gina sneak out onto the beach where the action heats up.

Gina pauses long enough to ask, "Where's your condom?"

"I left it at home," replies Ricky, "but that's okay. I'll pull out in time."

"I don't think that's such a good idea," says Gina.

"Come on, it will be fine. You know we both want this," implores Ricky.

Delivery suite, Thursday, January 27, 2013:

Little Ricky is born.

Never assume your partner will remove his penis from the vagina prior to ejaculation. You're asking him to stop the very activity that has brought him to the peak of arousal. If by some miracle of willpower he is able to withdraw before ejaculation, it certainly decreases your chances of pregnancy. However, this method is far from foolproof. A small amount of semen emanates from the penis prior to ejaculation, which may be sufficient for conception. If there is sudden ejaculation, even larger amounts of semen will be deposited into the vagina prior to his withdrawal. If you really want to avoid becoming pregnant, don't rely on withdrawal.

How good are over-the-counter spermicides?

Spermicides encompass creams, foams, jellies, suppositories, and films containing a chemical (usually Nonoxynol-9) that kills sperm. They are easier to use than physical barriers, but are less effective. Spermicides are 70–80 percent successful at preventing pregnancy. This means you have a one in five chance of becoming pregnant over the course of one year. Spermicides are most reliable when used with a condom or diaphragm. Allergic or irritant reactions sometimes occur with spermicides and may slightly increase the risk of a woman acquiring a urinary tract infection, yeast infection, or a condition called bacterial vaginosis (see chapter 5). Overall, adverse reactions are uncommon with only 3–5 percent of women discontinuing the use of a spermicide from one or more adverse reactions. If you note severe vaginal burning or itching, discontinue using them. In more recent years, both the Center for Disease Control and the World Health Organization have recommended against the use of spermicides. Perhaps most significant among their concerns is that it has been shown to increase the risk of HIV transmission.

The Right Fit

Beth is eighteen and about to leave for Penn State. Dr. Weston knows that Beth has been sexually active previously and asks her what she plans to do for contraception while at college.

"I assume I'll just use condoms," Beth says casually. "They've always worked before."

Dr. Weston replies, "So far you've been lucky, Beth. You should continue to use condoms

Why should I use the birth control pill?

Birth control pills, also referred to as oral contraceptives or "the pill," are extremely effective. When used properly, their success rate is 99 percent. Birth control pills work primarily by inhibiting ovulation but may also inhibit pregnancy through altering the quality of your cervical mucus and endometrium. They are easier to use and more convenient than barrier methods of contraception. Their contraceptive effect to prevent sexually transmitted infections, but condoms alone do not protect you well enough against pregnancy. If you really need to avoid pregnancy, which most women do while they're at college, you will need something more effective."

Beth acknowledges, "Yes, you're right. I really can't afford to get pregnant at this time in my life. I guess I'll try birth control pills."

Beth is a good candidate for birth control pills. She has plans that clearly do not include pregnancy for at least the next four years. Presuming she is healthy and conscientious about taking her pills, oral contraceptives are a good fit.

is easily reversible when you want to conceive. Modern pills, which contain lower doses of hormones than older versions, are usually tolerated quite well. In addition, the pill has numerous health benefits. Menstrual cycles are very regular on oral contraceptives and your menstrual flow will usually be lighter. The risk of iron deficiency anemia is reduced. Women with painful periods usually have fewer cramps while on the pill. The pill eliminates midcycle pain associated with ovulation. The lifetime risk of developing ovarian or endometrial cancer is reduced by as much as 40–50 percent.

Aren't birth control pills dangerous?

There are innumerable myths surrounding the birth control pill. Let's try to separate fact from fiction.

The most serious complication of oral contraceptives is deep vein thrombosis (DVT). In this condition, a blood clot develops in the deep veins of the leg. If a portion of this clot dislodges, it can travel to the lungs and cause a pulmonary embolus (blood clot in the vessels of the lung). This is a rare event, particularly with low-dose modern pills. However, women using oral contraceptives should call their doctor immediately if they develop severe leg pain, chest pain, or shortness of breath. Previously, there have been concerns regarding other cardiovascular problems such as strokes and heart attacks. Recent studies indicate no increased risk of these in otherwise healthy nonsmokers using low-dose oral contraceptives. Smokers have an increased risk of various cardiovascular complications, and oral contraceptives are not recommended for smokers over age thirty-five. Oral contraceptives may also accentuate the likelihood of an adverse cardiovascular event in women with additional risk factors for cardiovascular disease such as obesity, diabetes, poor lipid profiles (high cholesterol and triglycerides), and a family history of early cardiovascular disease.

Women who are prone to migraine headaches should use oral contraceptives with caution. Approximately 20–30 percent of women who get migraine headaches develop auras before their headaches. The aura is usually comprised of focal neurologic phenomena such as visual disturbances, unusual sensations, or confusing thoughts. Those who develop an aura before their headache have an increased risk of stroke when using oral contraceptives. While the absolute risk of this is very low, most physicians would recommend against using oral contraceptives in these women. Women who have migraine headaches without auras can try oral contraceptives. Presuming the frequency and severity of their headaches do not increase, they can continue using this method of contraception.

The greatest concern women have about the birth control pill is cancer. Most studies show that the pill does not increase the risk of cervical cancer. A review of studies from around the world suggests that women using oral contraceptives have a slightly higher detection of localized breast cancer (one that hasn't spread beyond the breast). It is difficult to know whether this is a real increase or just reflects earlier diagnosis among women who use birth control pills because these women are given regular breast exams and are more likely to

Before starting the pill, tell your doctor if you have a history of:

- *Blood clots in your veins*
- *Migraine headaches*
- *Hepatitis*
- *Vascular disease*
- *Smoking*
- *Unexplained vaginal bleeding*

undergo mammography. These same studies tend to show that women on the pill have a lower incidence of advanced breast cancer compared with nonusers. The small increase in breast cancer in women who use birth control pills disappears ten or more years after they stop, suggesting that there is little or no increase in the overall risk. Women who use the pill are far less likely to get endometrial and ovarian cancer. The decrease in ovarian cancer is particularly significant, since this is the most difficult gynecologic cancer to detect, often appearing in its advanced stages before being discovered.

Two other uncommon complications are worth mentioning. Women who are predisposed to high blood pressure may have a greater chance of developing it while using oral contraceptives. Oral contraceptives rarely induce the development of a liver tumor. The risk is approximately three women per one hundred thousand users.

Common myths about the pill:

- *It makes you gain weight.*
- *It causes cancer.*
- *It causes infertility.*

For most women who require reliable contraception, the benefits of the pill outweigh the risks. There are far greater risks associated with pregnancy. The birth control pill is not recommended for the following groups:

- Smokers over age thirty-five
- Women who have a history of uterine or breast cancer
- Women who have a history of active liver dysfunction such as hepatitis
- Women who have a history of vascular disease (blood clots, stroke, heart attack)
- Women who have unexplained vaginal bleeding

What are all the side effects from the pill?

Almost every symptom known to humanity has been popularly associated with the pill. In reality, 90 percent of women who try the pill do well with it. Common side effects include nausea, bloating, headaches, mood changes, breast tenderness, and bleeding between periods. Most side effects will decrease after the first few months. If they are particularly severe, the doctor can prescribe a different brand. One common myth is that oral contraceptives induce weight gain. Studies comparing birth control pill users and nonusers show that there is no difference in weight gain or loss with the two groups.

It is common to miss a menstrual period on the pill. This is a source of distress for the woman who assumes this means that she is pregnant. Actually her chances of pregnancy are less than 1 percent. In this case, there are no adverse consequences of missing a period. The lining of the uterus simply didn't thicken sufficiently for menstrual flow. If no pills were missed that month, the next pack can be started without concern. If pills were missed, your doctor should be consulted.

Are there any medications I can't take with the pill?

There are no adverse cross-reactions between the pill and other medications. However, some medications may decrease the efficacy of the pill or increase the chances of bleeding between periods. Drugs that have been associated with this include the following:

- Rifampin, ampicillin, and tetracycline—antibiotics
- Barbiturates, carbamazepine (Tegretol), phenytoin (Dilantin), felbamate (Felbatol), oxcarbazepine (Trileptal), topiramate (Topamax)—anti-seizure medications
- Phenylbutazone—anti-inflammatory drug
- Modafinil (Provigil)—sleep disorder drug
- Griseofulvin—antifungal medication

If you are taking one of these medications for a short period of time, it is probably safest to use a backup method of contraception such as the condom. That way you don't have to worry. If you will have to be on the medication for a long time, consult your gynecologist. In addition to the above medications, the herb St. John's wort, most commonly used for depression, also lowers blood levels of oral contraceptives and may interfere with their efficacy.

What should I do if I miss a pill?

It is not uncommon to forget a pill. Don't panic! Take two pills the next day, or as soon as you remember. Take them at different times of the day to reduce the likelihood of nausea. Expect spotting when you miss a pill. If you miss more than one pill, use a backup method of protection and call your doctor for instructions.

If you find yourself missing pills frequently, you should consider two other hormonal contraceptives that are similar to the birth control pill. NuvaRing is a small flexible ring containing estrogen and progesterone. You place it in the vagina where it remains for three weeks. At the end of three weeks you remove it for one week and then insert a new ring. It is more convenient than remembering to take a pill every day. The ring is not noticeable during everyday activities. It does not have to be removed before sexual activity, but if it bothers you or your partner during intercourse, it can be temporarily removed (just don't forget to put it back in afterwards). The thought of a foreign object in the vagina bothers many women, but in the original clinical trials more than 90 percent of women wanted to continue with the ring after the study. For further information, visit www.NuvaRing.com.

Another option for women who frequently forget pills is the birth control patch, Ortho Evra. The estrogen and progesterone are released from a skin patch that is replaced weekly for three out of every four weeks. The patch has fallen somewhat out of favor because of studies demonstrating a somewhat higher incidence of deep vein thrombosis compared with most birth control pills. However, the absolute incidence of DVT is still very low and much lower than the incidence of DVT in pregnancy. If remembering to replace a patch once a week is easier for you than remembering to take a pill every day, this may be an option for you.

Will I have trouble getting pregnant when I stop taking the pill?

Oral contraceptives do not adversely affect fertility. Infertility is a common problem, affecting one in five couples. However, studies comparing previous pill users and nonusers reveal no difference in pregnancy rates. In fact, one of the more common causes of infertility, endometriosis (see chapter 8), is relatively suppressed while using the pill.

Some birth control pills let you skip periods. Is there any reason not to use these?

Traditionally, oral contraceptives have been designed with inactive pills at the end of each pack in order to induce a menstrual flow. They were designed this way to mimic the natural menstrual cycle. In recent years, some manufacturers have designed oral contraceptive regimens that eliminate these inactive pills, thereby eliminating periods. Some of these (Seasonale, Seasonique, Jolessa, Quasense, Camrese) cycle off every three months, giving you four periods annually. One regimen, Lybrel, is designed to be taken continuously without cycling off.

Consider continuous oral contraception if you have:

- *Severe cramps with periods*
- *Migraine headaches*
- *Endometriosis*
- *Irritable bowel disorder*
- *Epilepsy*
- *Asthma*
- *Anemia*

There are definitely advantages to continuous oral contraception. The first and most obvious is that it is more convenient to have fewer periods. This may be especially important if your menstrual flow is heavy or you have severe cramps with your period. There are also medical conditions that sometimes worsen during a menstrual period such as migraine headaches, epilepsy, asthma, and irritable bowel disorder. Women with these problems may benefit from continuous birth control pill regimens. Anemia secondary to heavy menstrual flow will also be improved with fewer periods. Certain gynecologic conditions such as endometriosis can improve with the use of continuous oral contraception.

The hormones in continuous oral contraceptives are similar to those in traditional oral contraceptives, so you are likely to experience similar side effects with either regimen. The side effect that is much more common with continuous oral contraception is breakthrough bleeding, or bleeding when you don't expect it. This tends to dissipate with time but can be rather disconcerting while it is happening. If it is persistent, your doctor may recommend that you discontinue the pills for three to four days and then restart. This often solves the problem.

To be honest, we do not know if continuous oral contraception is more or less safe than traditional regimens. We can tell you that in the short term it is just as safe, but there are no long-term studies to evaluate risks that may accumulate over time such as cancer. At this point in time, it seems that most gynecologists feel that it is just as safe to use these products as traditional pills.

What is the minipill?

Is this just a smaller version of the real thing? Well, not quite. The minipill is an oral contraceptive containing only progesterone—the more common birth control pills have both estrogen and progesterone. It is often prescribed for women who should not take estrogen because they are prone to conditions such as blood clots. It is also safer in cigarette smokers over the age of thirty-five and women with either migraine headaches or high blood pressure. It is commonly used in women who are breast-feeding. Combination birth control pills (those containing estrogen and progesterone) decrease milk production in breast-feeding mothers, while progesterone-only pills do not, and they do not harm the baby. Minipills are also useful for women who experience estrogen-related side effects when using combination birth control pills. There are two main problems with minipills. First, they are not as effective as combination birth control pills. The failure rate is

1–5 percent. Second, erratic bleeding is common. This poses no danger but is rather disconcerting.

It is important to try and take the minipill at the same time, even the same hour, every day. If you are more than three hours late in taking the pill, take it when you remember, continue your normal pill schedule, and use a backup method such as a condom for two weeks. Missing minipills puts you at significant risk for pregnancy if a backup method is not used.

What is the "morning-after" pill?

Jill calls her sister Lauren in a panic. "Oh my God, I can't believe what I did last night!"

Lauren senses her sister's anxiety. "What did you do? It can't be that bad."

"I got a little drunk and ended up having sex without using a condom," Jill confesses.

"Well, you shouldn't get pregnant," says Lauren, trying to reassure her sister. "At least you're on the pill."

"That's the problem," explains Jill. "I was getting headaches from my birth control pills so I stopped taking them. Now what can I do?"

The passion of the moment took over, and you had unprotected intercourse. Or maybe you used a condom and it slipped off or broke, or used a diaphragm and it slipped out of place. Now what do you do? You may be a candidate for using hormonal contraceptives in the "morning-after" regimen (also called emergency contraception). Older morning-after regimens utilized pills that contained estrogen and progesterone, similar to, or in some cases the same as, birth control pills. More recent products such as Plan B and Next Choice provide progesterone-only tablets containing 1.5 mg of levonorgestrel, either as two .75 mg doses twelve hours apart or as a single dose. These emergency contraceptives alter the inside lining of the uterus, decreasing your chances of becoming pregnant. With hormonal regimens, it is recommended that you start your emergency contraceptive product within seventy-two hours after unprotected sex, ideally within the first twenty-four hours. The FDA places the effectiveness of these products at 89 percent. Women can now obtain progesterone-based emergency contraception such as Plan B without a prescription. The most common side effect from hormonal emergency contraception is nausea. Your doctor can prescribe an anti-nausea medicine to limit this. If you vomit within two hours of taking a dose, you should repeat another dose to ensure effectiveness (after taking medication to reduce the risk of nausea and vomiting).

A more recent emergency contraceptive is Ella (ulipristal acetate). It works primarily by delaying or inhibiting ovulation. It has the advantage of being effective for up to 120 hours (five days). Ella appears to be somewhat more effective than levonorgestrel-based products, but is somewhat more expensive and is available only by prescription.

Another alternative for emergency contraception is placement of an IUD within 120 hours of unprotected sex. This is very effective and provides the additional advantage of remaining in place for future contraception. The most significant limiting factors are cost (very expensive if you do not have coverage) and accessibility (must be placed by a healthcare provider with experience).

For more information on emergency contraception, call the emergency contraception hotline at 800-584-9911 or go to www.soc.ucsb.edu/sexinfo/article/emergency-contraception-pills-ecps-0.

The Right Fit

Beth returns home from her first semester at college. She is a little anxious because she and her boyfriend Danny have been having sex. Danny has always used a condom, but Beth keeps forgetting to take her pills.

Beth calls Dr. Weston. "This is a little embarrassing. You put me on the birth control pill but I keep forgetting to take it. Is there anything else that would make sense for me?"

"Actually," begins Dr. Weston, "there are many other products for you to consider. There is a vaginal ring called NuvaRing that works just like the birth control pill. You only need to remember to replace it once a month. There are also birth control patches which are changed weekly. Both of these would be easier for you to remember."

Beth isn't sure that she'll remember to change the patch or ring. She thinks a minute and then asks Dr. Weston, "My roommate has an IUD. Is that safe for someone like me?"

"Doctors previously didn't use IUDs in women who haven't had children," replies Dr. Weston, "but, these days we feel it is okay. The risk is low. There is another possibility that you should consider. A small rod called Implanon that releases hormones can be placed under the skin in your upper arm under local anesthesia. It can stay there for three years and won't require you to remember anything."

After thinking it through, Beth decides to try Implanon.

What is the birth control device that is placed in the arm?

Implanon (also known as Nexplanon—the same product but contains an ingredient that makes it visible on X-rays) is a single rod made of a flexible polymer (like plastic), approximately the size of a matchstick, that is implanted in the inner upper arm. It is generally not visible, although you can feel it since it is placed superficially under the skin. Implanon is injected with progesterone that gradually is released into the body. It is very effective at preventing pregnancy and has a failure rate of less than 1 percent. After being inserted under local anesthesia, the rod may be allowed to remain in place for three years. At the end of that time, it is removed under local anesthesia, and a new one can be inserted. Because it contains progesterone, it may cause some of the same side effects that occur with birth control pills: nausea, headaches, bloating, breast tenderness, and mood changes. However, the majority of women tolerate Implanon well, with few side effects. Norplant-2 is similar to Implanon, but it consists of two rods instead of one and remains effective for five years rather than three.

Implanon's biggest drawback is its high price and the erratic bleeding it can cause. Because it contains only progesterone, erratic bleeding is common, particularly in the first year of usage. Although the bleeding is not dangerous, some women will discontinue use of Implanon because of this side effect. There may also be an increased frequency of ovarian cysts with use of Implanon, so if you are a woman who has had recurrent ovarian cysts, this may not be your best choice for contraception. Contraindications to the use of Implanon are similar to those listed above for other hormonal contraceptives. In addition, there have not been enough studies looking at the use of Implanon in women who are severely overweight. If your BMI is greater than thirty-five (go to www.nhlbi.nih.gov/guidelines/obesity/BMI/bmicalc.html to calculate your BMI), you should consider an alternate method of contraception.

I hear that there are shots that prevent pregnancy. Is that true?

You heard correctly. A progesterone injection called Depo-Provera can be injected into the arm and will slowly release the hormone into the body. A shot administered every three months provides reliable contraception. Available for decades in this country, this hormonal preparation originally was not approved for contraceptive use because studies linked it to breast tumors in beagles. Subsequently, researchers found that it does not cause tumors in people. Others have raised concerns that women who use Depo-Provera for a long time may suffer loss of bone density. The risk appears to be small and in most cases bone density is recovered after women stop using it.

Side effects with Depo-Provera are similar to those of Implanon: nausea, bloating, headaches, breast tenderness, and mood changes. In addition, weight commonly increases by five to ten pounds. The most common reason for discontinuing the use of Depo-Provera is erratic bleeding. Adverse reactions may persist for as long as four months, since the progesterone is slowly released over the course of three months. Its contraceptive effect can persist even after it is discontinued. Therefore, it is not a good choice for those who plan to get pregnant in the near future.

Are IUDs safe?

The IUD, short for intrauterine device, got a bad reputation from the Dalkon Shield, a particular type of IUD that caused a high incidence of pelvic infections. The Dalkon Shield received much publicity, resulting in multiple lawsuits. The adverse publicity resulted in a decline in IUD usage, which is unfortunate, because it is a good choice for many women.

The IUD is a plastic device inserted into the uterus by a trained healthcare provider. It contains either copper (ParaGard) or progesterone (Mirena, Skyla). Periodically (every three years for Skyla, five years for Mirena, and every ten years for Paragard) it is removed, and a new IUD is inserted. When conception is desired, it is removed. The IUD is 98–99 percent successful in preventing pregnancy. Little is required of the woman, so it is convenient.

Sounds great! What's the catch? Well, IUDs can be rather expensive (six hundred dollars plus the cost of insertion) so you will have to check with your insurance company to see if it is covered. With insertion of an IUD there is a small risk of developing PID, or pelvic inflammatory disease. With every pelvic infection, there is a chance of developing scar tissue, called adhesions, which may in turn result in infertility or chronic pelvic pain. Women in a mutually monogamous relationship who are at low risk for contracting sexually transmitted infections have minimal risk of developing PID. The increased risk of PID is seen within the first three weeks of insertion. After that time, your risk for PID returns to what it was before insertion of the IUD. You can be screened for sexually transmitted infections and other conditions such as bacterial vaginosis (chapter 5) that may increase your risk of PID prior to insertion for reassurance.

IUDs may also alter your menstrual flow. There is a tendency for heavier menstrual periods with more cramps in the first three to six months after IUD insertion. This usually lessens over time, and in the case of Skyla and Mirena, menses may become infrequent or even cease altogether. In fact, both Mirena and Skyla can be used for women who have heavy menstrual periods to lessen their flow. Skyla is slightly smaller than Mirena so there may be less pain with insertion, but it must be changed in three years, whereas Mirena is approved for five. More serious complications of IUDs including expulsion (the IUD expelling out of the uterine opening), sepsis (infection spreading throughout the body), embedment (getting stuck in the wall of the uterus), and perforation (extruding through the wall of the uterus) are uncommon and should not dissuade you from choosing this as a method of contraception. In general, IUDs provide safe, reliable contraception. However, if you experience any of the following, contact your doctor immediately:

- Persistent pain very low in the abdomen
- Persistent fever
- Prolonged bleeding (more than a week) or a missed period
- Inability to locate the IUD's string, or feeling hard plastic when checking for the string

Although pregnancy rarely occurs if an IUD is in proper position, serious complications can result when it does. There is an increased risk of miscarriage, ectopic pregnancy, premature delivery, and uterine infection. If you miss a period while using the IUD, contact your doctor. If pregnancy is confirmed, he or she will recommend removal of the IUD. Although its removal increases your chances of miscarriage, it decreases the risks of serious complications late in the pregnancy.

For more information on IUDs, visit:

www.mirena-us.com

www.paragard.com

How can I tell if my IUD is in place?

Every IUD has a string attached to it. The doctor trims the string so that approximately half to one inch protrudes into the vagina from the cervix. Prior to intercourse, place a finger in the vagina and feel for this string, which feels like fishing line. First, locate your cervix, which feels like the tip of your nose. The string emanates from the opening of the cervix. If you feel a hard plastic piece, it indicates that the uterus has expelled your IUD. Expulsion most commonly occurs within the first few weeks after insertion, but it can happen at any time. Most women generally have no problems with the IUD. But if you can't feel your string, one of three events has happened:

- The uterus has expelled the IUD. It must be replaced.
- The string has simply retracted into the uterus, but the IUD remains in place. An ultrasound scan can confirm this diagnosis, and no

Does educating teens about contraception increase their likelihood of engaging in sexual activity?

Many parents assume that educating their teen about contraception is tantamount to giving them permission to engage in sexual activity. However, studies looking at this issue do not support that contention. The nonpartisan National Campaign to Prevent Teen and Unplanned Pregnancy found that "at present, there does not exist any strong evidence that any abstinence program delays the initiation of sex, hastens the return to abstinence, or reduces the number of sexual partners."

Mathematica Policy Research Inc. studied four abstinence education programs over five years. They concluded that the number of youth who remained abstinent, the average age at first sexual intercourse, and the number of sexual further treatment will be needed.

- The IUD has perforated the uterus—a very rare but potentially serious complication. It must be removed. Laparoscopy may be necessary. Contact your doctor if you cannot feel your string.

How do I know which method of contraception is best for me?

No single method of contraception is right for everyone. This decision must be made in conjunction with your doctor. Here are a few guidelines:

partners were almost identical for program and control youth.

Discouraging casual sex is an important role for parents and sex educators. The value of limiting sex to long-term committed, intimate relationships should be stressed. However, we must also prepare young people with appropriate information about contraception. Our experience as physicians has taught us that providing information regarding contraception does not significantly increase the likelihood of sexual activity, but it does prevent unwanted pregnancies and sexually transmitted infections.

- If you wish to avoid "artificial" contraception, natural family planning is your only choice. Keep in mind that it is the most difficult and least successful of contraceptive methods.
- If you are single and sexually active, hormonal contraceptives are probably your best choice, since they are very effective at preventing pregnancy. Unless you are involved in a stable, mutually monogamous relationship, condoms should also be used to protect you against sexually transmitted diseases. Smart phone apps like "myPill" can function as a daily reminder system. A daily reminder appears at a preset time that says, "Take a pill!" The reminder also can be sent via text or email.

It can also be set to remind users to replace their NuvaRing contraceptive.

- If you are notoriously unreliable in taking oral contraceptives regularly, the IUD and Implanon (or Norplant) are good choices. Once in place, these offer excellent protection and require little or no effort on your part.

- If your goal is to use the safest contraceptives with the fewest side effects, barrier methods are your best choice. However, you must combine multiple barrier methods to approach the effectiveness of hormonal contraceptives. Barrier contraceptives also tend to disrupt foreplay, so you must be highly motivated to use them effectively.

- If you have completed your family, sterilization (tubal sterilization or vasectomy) may be the best bet. Consider this only if permanent contraception is your goal.

How are abortions done?

There are two commonly used practices for electively terminating an early pregnancy. The first, a D&E, or dilation and evacuation, can be performed if the pregnancy is early (up to twelve to fourteen weeks from the last menstrual period). A D&E, also referred to as suction curettage, is usually performed as an outpatient procedure, either at a physician's office or surgical facility. The pregnancy is confirmed by a blood pregnancy test, a pelvic ultrasound, or both. The doctor administers a local anesthetic in or near the cervix. Sedatives may also be given. If the pregnancy is more advanced, general anesthesia may be administered. The doctor dilates the cervix and inserts a plastic tube that is connected to a suction pump. The pregnancy is then evacuated. After a period of observation (one to three hours), the patient can go home. A variable degree of cramping and bleeding will follow the procedure. Activities may be restricted after the procedure, although most can be resumed within a day or two.

"The topic of abortion evokes strong and varied convictions about the social order, the roles of women and men, human life and human responsibility, freedom and limits, sexual morality and the significance of children in our lives. It involves powerful feelings that are based on different life experiences and interpretations of faith and life in the world. If we are to take our differences seriously, we must learn how to talk about them in ways that do justice to our diversity. The language used in discussing abortion should ignore neither the value of unborn life nor the value of the woman and her other relationships. It should neither obscure the moral seriousness of the decision faced by the woman nor hide the moral value of the newly conceived life."

—Evangelical Lutheran Church in America

Dr. Thornton does not personally perform elective termination of pregnancy.

If the pregnancy is nine weeks or less, termination can be medically induced. Early pregnancy is highly dependent on progesterone, one of the ovarian hormones. Mifepristone (also known as RU-486) is an anti-progestational agent. Mifepristone interferes with early pregnancy by causing a separation of the placenta from the endometrium, softening the cervix, and inducing uterine contractions. Within forty-eight hours, misoprostol, a second medicine which heightens the uterine contractions, is given, whereupon the pregnancy is expelled, similar to a spontaneous miscarriage. Misoprostol can be administered vaginally, orally, or buccally (between the gum and cheek). Depending on the dose and route of administration, it may be given as early as six hours after the mifepristone. Some doctors will ask you to remain for four hours after administering misoprostol. If serious side effects occur, they are most likely to occur during this time. Other doctors may allow patients to self-administer the misoprostol at home. Side effects from the misoprostol include

However, if a woman has made the very difficult choice of terminating her pregnancy, he will refer her to a medical facility that can provide her with the necessary resources and emotional support. The information provided in this chapter is for educational purposes. It is not a moral statement either condemning or condoning elective termination of pregnancy.

nausea, vomiting, diarrhea, headaches, dizziness, chills or flushes, shivering, and fatigue. If these are severe, you should contact your doctor. You should also contact your doctor if heavy bleeding persists for more than twelve hours or if you have severe, unremitting lower abdominal pain. Complete expulsion of the pregnancy is often confirmed at a follow-up appointment. A D&E is performed if the abortion is incomplete. Medical abortion is 92 percent effective when your pregnancy is seven weeks or less.

Elective abortion of more advanced pregnancies (fourteen to twenty-three weeks from the last menstrual period) is accomplished by using agents that induce labor. This often includes a prostaglandin like misoprostol and an intravenous solution containing Pitocin, a hormone that causes uterine contractions. Labor-inducing abortions are usually performed in the hospital and may require an overnight stay. Side effects are similar to those mentioned above for misoprostol, although they may be more severe since multiple doses may be used and more severe cramping will be experienced when the pregnancy is advanced. Medications are given before and during the induction to decrease the severity of the side effects.

Some physicians perform an extended D&E on advanced pregnancies. In addition to suction curettage, special instruments are used to evacuate the pregnancy from the uterus. An extended D&E has several advantages over induced labor. The painful contractions of labor are avoided, as are the side effects from the prostaglandins. The procedure is also less time-consuming. If the physician is inexperienced, however, there is a significant risk of uterine perforation, hemorrhage, and incomplete evacuation of the pregnancy. With experienced healthcare providers, serious complications are rare. Pain that lasts for more than a day or two, heavy bleeding, fever, or nausea and vomiting should prompt you to call the gynecologist.

The effects abortion may have on your emotional state depend on your values, your circumstances, and your religious beliefs. Depending on your circumstances, consultation with a psychiatrist, psychologist, counselor, social worker, or religious leader may be beneficial.

Can I have a normal pregnancy after having an abortion?

Most physicians agree that an uncomplicated abortion will have no impact on subsequent pregnancies. There is always a small chance that a severe complication could have an effect on your future fertility, but this is uncommon. Few studies have looked at the effect of multiple abortions on fertility. Multiple abortions may increase the risk of pre-term birth in later pregnancies.

How is a tubal ligation done? Is it safe?

A common question is "How do they tie your tubes?" Actually, the term is a misnomer because tubes are not usually tied. Except for sterilization performed immediately after delivery, tubal ligations are done as outpatient surgery, utilizing laparoscopy. After administering anesthesia, the doctor expands the abdominal cavity by filling it with gas. A telescopic instrument is inserted through a tiny incision near the navel to permit a view of the pelvic organs. A section of one fallopian tube is grasped and is coagulated (electric current is passed through the tube), clipped, or banded. The doctor performs a similar procedure on the other tube. Depending on the technique used, a second small incision may be necessary. The incisions (less than one half inch in length) are easily closed. After a period of observation in a recovery area, the patient is discharged and may resume normal activities the following day.

Occasionally, the procedure cannot be completed through the laparoscope, and a larger incision is required to finish the operation, which might lengthen hospitalization and recovery. If this is unacceptable, let your doctor know in advance.

Recovery from laparoscopic sterilization is usually uneventful. It is common to experience discomfort in the shoulder for a day or two. The cause is actually residual gas in the abdominal cavity, but the brain mistakenly attributes it to the shoulder. The body will absorb the gas, and the symptom will disappear. If you experience nausea from the anesthesia or surgery, eat lightly until it clears, usually within twenty-four hours. Pain may be felt in the pelvic region or at abdominal incisions. Your doctor can give you prescriptions to relieve pain and nausea before you leave the hospital.

Complications with laparoscopic tubal sterilization are uncommon. They include bleeding and injury to other internal organs such as the bowel, ureters, and bladder, and their repair may require a more extensive operation. The possibility of complications should not deter a woman from choosing this operation, however, because they are rare.

The failure rate for tubal sterilization is less than 1 percent. When pregnancy does occur, there is a greater than normal chance that it will be a tubal one. Tubal pregnancies are life-threatening if not detected early. If you miss a period after undergoing tubal sterilization, contact your physician.

Essure is a procedure available as an alternative to laparoscopic tubal sterilization. An Essure-certified provider will introduce small inserts into your fallopian tubes through the vagina and cervix without requiring any incisions. The tips of the inserts remain visible so your doctor can confirm proper placement. Over the following three months, your body works with these inserts to create a permanent blockage of the fallopian tubes. Backup contraception is still required during this time. At the end of three months, your doctor will inject dye into the uterus and take an X-ray in order to confirm that blockage is complete. While the Essure procedure is fairly new (approved since 2002), it is just as effective as laparoscopic tubal procedures, eliminates the need for incisions, and can often be done as an outpatient procedure in the office. For more information, visit www.essure.com.

> ## Proceed with caution!
> *If there is any chance at all that you may want to conceive down the road,* do not *get an elective sterilization procedure. Do not assume that you will be able to reverse the procedure.*

Can my tubes be put back together?

A tubal sterilization should not be considered reversible. If there is any chance that you might want to become pregnant in the future, tubal steriliza-tion should not be performed. Having said that, we realize life doesn't always lead down expected paths. Loss of a child or a second marriage often motivates women to try to get their tubal sterilization reversed.

To rejoin the severed tubes, infertility specialists perform tubal reanastomosis. For this operation to be successful, a large proportion of the tubes must be healthy. If there is sufficient tubal length to allow the procedure, success rates are 50 percent. If the tubes are beyond salvage, you should consider in vitro fertilization. In this procedure, your eggs are retrieved from the ovary, fertilized outside the body, and then introduced into the uterus, bypassing the tubes.

Why have my periods been irregular since my tubal sterilization?

Although it often seems that there is a change in one's menses in the years following a tubal sterilization, most investigators who have looked into this question have not found a greater incidence of menstrual abnormalities among women who have undergone that operation. One reason for the apparent rise in problems following tubal sterilization is that most women undergo tubal sterilization in their middle to late thirties, a time when periods normally start to exhibit more variation.

Is it better for my husband to have a vasectomy than for me to undergo a tubal sterilization?

Jenny is forty-two and has a healthy, stable marriage with her husband George. She has three children who are all doing well and doesn't plan on having any more children. She is thinking about getting a tubal steriliza-tion procedure when a thought pops into her head. Wait a minute! Why am I doing this? Why is it that the woman always has to bear the brunt of everything? I was the one who took birth control pills all those years and I was the one who went through three pregnancies. I mean, I'm not complaining. I would do it all again, but isn't it time that George assumed responsibility?

Jenny discusses this with George over dinner. George agrees that they won't have more children and should do something more permanent, but isn't thrilled with the prospect of getting a vasectomy. The thought makes him feel somewhat emasculated. After all, isn't that going to interfere with his ability to have sex?

The scenario above is very common. Often it is assumed that women should get a tubal sterilization procedure if permanent contra-ception is desired. However, vasectomy is an easy, effective alternative that should certainly be considered. A vasectomy is easier than a lapa-roscopic tubal sterilization procedure but no easier than the Essure procedure. Most of the male reproductive tract is outside the body, making it more accessible. Sperm is made in the testes and then trans-ported through tubes called the vas deferens. Under local anesthesia, they can be easily cut and sealed, thereby preventing the release of sperm from the testes. Minor swelling and discomfort are typical, but serious complications or side effects are rare.

The main drawback of vasectomy is that, unlike tubal steriliza-tion, it is not immediately effective. A backup method of contraception must be used until the doctor determines that no sperm are present on semen analysis. This may take as long as several months.

Men often avoid vasectomy because of the misimpression that it will interfere with sexual performance or enjoyment. Vasectomy does not interfere with arousal, erection, or ejaculation.

Vasectomy is very reliable, with a failure rate of less than 1 percent. Although putting the tubes back together may be successful, you should not consider vasectomy reversible.

If I'm in menopause, can I still get pregnant?

First, make sure you're really in menopause. You may think you are menopausal if you are over forty and not having menstrual periods. However, it is possible that your cycle is "out of sync" but your ovaries are still active. If this is the case, you might still ovulate and conceive. If you are not having menstrual periods and are experiencing hot flashes, it is probable that you are menopausal. This can be confirmed through measuring hormone levels. Once menopause is confirmed, continue to use a method of contraception for at least another six to twelve months. Occasionally, a woman will still manage to ovulate within this time—a kind of last hurrah.

4

SEXUAL RELATIONS

Why does it hurt when I have sex?

It doesn't seem fair. Your reproductive organs cause you grief your whole life. Your menstrual period disrupts your life at the most inopportune times. On top of that, cramps come with it. There is a litany of things that can go wrong with the reproductive organs. At the very least, you deserve to get some pleasure from them. Isn't that where sex enters into the picture? You hope so. Therefore, it is particularly distressing when you experience pain during sexual encounters. What should be intimate and pleasurable is transformed into a frightening, painful experience. This extends beyond the physical pain to affect your emotional well-being. If the problem is recurrent, it may also strain a relationship.

If intercourse is painful, seek help. You must overcome any embarrassment you may have about discussing this with your doctor. Trust us: Your problem is not unique, and the doctor can't help you if you don't ask.

There are numerous causes for painful intercourse. We'll start our discussion with the most common causes and gradually work our way toward those that are more obscure.

The most likely cause for discomfort in the vagina during intercourse is insufficient lubrication. Vaginal lubrication naturally happens as sexual arousal occurs; the vagina moistens with secretions produced by the vaginal walls. Without adequate foreplay, lubrication will not occur. Some men think getting undressed constitutes ample foreplay, so you might have to give your partner a clue as to what is required for you to become stimulated. Sexual arousal is more difficult when you are anxious, so try to initiate sex in a relaxed setting.

Vaginal dryness is normal at some points in life. The weeks immediately following childbirth are one such time. If you breast-feed your infant, dryness will continue longer. As your estrogen production resumes, the problem will correct itself. You will also develop vaginal dryness at menopause. Estrogen replacement will help, if you choose to pursue hormone replacement therapy (see chapter 13). Vaginal moisturizing creams (Replens, Gyne-Moistrin, Luvena, and RepHresh) can be purchased over the counter for generalized vaginal dryness. However, if your problem is painful intercourse, you should use a lubricant. Lubricants can be purchased over the counter without a prescription. The cheapest is ordinary K-Y Jelly (or a generic version of K-Y), which gynecologists often use for examinations. All lubricants are water-based preparations that do not stain and clean up readily. K-Y and other manufacturers have added additional ingredients that supposedly enhance your sexual experience. Keep in mind that these products will be more expensive and that there is a possibility of you having either an allergic or irritant reaction from the additional chemicals. Do not use petroleum or oil-based products such as Vaseline, particularly if your partner uses latex condoms, because petroleum jelly dissolves latex.

Vaginitis, inflammation of the vagina, is another common cause of painful intercourse. Suspect an infection if you have vaginal burning or itching. An unusual discharge or odor may also be present. Although the infection may begin in the vagina, it can spread externally to create vulvitis, inflammation of the vulva. Yeast infections are notorious for causing inflammation of both the vagina and the vulva. Other infections cause ulceration of the vulva or opening of the vagina. Herpes and syphilis can both do this. Of the two, herpes is more likely to cause painful open sores that prevent intercourse. Genital warts (condylomata) commonly affect the external genitalia and can produce irritation. We will discuss these infections in more detail in chapter 5.

Vulvar inflammation and sensitivity (see chapter 11) can also arise from an irritant or allergic reaction. A few suggestions are worth emphasizing. Use only mild soaps without deodorants, scents, and dyes (a good choice is hypoallergenic Aveeno). Use white, unscented toilet paper. Wear white cotton underclothing, and wash your underclothing with mild detergents.

Various dermatologic diseases produce vulvar inflammation, making intercourse painful. The doctor diagnoses these either by their appearance or with a skin biopsy, which can be done in the office under local anesthesia. Your gynecologist or dermatologist can treat these with anti-inflammatory creams or ointments to reduce the inflammation.

Vaginismus, a painful spasm of the vagina that precludes intercourse, may also cause pain on attempted entry. Muscles at the opening of the vagina often tighten in anticipation of pain. If you have experienced painful attempts at intercourse previously or have been sexually abused, this is more likely to happen.

The good news is that you can learn to control these muscles. Place one finger into the vagina and attempt to contract the muscles around your finger. Now concentrate on relaxing the muscles. Continue to do this until you achieve control. Once you have established control, introduce a second finger and repeat the sequence. Finally, overlap three fingers (place your second and fourth fingers under your third finger). When you can successfully introduce three overlapped fingers and still relax your muscles, intercourse should be possible. It is important not to attempt intercourse prior to this point. If you try too soon, you will feel pain, which makes it more difficult to learn vaginal muscle relaxation.

Some women prefer to use vaginal dilators for their relaxation exercises. They are available in sets of graduated sizes. Dilators can be purchased through your doctor's office, directly from a manufacturer (Syracuse Medical Devices), or online (www.middlesexmd.com, www.vaginismus.com). You should insert a size that can be placed in the vagina without pain. Use a water-based lubricant such as K-Y Jelly when introducing the dilator and leave it in place for five to fifteen minutes. Every three to four weeks, transition to the next largest dilator.

Before attempting intercourse, concentrate on sexual foreplay to help with vaginal lubrication and relaxation. Digital stimulation, with your partner placing his fingers in your vagina, is helpful. See if you can relax your vaginal muscles while your partner puts his fingers in the vagina. You can then attempt intercourse. Don't hesitate to use a lubricant, and lower yourself from above onto his penis. That way you have control over the degree of penetration. You can lower yourself slowly, stopping intermittently to relax the vaginal muscles.

Sometimes, the opening of the vagina is partly closed by the hymen, a ring of tissue located at the entrance to the vagina. Your doctor can assess this and instruct you on how to stretch the hymenal ring, using your fingers or vaginal dilators. If this is unsuccessful, the doctor can make small incisions (after injecting an anesthetic) to open the hymenal ring.

A cyst or abscess in the special glands located between the labia, at the entrance to the vaginal canal in what is called the vestibule, can cause pain with attempted entry into the vagina. They can be treated with warm compresses, incision and drainage, or removal. Vulvar vestibulitis, a local or generalized inflammation limited to the vestibule, can also be the problem. The inflammation is often overlooked on examination but causes intense pain when touched. Vestibular disorders are discussed more thoroughly in chapter 11.

> **Do not wait!**
>
> *If sexual activity is painful, seek help. You can certainly try easy things such as adding lubricants and changing positions, but if that fails, make an appointment with your gynecologist. The quality of your current sexual experiences impacts future sexual satisfaction. If sex is painful, pretty soon you will no longer desire sex. You may also develop problems with arousal and orgasm.*

Urinary tract infections occasionally cause painful intercourse, but not usually. The bladder and urethra lie in direct proximity to the vagina. The opening of the urethra, called the urethral meatus, is located immediately above the vaginal opening. Inflammation associated with cystitis (bladder infection) or urethritis (urethral infection) may cause pain either with initial penetration of the vagina or during intercourse. Other common symptoms of urinary infections include frequency (you feel as if you have to run to the bathroom every five minutes), urgency (you feel as though you'd better get there quickly or have an accident), and pain or burning when you urinate.

Pain that occurs with deep penetration is the most serious problem, as it may represent a disorder of the internal reproductive organs. Uterine infections (not to be confused with vaginal infections) may cause pain with deep penetration. Treatment consists of antibiotics. Other uterine problems such as fibroids (noncancerous tumors in the wall of the uterus) and adenomyosis (a condition in which the inside lining of the uterus grows into the wall of the uterus) may create pain when the penis hits the cervix. Ovaries are very sensitive, and cysts or tumors of the ovaries increase the likelihood of experiencing pain with deep penetration. Endometriosis (see chapter 8) and pelvic adhesions also create pain felt deep in the pelvis. A thorough examination and pelvic ultrasound are warranted when there is deep pelvic pain during intercourse. If the results of the tests are normal, you should try different positions. You may have less pain if you control the degree of penetration by positioning yourself on top during intercourse. If the problem is persistent and severe, you should consider laparoscopy. During laparoscopy, your doctor inserts a telescopic instrument into the abdomen under anesthesia in order to get a direct look at your pelvic organs.

Rarely, pain in the vagina results from scarring related to previous vaginal surgery or injuries incurred during childbirth. These areas may stretch and become less painful with time. Anesthetic creams or lubricants may help. Experiment with different positions during intercourse. If the vagina is narrowed, vaginal dilators can be used to increase the width of the vagina (see page 87). Surgery is indicated if no improvement is seen over time. There is always a small chance that the operation will produce scarring that might worsen the condition. Therefore, it is best to pursue the conservative options before proceeding with surgery.

Finally, emotional factors can influence sexual response. Problems within a relationship, depression, anxiety, and emotional or sexual abuse all interfere with the natural sexual response, inhibiting relaxation of the muscles at the opening of the vagina and decreasing vaginal lubrication. The lengthening of the vagina that occurs with a normal sexual response may be inhibited, allowing the penis to hit sensitive structures deep within the pelvis. All of these can produce pain, which causes more emotional distress, further restricting the natural sexual response. A vicious cycle develops, which becomes progressively harder to break. Depression or anxiety that interferes with your sex life warrants evaluation by a psychologist or psychiatrist. A strained relationship may benefit from marriage counseling. Deal with the problem, and seek help early before it becomes overwhelming.

Why don't I have orgasms?

We're presuming that you see this as a problem. Lack of an orgasm is a problem only if you or your partner perceives it as one. For many women, orgasm is not a primary endpoint when it comes to sexual activity. A desire for increased emotional closeness and intimacy is often the primary motivation for pursuing or initiating sexual activity. Having said that, approximately 90 percent of women can experience orgasm. The inability to achieve one frequently relates to misconceptions about the normal sexual response. Classically, this response is defined by the four stages described below. However, many women do not move progressively and sequentially through all of these stages or even experience all of these stages.

Stage I: Motivation, Excitement, and Arousal Initially a woman must have motivation to instigate or agree to sexual activity. This may encompass a desire to receive and share physical pleasure or emotional closeness to her partner. It may be an expression of love or arise from a desire to please her partner. As motivation is maintained, a woman will find and consciously focus on sexual stimuli that lead to sexual arousal. With increasing excitement, the clitoris enlarges and hardens. The clitoris is a swelling located immediately above the vaginal and urethral openings. There is a "hood," or fold of tissue, overlying it that often retracts during this phase, making the clitoris more accessible. The clitoris is far more sensitive than any other structure in the genital region and is almost always responsible for initiating orgasm. Difficulty achieving orgasm is most typically the result of insufficient stimulation of the clitoris. Women generally require prolonged stimulation of this and other erogenous areas in order to experience orgasm. Occasionally, the clitoris is so sensitive that direct stimulation is painful. This can be overcome by stimulating the tissues adjacent to the clitoris while avoiding direct contact.

Explore your body to identify other areas that arouse you. Pleasurable places may include the breasts (particularly the nipples), ears, neck, vagina, buttocks, anus, thighs, and feet. You must communicate with your partner and direct him to the areas that provide pleasurable sensations for you. This is no time to be shy; assertiveness in the bedroom has its distinct rewards. Men often become excited and experience orgasm quickly. He needs to understand that this is not a race. Tell him that he needs to be more attentive for an extended time before and after intercourse. Try to have sex in a relaxed setting when neither of you are pressed for time. Leave your stress and tension at the bedroom door. Try to let your mind focus on the pleasurable sensations you are experiencing, not on whether Billy did his homework and Susie finished her piano practice.

During the excitement phase, the vagina moistens with secretions. Blood begins to engorge the internal and external genitalia, which may be noticed by swelling of the labia. The vagina begins to lengthen and expand to readily accept the penis. The uterus swells and rises from its usual position. The nipples may become erect and more sensitive to stimulation.

Stage II: Plateau Phase During this phase, excitement continues to build. Continued stimulation allows sexual excitement and pleasure to become more intense, triggering the desire for sex itself. The pelvic structures become further engorged. The vagina continues to expand. At this point, the clitoris retracts under its hood. The breasts expand and nipple erection is maintained. Muscular tension increases along with the heart rate, blood pressure, and respiratory rate. If sexual response stops at this phase without progression to orgasm, congestion of pelvic blood vessels can occur. This may cause pelvic soreness or aching and sometimes backache. It can be relieved by continuing stimulation until orgasm is reached.

Stage III: Orgasm The peak of the cycle brings extremely pleasurable sensations in association with rhythmic contractions of the vagina and uterus. There is a feeling of increased sexual awareness in the area of the clitoris which spreads upward with a suffusion of warmth that spreads from the pelvis throughout the body. The anal muscles tighten, and the toes may curl. Muscles throughout the body may contract involuntarily, causing pelvic thrusting and spastic movements of the neck, hands, arms, feet, and legs. After a short period of time this abates, and muscular tension relaxes.

Stage IV: Resolution Following the orgasm, a woman may return to the plateau phase. If stimulated at this time, she may again achieve orgasm. Some women will experience multiple orgasms during sex. If there is no further stimulation, the pelvic organs and genitalia return to their pre-aroused state. At this point, many women do not enjoy further physical stimulation.

There is tremendous variability in sexual responsiveness. Orgasms may be experienced at varying levels of intensity, and not all sexual encounters will culminate in orgasm. Sexual intimacy should be about love and sharing, not performance. Focusing on performance produces tension and anxiety that decreases the chances of having a fulfilling sensual experience.

If you can't allow yourself to relax and enjoy the pleasurable sensations provided through sexual stimulation, your chances of reaching orgasm are diminished. Your inhibitions may result from a misconception that sex is "dirty." This is often the message that parents inadvertently (or not so inadvertently) transmit to their children. Some mothers have told their daughters that sex is a duty, performed for the man's enjoyment and not the woman's. This misimpression doesn't change overnight. However, with a supportive partner, you should be able to gradually allow yourself to experience the pleasure you deserve. If you still have difficulty, consider sexual counseling.

Drugs, alcohol, and certain medications may decrease your ability to become sexually aroused and reach orgasm. Alcohol may initially lower your inhibitions and therefore increase your ability to enjoy sex. However, it depresses the central nervous system and ultimately decreases response to sexual stimulation. Some medications decrease libido (sexual desire) or sexual responsiveness. Check with your physician if you are taking medications and have this problem. The *Physicians' Desk Reference* will state whether decreased libido is a side effect.

Certain medical disorders, such as depression or anxiety, may interfere with your sexual responsiveness, as do chronic medical illnesses. Lowered hormone levels experienced by nursing mothers may decrease sexual arousal, and chronic fatigue and sleep deprivation play their part as well: "I don't see him getting up to nurse the baby." Lowered hormone levels during menopause may decrease libido. Hormonal replacement, particularly if testosterone is included, can help (see chapter 13).

In recent years there has been a great deal of interest in finding medications that will treat female sexual dysfunction. Two of the more common medications looked at are sildenafil (Viagra) and bupropion (Wellbutrin). While Viagra, Cialis, and Levitra have been very successful in treating male erectile dysfunction, their place in treating female sexual dysfunction is cloudier. Studies are very mixed in their results. If there is a role for sildenafil in women, it would be for the treatment of disorders of arousal or orgasm, where there are at least some studies suggesting a benefit. Bupropion has mostly been studied in conjunction with sexual dysfunction related to SSRI antidepressants. Again, the studies show mixed results, but it would not be unreasonable for a doctor to add bupropion to a patient with sexual dysfunction who is on an SSRI antidepressant. Phentolamine, apomorphine, and prostaglandin E1 are other drugs under investigation. L-arginine and yohimbine are used in the complementary and alternative community for sexual dysfunction and theoretically should have some benefit in treating disorders of arousal or orgasm. Pharmacists will sometimes compound a cream with these ingredients, with or without sildenafil, for direct application around the clitoral region.

Does Kelly Need a Sex Therapist?

Kelly and Marie have been best friends since high school. They are both married, Marie for five years and Kelly for three. They live at different parts of the city but meet every Tuesday at the Olive Garden for lunch. Today, there is an awkward silence. Marie senses that something is wrong with her friend, who is usually quite chatty.

"What's on your mind?" asks Marie.

"What do you mean?"

"I've known you for ten years. You can't fool me. I know when something is on your mind."

Kelly seems hesitant. "Okay, can I ask you a personal question?"

"Sure, fire away," Marie blurts out, not knowing exactly what to expect.

Kelly summons a bit of courage and asks, "Do you enjoy sex?"

"Of course," responds Marie, "doesn't everybody?"

"I don't know. I mean, maybe."

Marie is a little perplexed. "There isn't really a maybe. Either you like sex or you don't."

Kelly thinks a minute before responding. "Well, I like being with Bill when we're in bed together. I like being close to him. But when it comes to sex, he gets excited very easily and next thing I know we're done. I don't think I've ever had an orgasm."

"Well, that's men for you," says Marie. "Wham bam thank you ma'am. You have to tell him to slow down and pay more attention to you and your needs. Do you get orgasms when you masturbate?"

"Oh Lord, I would never do that!" Kelly blushes.

"Really?" Marie is skeptical. "We live in the twenty-first century, not Victorian England."

"Well, you've known me for a long time," Kelly says, a bit defensive. "I was raised in a strict Catholic home. Sometimes I get anxious just thinking about sex."

Marie doesn't know how to respond, but offers, "Maybe you should see somebody about that."

So what do you think? Does Kelly need a therapist? Well, maybe. She may be content with the level of intimacy provided in her current sexual encounters with Bill and derive satisfaction from the pleasure it brings her husband. However, if she wants to experience more intense sexual pleasure herself, she will have to overcome her anxiety and fear of losing control as well as any inhibitions she may have regarding various types of sexual activity. She will also have to get to a point where she feels comfortable communicating her physical needs with Bill. Certainly a therapist, perhaps a sex therapist or couples therapist, can help her.

Where is the "G-spot"?

Okay, you got us. This is not a frequently asked question, but it was too good to pass up. One can't talk about orgasm without at least mentioning the famous "G-spot," or Grafenberg spot. This is a swelling in the upper front section of your vaginal wall that is reputed to create orgasmic arousal. Stimulation of this area is thought to elicit a "vaginal orgasm." Some physicians do not acknowledge the existence of the G-spot. They feel that vaginal stimulation indirectly transmits neural impulses through the clitoris to induce sexual excitement. Finding the G-spot is certainly not critical for a fulfilling sexual experience. Nevertheless, think of all the fun you will have trying to locate it.

Why don't I have any sex drive?

Betty is a fifty-six-year-old postmenopausal woman who loves her husband and wants to be intimate with him, but she has no sex drive. What's going on here? What can she do to get her sex drive back? There must be a problem with her hormones, right?

Well, not necessarily. Emotional intimacy is the most important aspect of a fulfilling sex life. Television, movies, and the burgeoning influence of pornography have removed emotional intimacy from sex and promoted it more as a pleasurable diversion. Ideally, sex is about two people wanting to be in perfect union with one another, wanting to become a part of each other. You and your partner must make time for each other and engage in activities together that reinforce emotional attachment. Often this intimacy was built around raising children together. Intimacy diminishes as children achieve independence and move out of the house. Without realizing it, you and your partner grow apart as each person pursues their own interests. You and your partner must intentionally find common activities and goals that will foster togetherness. You have to do things for each other to strengthen your relationship.

With the frantic pace of couples' lives today, it is difficult to find time to relax and reach the degree of intimacy necessary for romance. Work may leave either partner stressed or exhausted. It's unrealistic to expect a sex drive to thrive under those circumstances. You must make time for one another. A vacation away from work with just the two of you is ideal. It gives you the opportunity to forget all the complications of your life and to focus on each other. If that much time away is not possible, aim for a weekend or even just a day.

Another strategy for jump-starting your sex drive is devoting more time to thoughts and activities that enhance sex. Men usually spend more of each day thinking about sex than women do. It's no wonder they are often raring to go. Discover (or rediscover) activities that sexually arouse you. Sometimes reading romantic or erotic novels or magazines will intensify your sexual drive. Sexual fantasy may also heighten your desire for an encounter. It is unrealistic to spend your entire day without sexual thoughts and then to expect to instantly turn on your libido when needed.

Decreased frequency of sexual encounters ultimately decreases your desire for more sexual encounters. In other words, the less sex you have, the less you will want it. Obviously, making a concerted effort at increasing the frequency of sexual encounters with your partner (even if at first you are not so inclined) will solve this problem. Increasing your sexual experiences through masturbation is another alternative that may help resolve this dilemma.

Fear is a great libido killer. If you're afraid of getting pregnant, consult your doctor for a contraceptive that ensures adequate protection. A fear of being hurt may stem from misconceptions regarding sex. Educate yourself regarding sexual techniques, and advise your partner of your concerns so that he will be more sensitive to your problem. If you have experienced pain during sexual encounters, see your gynecologist prior to attempting intercourse again. Tell your partner about any psychological fears, such as a fear of losing control or of being emotionally hurt. Consultation with a therapist may be useful.

Iron deficiency and hypothyroidism are medical conditions that may cause fatigue and also zap your sex drive. If fatigue extends to the other areas of your life, a good physical exam and possibly some lab work should be scheduled. But if you have unlimited stamina yet simply no interest in sex, it is unlikely a physical disorder is causing the problem. Depression is associated with decreased libido and must be treated if sexual desire is to resume. Some medications decrease libido as a side effect. If the problem appears to coincide with starting a particular medication, check with your doctor. Perhaps substitutes are available.

Probably the least common cause for decreased libido is a hormonal disturbance. Estrogen may influence sex drive, but the most important hormone linked to sex drive is testosterone. You may be thinking, *Wait a minute, isn't testosterone a male hormone?* Yes, but women also produce testosterone from their ovaries, as well as other androgens from their adrenal glands. Testosterone is also thought to play a role in sexual arousal and vaginal lubrication. It is uncommon for young women with functioning ovaries to have decreased testosterone levels, but they may occur in women who use oral contraceptives. This problem may be overcome by changing to a different formulation or by adding a small amount of transdermal testosterone.

There is also an age-related decline in testosterone levels across the reproductive years; by the time women reach their late forties, their blood testosterone levels are approximately half what they were in their twenties. A decrease in estrogen and testosterone after menopause may also lower libido. If estrogen replacement does not solve the problem, you should consider adding a small amount of testosterone to your hormonal regimen. We will discuss the pros and cons of testosterone supplementation in women in chapter 13.

Will my sexual pleasure decrease after a hysterectomy?

After a hysterectomy, uterine contractions will no longer occur during orgasm. Very occasionally, some women may experience a decrease in enjoyment from this change. Most sexual arousal, however, is generated through either direct or indirect stimulation of the clitoris and is not altered by a hysterectomy. A slight shortening of the vagina results from a total hysterectomy but is usually inconsequential to successful intercourse. A hysterectomy without removal of the ovaries does not alter hormone production. If the ovaries are removed at the time of hysterectomy and hormone replacement is not begun, vaginal dryness and problems with libido can arise. Occasionally, postoperative adhesions (scars) at the top of the vagina will cause painful intercourse during deep penetration. This condition is uncommon and can often be overcome by changing position during intercourse or limiting the degree of penetration. In severe cases, surgery may be required to release the adhesions.

Psychological factors can play a positive or negative role in your sex life after hysterectomy. It has been our experience that hysterectomy often has a positive psychological impact. Often much distress has been associated with the uterine disorder. You may have had a long-standing history of prolonged or erratic bleeding. Your condition may have caused chronic or recurring pelvic pain. A multitude of treatments may have been attempted without success. After a hysterectomy, life can return to normal and your interest in sex returns. Strained interpersonal relationships also improve with resolution of your long-standing ailment. If a fear of pregnancy has been restricting your ability to relax and enjoy sex, you may find greater sexual freedom after the hysterectomy.

For some women, however, losing the capacity for childbearing may be difficult to accept. If this is the case, a hysterectomy can have a profound emotional impact that diminishes sexual responsiveness. You may be able to overcome this problem on your own, but don't hesitate to consult a therapist if you cannot resolve these feelings. It is important to discuss these feelings with your partner. His support, along with the reassurance that he still finds you desirable, may help.

In our experience, a hysterectomy usually does not have a significant impact on sexuality. If your sex life was excellent before the hysterectomy, it will probably remain so after. If it was lousy before, it's not likely to improve because of the surgery. Don't let worries about sex become overriding if a hysterectomy is necessary.

Is oral sex dangerous?

Many sexually transmitted infections can be transmitted through oral sex. However, considering the high prevalence of sexually transmitted infections, oral infections are uncommon. Prevention of oral→genital and genital→oral STI transmission is discussed in chapter 5 (see page 131). As a rule, if either you or your partner notices an unusual lesion (a wart, ulceration, or skin change) or a discharge, sexual contact of any sort should be put on hold until you find out what's wrong. If a sexually transmittable infection is diagnosed, ask your doctor about any restrictions that may apply regarding sexual activity. Do you need to refrain from all sexual practices while undergoing treatment? Does your partner need to be examined? Will there be any restrictions after treatment? How soon after treatment can you resume normal sexual practices?

Assuming that both of you maintain proper hygiene, there is no danger to you or your partner from oral-genital sex. The mouth and the vagina are both laden with bacteria, but not the types detrimental to health. There is no harm in ingesting either vaginal secretions or semen.

Is anal sex safe?

Lynn and Jeff are lying together in bed, basking in the afterglow of fulfilling sex. They are content, snuggling in each other's arms when Jeff breaks the silence.

"We should try anal sex sometime."

Lynn is a bit shocked. "What? Are you kidding me?"

"No, really," continues Jeff. "Everyone is doing it."

"Who is everyone?" replies Lynn. "I think you've been watching too much porn."

Jeff persists. "I know lots of people who have done it."

Lynn is not so sure. "It sounds dirty to me, and seems like it would hurt."

"We can look it up on the Internet," suggests Jeff. "There must be ways of doing it that won't hurt."

"I'll look at it," concedes Lynn. "But I'm not making any promises."

Whether you are curious like Jeff or wary like Lynn, questions about anal sex have become progressively more common, especially from women in their twenties and thirties. What once was considered taboo is now reasonably common. Studies from the early '90s found that 20 percent of heterosexual couples engaged in at least one episode of anal intercourse. In more recent reviews of sexual behavior that number has increased to 35–45 percent. The increased tightness associated with the anal canal often provides greater tactile pleasure for men. The experience for women is more diverse, ranging from painful to pleasurable and exciting. It is unusual for women to achieve orgasm through anal intercourse alone without simultaneous stimulation of the clitoris or G-spot.

Precautions must be taken. Extra attention to hygiene in the anal area is a must. In addition, a woman should use an anal douche or enema prior to anal intercourse in order to evacuate stool from the lower rectum. This can be accomplished by emptying a Fleet enema bottle and filling it with warm water. Most women will do better if they gradually work their way up to intercourse by first employing finger play or using graduated sizes of vibrators or butt plugs. Perianal massage can also be used to help relax the anal sphincter muscles prior to penetration. There is no natural lubrication produced by the anus, so use of a lubricant is an absolute must.

Anal intercourse is considered a high-risk sexual behavior when employed outside of a long-term mutually monogamous relationship. The anal and rectal tissues are easily injured, creating microlacerations (tiny tears) which may lead to anal fissures. More importantly, it is very easy to transmit sexually transmitted infections (STIs) through the tiny tears and abrasions. All of the STIs that are transmitted through vaginal intercourse can be transmitted through anal intercourse. Anal intercourse poses the highest risk of transmitting HIV of all sexual behaviors and there is a very high transmission rate of HPV, which increases the risk of anal cancer. Condoms are highly recommended and once there has been penetration of the anus, a penis or sex toy should not be introduced into the vagina. Doing so will introduce fecal bacteria into the vagina, upsetting the normal balance of bacteria and increasing the risk of vaginal infection.

For additional information regarding sex education or sexual dysfunction, consider contacting the following agencies:

American Association of Sex Educators, Counselors, and Therapists: www.asect.org

SexEd Library: www.sexedlibrary.org

5

PELVIC INFECTIONS

Why does my vagina itch?

Vaginal and vulvar infections commonly cause itching or burning. Infections that are commonly associated with this include yeast, trichomoniasis, genital warts, and herpes infections. We'll discuss these one by one. Bacterial vaginosis will also be discussed, although it is not really an infection and more typically causes an increased, foul-smelling, "fishy" discharge without much else in the way of symptoms. First, however, you should know that irritant and allergic reactions account for many cases of external itching. If the doctor cannot identify an infectious source for the problem, it is typically caused by one of the following common irritants and allergens:

- *Soaps that have deodorants, dyes, or scents*: Your best bet is to stick with a mild soap such as Neutrogena or Aveeno.
- *Toilet paper with dyes or scents*: Forget that fancy stuff. Use white, unscented toilet paper.
- *Powders, talcs, and feminine hygiene sprays*: Don't buy into those mother-daughter feminine hygiene moments on TV. You're more likely to create problems than to solve them with those products.
- *Clothing detergents and fabric softeners*: All of that neat stuff they put into detergents to whiten, brighten, and dissolve stains can be quite irritating to your genitalia. Wash your underwear in mild detergents and rinse them well after washing.

- *Contraceptive products*: Spermicides, condoms, and diaphragms may cause irritation. Chapter 3 presents alternatives to consider if you have this problem.
- *Deodorant pads and tampons*: Again, unscented products are preferable.
- *Nickel*: From piercings.

Irritant reactions occur immediately upon contact with the offending substance. Allergic reactions may be immediate but usually become more evident hours or days later. Redness and swelling or a rash may be present. If no warts or ulcerations are detected on examination and no infection is identified, an irritant or allergic reaction (also called contact dermatitis) is assumed to be the cause of your discomfort. Your doctor can give you an anti-inflammatory cream (hydrocortisone or something stronger) to resolve the inflammation.

The problem will persist if the offending substance is not eliminated. Wear only white cotton underwear, and if you wear pantyhose, make sure they have a white, cotton insert. Cotton breathes, whereas synthetic fabrics trap moisture that increases your chance of experiencing irritation and infection. Avoid tight pants for the same reason.

Over-the-counter products that treat minor vaginal irritation usually have hydrocortisone or benzocaine as the active ingredient. Avoid the temptation to use these without being evaluated. Serious conditions may be overlooked if you are not examined.

A chronic skin condition, referred to as vulvar dystrophy (ex. lichen sclerosis, squamous cell hyperplasia), can cause burning or itching in the vulvar region. Skin changes may include thinning or thickening as well as color changes; the skin is usually whiter than normal. In more advanced stages, the opening of the vagina may narrow and ulceration may develop. Your doctor will prescribe a cream or ointment to decrease the itching and prevent worsening of the condition. Treatment must be long-term, and periodic visits are necessary (approximately every three to six months) to monitor the condition. In severe cases in which ulceration has developed, surgery may be required to remove the abnormal skin. Chronic skin conditions that affect other areas of the body, such as psoriasis, may also involve the vulvar region. These skin diseases are usually treated by a dermatologist.

Vulvar cancer may also cause itching (see chapter 11).

Why do I keep getting yeast infections?

In asking this question, you probably think that you're the only person in the world getting recurrent yeast infections. Actually, yeast infections are quite common, and it is not unusual for women to get them again and again. Yeast and fungi live all around us. They exist in our environment and in our food and are not generally acquired through sexual activity. Where does yeast prefer to live? Ideally, it prefers a moist, dark environment. The vagina certainly fits that description.

If you think you have a yeast infection (also referred to as Candida vaginitis or monilial vaginitis), your best bet is to see the gynecologist. Commercials for antifungal creams have misled women into thinking that vaginal burning, itching, and discharge always come from yeast infections. However, your symptoms may not be related to yeast. Other types of vaginal infections and other disorders can create similar symptoms. (We discuss infections in this chapter; other vaginal and vulvar conditions are addressed in chapter 11.) If you or your doctor treat your infection without pursuing appropriate diagnostic techniques, you may be treating the wrong problem. All the antifungal medication known to modern medicine won't help if the problem doesn't stem from a fungus. Treating without an appropriate diagnosis can make it

> **Do not treat yourself!**
>
> *Many women assume that all genital itching is a yeast infection. Women commonly treat themselves with over-the-counter products for their presumed yeast infection, and then call the doctor when it hasn't cleared. Whenever possible, get evaluated by a healthcare professional first. It is important to determine if your itching is really caused by yeast or if there is some other reason for the symptom.*

more difficult to accurately assess your condition later, should your symptoms persist. If you can't see the doctor, then use an over-the-counter test (ex. SavvyCheck) that specifically tests for yeast prior to using an antifungal medication. Avoid the temptation to treat yourself or to let your doctor treat you by phone if the problem is recurrent. You may have an atypical strain of yeast (see below) or a condition other than yeast. If there is severe external burning or itching, your doctor can also prescribe an anti-inflammatory cream similar to hydrocortisone for immediate relief.

Once it is determined that your repeated infections are caused by yeast, we're back to your initial question: Why? Use of antibiotics often induces yeast infections in women. They can decrease the normal bacteria in the vagina, allowing yeast to become dominant. Some women notice a pattern of developing vaginal yeast infections every time they take antibiotics. If this is true for you, it is reasonable to use an antifungal medication following the antibiotics. If you need to be on antibiotics continually, you may need to take an antifungal medication regularly, once or twice per week.

A small percentage of women have yeast infections related to diabetes. Diabetes elevates the sugar level in vaginal secretions, thereby providing an increased food source for the yeast. If you recurrently get yeast infections, check with your primary care doctor to see if you have been screened for diabetes in the recent past. If not, he or she can do so.

The immune system helps fight fungal infections. When this system is compromised, yeast infections persist, recur, or spread to other areas of the body. Drugs that can compromise the immune response include those used in chemotherapy and high doses of cortisone-like steroids. Diseases that compromise the immune defenses, such as leukemia and AIDS, can also set the stage for chronic or repeated yeast infections. If you or your physician has reason to suspect the presence of one of these diseases, appropriate tests should be ordered. However, remember that these conditions are very uncommon whereas recurrent yeast infections are very common. Most people with repeated yeast infections do not have a serious underlying illness.

Physicians have debated over the years whether taking oral contraceptives increases the chance of developing vaginal yeast infections. If you are having difficulty with yeast infections and are using oral contraceptives, consider stopping them for several months—but only if you can reliably use an alternative method of contraception. If the yeast infections disappear, consider discontinuing oral contraceptives and permanently using a different method.

Most of the time, no reason can be found to explain recurrent yeast infections. However, following these general rules will decrease the likelihood of contracting vaginal infections. Keeping the genital area dry is of paramount importance. You should wear only loose-fitting clothing and cotton undergarments. Synthetic fabrics don't breathe, and tight clothes trap moisture (remember, yeast likes moisture). If you wear pantyhose, choose a style with a cotton insert. After you shower or bathe, use a blow-dryer to ensure that the genital region is dry. Try not to sit around in a wet bathing suit or workout clothes for a prolonged time. After you swim or work out, use the blow-dryer and change into dry clothes. Avoid foods containing sugar and sweetened drinks (yeast loves sugar).

Are yeast infections dangerous?

Your vaginal yeast infection poses no danger to you. The infection does not involve the uterus, fallopian tubes, or ovaries. There is no adverse impact on fertility or childbearing. Vaginal yeast infections do not cause pelvic adhesions or chronic pelvic pain.

Some books propose yeast as a cause for every disorder known to humanity. We have our doubts. Infections spread through the bloodstream are rare, usually affecting only those with a weakened immune system. In a few rare situations, a woman develops an allergic response to yeast. But in general, you can conclude that your yeast infections cause no harm.

How are yeast infections treated?

There are numerous medications designed to treat vaginal yeast infections. Many of these (Monistat, Gyne-Lotrimin, Vagistat-1, Femstat) are available over the counter. All of them work at least 80 percent of the time. After a yeast infection has been confirmed, it is fine to use one of these products. Other antifungal preparations are obtained by prescription. Examples include Terazol (available as a cream or suppository) and Diflucan (a single dose pill). If your partner seems fine and has no genital rash or itching, he doesn't need treatment.

Antifungal medications come in a variety of forms. There are creams, suppositories, and tablets. Length of treatment varies from one to seven days. Every physician has a preference, although the method of administration doesn't seem to substantially affect the success rate. It makes sense to use a cream to treat external itching or burning, but an antifungal product must also be taken orally or vaginally. Diflucan (fluconazole) is the only approved oral medication for vaginal yeast infections. It is taken as a one dose tablet, certainly the most convenient of the regimens. Its main downside is a 15 percent incidence of headache or gastrointestinal distress, usually minor, for women who take it. Diflucan interacts adversely with certain medications. If you take other medications, check with your physician before starting Diflucan.

Treating recurrent yeast infections can be exasperating. Current laboratory techniques allow physicians to identify particular strains of yeast. The most common yeast, Candida Albicans, accounts for approximately 80 percent of all yeast infections and will respond to most antifungal treatments. However, there are atypical yeasts that are more difficult to treat. Most of the atypical yeasts will not respond to over-the-counter antifungal products or Diflucan. Your physician may have to prescribe an antifungal for a more extended period of time. Another product that works reasonably well against atypical yeast is boric acid vaginal suppositories (600mg) used twice daily for two weeks. Some physicians will obtain swabs from multiple areas (mouth, rectum, and vagina) to find a possible source for recurrent infection.

However, the testing can get quite expensive. Most physicians take a more pragmatic approach, using suppressive therapy in which you take an antifungal medication once or twice weekly for several months or longer. If your partner has a rash or itch, he should be examined and treated also.

For more information, consult www.emedicinehealth.com/vaginal_infections.

Will yogurt or other natural products keep me from getting yeast infections?

The idea that yogurt (taken either orally or vaginally) can prevent vaginal infections derives from the presence of lactobacillus in the yogurt. Lactobacillus acidophilus is normally the predominant bacteria of the vagina. When the population of lactobacilli decreases, other organisms such as yeast have an opportunity to overpopulate the vagina. However, certain strains of lactobacillus are necessary to restore a healthy balance of bacteria in the vagina. Strains that produce hydrogen peroxide should be present. Very few brands of yogurt contain peroxide-producing lactobacillus acidophilus. Others contain lactobacillus acidophilus but are contaminated with unwanted bacteria.

Probiotics are an intriguing approach to restoring the natural balance of bacteria in the vagina. Probiotics introduce healthy bacteria. They are mostly used for gastrointestinal disorders, but may also be useful for the prevention of vaginal disorders such as yeast infections and bacterial vaginosis (BV). Most probiotics are limited in their effectiveness because they do not contain hydrogen peroxide-producing lactobacillus species, and those that do are usually found outside of the United States. However, there are some well-designed studies showing efficacy with currently available products and there is little downside in trying them. Probiotics designed for vaginal health and the prevention of yeast and BV include the oral capsules RepHresh Pro-B, Provella, Fem-Dophilus, and Pearls YB and the vaginal capsules Vivag and Ecovag. Most probiotics do not require a prescription so you can purchase them online or over the counter.

There are many natural antifungals like garlic, caprylic acid, pau d'Arco, oregano oil, coconut oil, olive leaf, goldenseal, and colloidal silver, just to name a few. While these may have some efficacy against Candida, their antifungal action is usually too weak to prevent recurrent infections in those women who are predisposed. Homeopathic products are another common "natural" approach to treating yeast infections. They are not harmful, but there is no evidence-based medicine to support their use. Boric acid capsules (mentioned above for the treatment of atypical yeast) administered vaginally is effective for preventing recurrent yeast infections. After being used twice daily for two weeks, boric acid capsules can be used once or twice per week on an ongoing basis in order to prevent future infections.

Before we continue our discussion on pelvic infections, let's have a little fun. Take the STI quiz below to see how much you already know about pelvic infections.

How Much Do You Know?

1. You can get an STI by all of the following ways except:
A. Oral sex
B. Sex without a condom
C. Sex with a condom
D. Reading a romance novel

2. Which of the following is not an STI?
A. Sagittarius
B. Trichomonas
C. Chlamydia
D. Hepatitis B

3. Herpes is:
A. A virus for which there is a treatment but no cure

B. Transmitted by sitting on a public toilet seat
C. Always prevented by using condoms
D. The name of my Aunt Patsy's cat

4. Trichomonas causes:
A. Infertility
B. A pelvic tumor
C. A foul-smelling vaginal discharge
D. Hiccups

5. Gonorrhea is:
A. A particularly virulent form of diarrhea

B. The Greek God of STIs

C. The illegitimate child of a former president

D. A bacteria that can cause pelvic infection

6. Pelvic infection can cause all of the following except:

A. Pain

B. A brain tumor

C. Infertility

D. No symptoms at all

7. Condoms may not protect against which STIs:

A. Herpes, HPV, and syphilis

B. HIV

C. Gonorrhea and chlamydia

D. Trichomonas

8. Which is true of HIV?

A. It only occurs in homosexuals and drug addicts

B. It may cause AIDS

C. It is transmitted through kissing

D. It can be successfully treated with antibiotics

9. What is the prevalence rate of HPV in single, sexually active populations?

A. 20 percent

B. 35 percent

C. 40-60 percent

D. What's a prevalence rate?

10. HPV can cause all of the following except:

A. Genital warts

B. Cervical cancer

C. Warts on your larynx

D. The common cold

How Much Did You Know?

1.D 2.A 3.A 4.C 5.D 6.B 7.A 8.B 9.C 10.D

How many correct answers did you get?

9-10: Excellent! You have the knowledge. Go and use it well.

7-8: You still have a lot to learn. Read this chapter carefully.

6 or less: You're in big trouble. Return to sex education 101 and this time, listen and take notes.

I have discharge but no itching or burning. Is that normal?

It is normal to have a vaginal discharge. The vagina and cervix produce secretions. These secretions, along with vaginal bacteria and exfoliated vaginal cells (surface cells of the vagina that have been shed into the vagina), create a normal discharge. The normal vaginal discharge is clear or white. It should not be particularly clumpy or exceedingly runny, and it should not have an unpleasant odor. It's normal for the discharge to increase in the middle of your menstrual cycle.

If you notice an increase in the amount of discharge, a foul odor, or a change in the color of the discharge, make an appointment to have it evaluated. This change may signal a vaginal infection that should be treated. Yeast infections produce a secretion similar to cottage cheese in texture. Usually it is white and does not have a foul odor.

Two other vaginal conditions frequently cause an increased discharge. Both usually produce a profuse, foul-smelling discharge, but they may not be associated with burning or itching. Your only clue may be the increased discharge or odor. The most common of these is bacterial vaginosis (BV), which is actually more common than yeast infections. Most of the time BV presents without significant signs of inflammation. The most common symptom is an increased discharge with a foul, "fishy" odor. BV may increase the risk of preterm labor and premature rupture of membranes in pregnant women. Women with PID (see below) also commonly have coexisting BV. The condition is caused by a decrease in the number of lactobacilli (the usual dominant bacteria of the vagina), allowing an increase in the population of other bacteria that are normally absent or present in small numbers. The best known of these is called Gardnerella, but Gardnerella is only one of a number of bacteria that overpopulate the vagina in this condition. The foul odor is caused by substances called amines, which are released by the bacteria. The doctor can easily diagnose the condition by looking at vaginal secretions through a microscope. This test is referred to as a wet prep. He or she can also check the vaginal Ph (increases with BV), perform a "sniff" test (detecting an odor after adding potassium hydroxide to a sample of your discharge), and obtain a swab to be sent to a laboratory, which can determine if bacteria are overgrowing at the expense of lactobacilli. Your physician may also use a rapid test called BVBLUE that detects BV.

The doctor will prescribe an antibiotic that selectively decreases the bacteria that have overpopulated the vagina. This gives our friend lactobacillus the chance to reassume its dominant position. The three antibiotics usually used for this are metronidazole (Flagyl), tinidazole (Tindamax), and clindamycin (Cleocin). Metronidazole and clindamycin are available in oral and vaginal preparations. The vaginal preparations are less likely to have side effects but are messier. Tinidazole is newer and sometimes reserved for those patients who do not respond to metronidazole or clindamycin. When using metronidazole or tinidazole, avoid alcohol. This is important! You *will* get sick with nausea and vomiting if you combine alcohol with these antibiotics. With BV, there does not appear to be a higher success rate if your partner is also treated, and most doctors won't do so unless you seem to have frequent recurrences.

Some patients will develop frequent recurrences of BV. This can be approached with longer courses of treatment with the antibiotics mentioned above. Boric acid capsules may also be effective using the same regimen described earlier for yeast infections. There is some evidence that probiotics (refer to the discussion above on yeast) may also be effective in reducing recurrences of BV. Using RepHresh vaginal gel after your period has finished and after sexual intercourse may help restore the vaginal Ph in women with BV.

Another vaginal infection commonly associated with a profuse, foul discharge is trichomoniasis. It is caused by an organism called trichomonas, which produces a green-yellow discharge, itching or burning, and a foul odor. It, too, is easily diagnosed by a physician using a microscope to analyze vaginal discharge or through a swab sent to the laboratory. Metronidazole and tinidazole are used to treat the infection. Since it is usually acquired through sexual transmission, your partner should be treated to prevent reinfection.

Aerobic vaginitis, desquamative vaginitis, and lichen planus are other conditions that lead to an increased vaginal discharge, often with significant inflammation of the vagina, and even ulcerations. Unlike bacterial vaginosis, they do not usually present with a foul odor. Due to the significant inflammation they cause, they may also present with painful intercourse as the primary symptom. In the absence of yeast and trichomonas, which are easily diagnosed, severe inflammatory vaginal changes should lead your gynecologist to suspect one of these more obscure conditions. These conditions are not well understood and treatment can be more difficult. Treatment may include a vaginal antibiotic cream (Clindamycin 2%) for two weeks or more, an oral antibiotic, or vaginal (or oral) steroids.

What is PID?

PID, or pelvic inflammatory disease, is an infection of the uterus, fallopian tubes, and ovaries. It is more serious than the vaginal infections described in the previous section. Infection involving the uterus, tubes, and ovaries can create adhesions that produce infertility, tubal pregnancy, or chronic pelvic pain. Severe PID may even develop into a pelvic abscess (collection of pus) that requires drainage or more aggressive surgery. The baby of an infected mother can develop conjunctivitis (an eye infection) or pneumonia.

PID usually begins as an infection of the cervix caused by either gonorrhea or chlamydia (or both), which are sexually transmitted organisms. Cervical infection may produce a discharge from the cervix, but commonly it has no associated symptoms. If untreated, the infection can spread into the uterus and through the fallopian tubes. The most common symptom experienced once the infection has ascended is pelvic pain. If the infection is severe, fever, chills, nausea, and vomiting may accompany it. Other symptoms associated with PID include yellowish vaginal discharge, painful urination, and abnormal vaginal bleeding. These other symptoms, without accompanying pelvic pain, however, are more likely related to other gynecologic disorders. Other possible sites of infection include the rectum through anal intercourse, the urethra because of its proximity to the vagina, and the mouth through oral sex.

When your doctor suspects the presence of PID, he or she will perform a pelvic examination. If you have PID, your pelvic exam will be painful. However, your gynecologist cannot make an accurate assessment without performing this examination. A pelvic ultrasound may also be ordered to detect other possible causes for pelvic pain such as ovarian cysts and tumors or the presence of a pelvic abscess. Other laboratory evaluation includes blood work and a urinalysis or urine culture to rule out a bladder infection as the source of your pain.

PID is treated with antibiotics that will eliminate both gonorrhea and chlamydia, which frequently coexist. The duration of treatment will vary depending on the severity of the infection. If the infection is mild, you will be treated as an outpatient. It is critical that you complete your entire course of antibiotics. It is tempting to stop treatment once you feel better. However, incomplete treatment can result in persistent infection. You may be admitted to the hospital if you have one of the following conditions:

- Severe infection (as evidenced by the amount of tenderness present, the level of your fever, and your white blood cell count—the cells that fight infection)
- Nausea and vomiting
- A pelvic abscess

When admitted, you will receive intravenous antibiotics. Once it is apparent that the infection is responding to the antibiotics, you will be discharged and can complete the antibiotics at home. If there is an abscess, it may have to be drained by insertion of a catheter or by surgery.

If your partner has signs of infection, such as penile discharge or burning, avoid sex until his problem is evaluated. If it is determined that he has either gonorrhea or chlamydia, you must also be evaluated and treated. Similarly, if you are diagnosed with either infection, he also needs to be treated. Abstain from sexual contact until both of you have completed the entire course of antibiotics and your doctor has determined that your infection has cleared. If it is possible that you contracted the infection from someone other than your current partner, that person must also be notified and sent for evaluation. If you are treated for gonorrhea or chlamydia, your doctor may suggest undergoing tests for other sexually transmitted diseases.

Is there any good news about this disease? Yes—it's preventable. Until you have a mutually monogamous relationship—lasting for years, not months—condoms should be used every time you have intercourse, even if you are using other contraceptives. (See chapter 3 for an in-depth look at condoms.) If your partner won't use a condom, use the female condom. If he still refuses, ditch him. That may seem drastic, but your health is more important than his ego.

In the Locker Room

Jen, Liza, and Sara, three college coeds, made a pact. Without fail they meet at University Fitness on 12th St. for a solid workout every Tuesday and Thursday morning. After finishing their workout, they hit the showers to freshen up before heading off to classes. As often happens, the conversation turns to boys.

Amidst the banter Jen blurts out, "Ben and I have started to have sex."

Liza responds, "Really, it's about time. You've been seeing him forever."

"Not really," Jen counters defensively. "We've been going out about six months now."

Sara decides to chime in. "Yeah, but in today's world, that's an eternity. Did he use a condom?"

"No," Jen says nonchalantly. "I don't need to worry. I'm on the pill." Shaking her head, Liza admonishes her friend. "You may not get pregnant, but you're going to get an STI."

Jen doesn't seem to understand what her friend is worried about. "The only other person I have been with is Charlie in high school, and Ben has only had two partners in the past. He says that he is clean so I don't think it's a problem."

"Jimmy won't use a condom," Sara adds. "He says he doesn't feel things as well when he wears a condom, so he refuses to use one."

Liza is amazed at her friends' ignorance. "Both of you are crazy. You need to use a condom every time. You're not just having sex with your current boyfriend. The way I see it, you're having sex with everyone they were with before you, and I'm not going to stay with any boy who won't use a condom. No condom means no sex. No exceptions! If he won't do that for you, then he's not worth having as a boyfriend."

Liza has the right idea. As doctors, we are constantly amazed at the number of young men and women not using condoms. Many, but not all, STIs are prevented with consistent use of condoms. Even if a woman plans to use condoms reliably, she should ask every new partner about their STI history. She should also specifically inquire about any skin lesions (bumps or ulcerations that could represent genital warts or herpes respectively; both transmittable despite using condoms). Prior to the onset of sexual activity, both partners in a new relationship should undergo STI screening. Women should see their gynecologist and men should ideally see an urologist, although some primary care doctors may be able to do this screening.

How can I tell the difference between a bladder infection and other pelvic infections?

Since the bladder is located next to your reproductive organs, it can be difficult to distinguish bladder problems from vaginal or uterine infections. Bladder infections, also called cystitis, are fairly common in women. The urethral opening is located immediately above the vaginal opening, making it easy for vaginal bacteria to enter the bladder.

You may have pelvic pain just above your pubic bone with a bladder infection. More typical symptoms include the following:

- Urinary urgency: It seems that you have to race to the bathroom.
- Frequency: You experience a marked increase in frequency of urination.
- Dysuria: You feel pain or burning with urination.

You may have only one of the symptoms or all three. If you see blood in your urine, don't panic. Bloody urine is common with bladder infections. The diagnosis of cystitis is obtained by urinalysis or urine culture. Treatment consists of antibiotics. Whenever possible, a urine culture should be obtained before starting antibiotics to confirm the diagnosis and to show which bacteria are causing the infection.

Occasional bladder infections should not be alarming. However, if they don't seem to respond to the antibiotics or occur more than three times per year, you should consider seeing a urologist for further evaluation.

Do people still get syphilis?

At one time in history, syphilis was extremely prevalent. With the arrival of penicillin, the number of cases decreased dramatically. However, it remains a dangerous, sexually transmitted infection.

Syphilis starts as a single, painless sore (in contrast to the herpes sore, which is painful), called a chancre. Common sites of infection include the genitalia, anus, and mouth. The chancre exists for one to five weeks and then disappears without a trace. If the mucous membranes (which line the mouth, the vagina, and the anus) or broken skin of a sexual partner contacts the chancre, the infection will be transmitted. In women, the chancre is often hidden in the vagina, preventing early detection of the disease. If it goes undetected in this early stage, the disease will reappear as a rash, often accompanied by a flu like illness. The disease then undergoes a period of latency with no symptoms. It can remain latent or reappear years later, causing serious problems with the heart, blood vessels, and nervous system.

The diagnosis of syphilis is usually made through a blood test. If a chancre is present, the organism can be detected by sending a swab from the fluid of the chancre. Treatment with antibiotics will cure the disease in its early stages. More advanced disease may be difficult to eradicate.

Syphilis can be transmitted during pregnancy from the mother to her fetus. Infection can cause miscarriage, stillbirth, and developmental problems for the baby. Because of this, all pregnant women should have a blood test for syphilis early in pregnancy. If syphilis is detected early, treatment can be instituted, thereby protecting the baby.

When an individual is diagnosed with syphilis, all current and past sexual partners must be examined and tested. Testing for other sexually transmitted diseases should also be performed. Your best protection against syphilis is to avoid sexual contact with multiple partners. Condoms afford some protection, but only if the chancre is covered by the condom. Examination of a potential sex partner may also reveal a chancre as well as certain additional STIs such as herpetic blisters, ulcerations, or genital warts. If you see any skin lesions, abstain from sexual contact until the potential partner has been evaluated by a healthcare provider skilled in the detection of STIs.

I have bumps that feel like warts. What are they?

You may be feeling genital warts, but other structures are often confused with warts. It is common to find pimples or cysts on the external genitalia. Sweat glands and sebaceous glands (glands that secrete an oily substance) are located just under the skin. When the ducts of these glands become obstructed, as they often do in the genital region, small pimples or cysts form, which feel

Check it out!

Many external lumps and bumps are nothing to worry about, but some will turn out to be genital warts. These have a way of spreading exponentially, especially if you shave your pubic area. If you discover a skin bump, do not shave and make an appointment with your gynecologist.

like bumps. You may also feel extra folds of labial skin or remnants of the hymen ring.

The most common warty lesions of the genitalia are genital warts, also called condylomata. Their formation is induced by a virus called HPV, or human papillomavirus. This sexually transmitted virus infects the vulva, vagina, cervix, and anus. It can also reside in the mouth or throat, in this case being acquired through oral sex. HPV viruses are categorized as low risk or high risk. Low-risk strains of HPV are responsible for genital warts. High-risk strains of HPV can cause atypical changes that ultimately lead to cervical, vaginal, vulvar, or anal cancer (with cervical cancer being the most common). Prior to the advent of HPV vaccines, the prevalence of HPV in single, sexually active populations was 40–60 percent, and the overall lifetime risk of acquiring HPV was 80 percent. Most people who acquire HPV are asymptomatic. Younger women (especially those in their teens and twenties) will usually develop an immune response that clears the virus within one to two years.

Low-risk HPV virus can induce genital warts within weeks, months, or occasionally even years of viral transmission. It is difficult to pinpoint the actual date of the initial infection for that reason. You may be the first person to detect the warts, or they may be discovered during a routine gynecologic examination.

Once discovered, warts are treated in a variety of ways. Doctors commonly use one of two chemicals, podophyllin or trichloroacetic acid (TCA), to destroy the warts. Podophyllin is applied to external warts but not to vaginal or cervical warts. It is not used during pregnancy because of concern that it might cause harm to the fetus. Repeated applications may be required. A podophyllin preparation (Condylox or generic podofilox) is also available by prescription for self application. The solution is applied to the warts with a cotton-tipped applicator for three days, followed by four days without the medication. This one week cycle may be repeated up to four times. A topical cream called Imiquimod (Aldara, applied three times per week for up to sixteen weeks, or Zyclara, applied daily for up to eight weeks) is also used for the treatment of external and perianal warts. Imiquimod does not appear to have any direct antiviral effects but rather modulates the local immune response, enhancing your body's ability to clear the virus. Use these regimens only with the supervision of your doctor to ensure proper application.

Efudex (Fluorouracil) cream is sometimes used to treat vaginal warts. The cream is inserted with an applicator. Great care must be taken to keep Efudex from touching the external skin of the labia and vulva. It can produce severe inflammation and ulceration. Some physicians recommend covering the labia and vulva with petroleum jelly to protect them against cream that may leak from the vagina.

Interferon is another drug used in the treatment of genital warts. Interferons are naturally occurring proteins that the body produces to fight viruses. In this regimen, extra interferon is administered to help the body fight the HPV virus. Interferon can be given intramuscularly or injected directly into the warts by your physician.

Other treatments for genital warts include these:

- Cryotherapy: freezing the warts
- Cautery: burning the warts
- Laser: vaporizing the warts with a high-energy beam
- Excision: surgically removing the warts

The best type of treatment is determined by the number, size, and the location of the warts. If there are just a few, chemical treatment is usually chosen. If the warts are numerous, large, or resistant to medical treatment, a more aggressive approach is taken. Sometimes these procedures can be performed in the doctor's office under local anesthesia. Others may require general anesthesia in an operating room as outpatient surgery.

Genital warts tend to increase in size during pregnancy. Sometimes they can be treated during pregnancy. If they are extensive, though, the doctor may wait until after delivery to treat them, since the HPV virus does not adversely affect the progress and development of the pregnancy. Rarely, newborns will acquire HPV virus from their mother during delivery and develop laryngeal warts.

A frustrating aspect of genital warts is that recurrence is common. Although the warts have been treated, the HPV virus remains in the surrounding "normal" tissue and can induce the formation of new warts. In contrast to bacteria, viruses cannot be eliminated with antibiotics. With repeated treatment, however, you should eventually be able to eradicate recurrent warts.

If you have genital warts, your partner should also be evaluated. This is best done by a urologist, a doctor who treats problems involving the male genitalia. Previous partners should also be notified, if possible. If you suspect that you or your partner may have genital warts, avoid sexual contact until the warts have been treated and completely removed. Although using condoms during sex decreases the risk of transmitting the warts, it doesn't eliminate it. HPV is transmitted through direct skin to skin contact and a condom only covers part of the male genitalia (or female genitalia in the case of the female condom).

Receiving the diagnosis of genital warts can be quite disconcerting. Try to remember that this is an extremely common infection. Although the HPV virus can induce abnormalities, it is almost always detectable with regular exams. The virus and warts do not infect the uterine cavity, fallopian tubes, or ovaries. There is no adverse effect on fertility. The virus resides locally and creates no problems elsewhere in the body.

Two vaccines have been developed for the prevention of HPV. One of these vaccines, Gardasil, is very effective at preventing genital warts. Although it does not vaccinate you against all of the strains which might cause this problem, it has been shown to be at least 90 percent successful at preventing genital warts. It is currently recommended that all girls and boys be vaccinated in their early teens. Insurance carriers will usually cover this vaccination up through age twenty-six. However, we recommend that you get vaccinated if you are single and sexually active regardless of age. The vaccination may not be as effective in older individuals (participants in the original trial ranged from eleven to twenty-six years in age), but it is extremely unlikely to be dangerous in older individuals and may still provide some protection for this very common sexually transmitted infection.

High-risk HPV viruses can be oncogenic (cause cancer) and will be discussed in chapters 9 and 11.

What is that painful sore down there?

Cue the Commercial

A wholesome-looking couple emerges. They are riding bikes, conveniently stopping for our benefit. "I have herpes," says the woman rather cheerfully. "And I don't," adds her partner. "And we want to keep it that way," they both announce. "So I take Valtrex every day," the woman proclaims.

This commercial is interesting from several perspectives. You have to be impressed with how cheerfully the woman announces her herpes. There should be no stigma attached to herpes, but I doubt most people are thrilled to have it. Nevertheless, daily use of antiviral medication like Valtrex (valacyclovir) is very effective at suppressing herpetic outbreaks and transmission to sexual partners. Every couple should get tested for Herpes 2 antibodies through blood work prior to engaging in sexual activity. If one of the partners tests positive and the other negative, daily antiviral medicine should be started in the positive individual. This is important even if condoms are used, since condoms will reduce but not eliminate transmission of herpes.

Painful blisters and ulcerations involving the external genitalia may represent a herpes infection. These may occur in conjunction with, or be mistaken for, other infections, so examination and laboratory tests are necessary to obtain an accurate diagnosis. Herpes is a virus that produces blisters and open sores. It commonly infects the genital area, usually through direct sexual contact with an infected partner. Other areas that may be infected include the buttocks, fingers, mouth, and eyes. Two types of herpes commonly cause these infections. Herpes simplex type 1 usually causes oral herpetic lesions, more commonly referred to as fever blisters or cold sores. Herpes simplex type 2 more commonly causes genital herpes. Either type of virus can infect the genitalia. Infection is acquired from active virus found in the blisters or ulcerations. Transmission is usually through one of the following mechanisms:

- Direct contact of your genitalia with the active lesions of a partner
- Autoinoculation—spread of the virus by your touching an active lesion (such as a fever blister) and transferring it to the genitalia
- Oral sex with a partner with oral herpes

Unfortunately, transmission may also occur from an asymptomatic individual—in other words, a person who has no evidence of active infection. Contrary to what many people think, there is no evidence suggesting that the virus is acquired from toilet seats, hot tubs, or swimming pools. Initial infection, also called the primary infection, is likely to be the most severe. Blisters appear, often in groups, at the infected site. The blisters open, forming painful ulcerations. A primary infection may also cause flulike symptoms including fever, fatigue, and muscular aches. Swollen structures in the groin represent enlarged lymph nodes. Urination can be painful as urine touches the open sores. The doctor diagnoses herpes by swabbing the herpetic lesions and sending it to a lab for testing. An asymptomatic carrier of herpes can be diagnosed through a blood test that looks for antibodies to this virus. Even without treatment, the open lesions dry up and gradually disappear over several weeks. However, most doctors will prescribe an antiviral medication. The most commonly used medications are acyclovir (Zovirax), famciclovir (Famvir), and valacyclovir (Valtrex). All of these medications shorten the amount of time required for the lesions to disappear. They are administered orally or as an ointment applied directly to the lesion. Using a blow-dryer several times daily keeps the lesions dry and helps them disappear more quickly. If your lesions cause painful urination, consider voiding in a sitz bath. If the pain associated with the infection is not controlled with over-the-counter analgesics, ask your doctor to prescribe a stronger pain reliever. If you must touch the lesions, use a glove or finger cot (a latex sleeve that slides over a finger to protect it). Also wash your hands thoroughly whenever you may have come in contact with a lesion. Use separate washcloths and towels for bathing while the lesions are present. If you share a bed, wear pajamas while the infection is active. There is no need to wash your clothes or bed linens separately.

Antiviral medications do not clear up the virus completely. After the initial infection, the virus recedes into the nerve cells that supply sensation to the affected area. If the virus becomes reactivated, a recurrence, or secondary infection, will occur. Recurrences appear in the location of the primary infection. However, the lesions are fewer and less severe. Secondary infections usually disappear within a week, often lasting three to five days. Most recurrences follow the primary infection by three to twelve months. Many women never have a recurrence. Others get an outbreak many years after the initial infection. Recurrences are more common during times of stress or fatigue and when the body is fighting another infection, such as a cold or flu. Sometimes there is forewarning in the form of tingling or itching at the site of recurrence before the lesions appear. If antiviral medication is given at this time, a recurrence may be abated or its duration limited. If you get frequent or severe outbreaks, you may be a candidate for taking daily antiviral medication as a preventive measure. Daily administration of an antiviral medication can significantly decrease the frequency and severity of recurrent outbreaks. The medications are usually tolerated well, and serious adverse reactions are uncommon. Daily antiviral medicine will also significantly reduce the risk of transmission to a sexual partner (keeping in mind that a large number of transmissions occur even when there are no visible skin lesions).

Recurrences during pregnancy are fairly common. They do not pose any harm to the developing baby or interfere with pregnancy. However, active lesions at the time of birth are a cause for concern. Contact with lesions during delivery can produce serious problems for the baby, including skin infection, blindness, damage to the nervous system, and even death. If signs of a herpetic infection appear near the end of your pregnancy, contact your obstetrician immediately. If an active infection exists when you go into labor or when your membranes rupture (signaled by a gush of fluid), the doctor will deliver the baby by cesarean section to avoid exposing the baby to the herpes virus. Most women with a history of herpes will not have active lesions at the time of delivery and can undergo normal vaginal delivery without concern. If your primary infection occurs near the time of delivery, your risk of transmitting the virus during delivery is much higher. In this case, your doctor may perform a cesarean section even if you have no remaining active lesions. Some obstetricians may recommend that you take an antiviral medication such as acyclovir in the last month of your pregnancy in order to reduce the risk of transmission to your baby during delivery.

The best way to reduce the chance of getting herpes is to avoid sexual contact with anyone who has active herpetic lesions. Condoms do not reliably prevent transmission of the virus, since they do not provide complete coverage of the external genitalia. You must have open communication with your sexual partner. You have to directly ask him if he has ever noticed blisters or sores on his genitalia. If you or your partner has herpes, avoid sex until any scabs have disappeared. If either of you has a "fever blister," avoid contact with the sore—no kissing, touching the mouth, or oral-genital contact—until the lesion has completely disappeared for several days. Since herpes can be transmitted from an asymptomatic individual, it is reasonable to ask a prospective partner to get a blood test for herpes. If the test is positive for herpes type 2 (almost everyone tests positive for herpes type 1, the type that causes oral fever blisters), you should ask that partner if he is willing to take a daily dose of Valtrex in order to lower the risk of transmission.

Several alternative medicines have been investigated as options for treatment or suppression of genital herpes including lysine, zinc, echinacea, eleuthero, and bee products. There have been very few well-designed studies to support the efficacy of these options. However, one study did show that propolis, a substance that bees produce from certain tree saps, improved healing time compared with acyclovir. These products are considered nutritional supplements, not drugs, so they are not subject to FDA approval. You can purchase them in stores or online.

For more information concerning herpes, contact the following:
www.cdc.gov/std/herpes/stdfact-herpes.htm
www.marchofdimes.com/pregnancy/genital-herpes.aspx

Can women get AIDS?

AIDS, or acquired immunodeficiency syndrome, was originally associated with male homosexuality, intravenous drug abuse, and blood transfusions. Many people were unaware or unwilling to accept that HIV (human immunodeficiency virus) is transmitted through heterosexual encounters. Heterosexual women constitute a significant proportion of the AIDS population. It is estimated that four hundred thousand women above the age of fifteen are living with HIV or AIDS in America. Accepting this and understanding how to prevent HIV transmission are critical.

HIV is transmitted through intimate contact with the infected body fluids (semen, vaginal secretions, blood) of another person. It is acquired through any of the following mechanisms:

- Sharing the needle of a drug abuser infected with HIV
- Having sex with a person who is infected (the most common route of transmission)
- Receiving a blood product contaminated with HIV

Blood transfusions received before 1985 carried a greater risk of HIV contamination. Since then, blood banks have routinely screened their supplies for HIV, and the risk is exceptionally rare (approximately one case per 1.5 million units of blood). However, if you plan to undergo surgery, you can ask your doctor if you can give your own blood or designate a blood donor prior to the surgery.

You cannot contract the HIV virus through casual contact with an infected individual. It is not transmitted from sharing food, drinks, bathing facilities, pools, or hot tubs with an infected individual. It is not contracted through kissing an infected individual or coming in contact with his or her sweat or tears.

AIDS does not develop immediately after HIV infection. The HIV virus attacks the immune system, and it may be months or years before symptoms develop from the virus. Eventually, though, the infected person becomes weaker and develops infections and unusual types of cancer. When these occur, the diagnosis of AIDS is made. Many people die from AIDS, especially in foreign countries where there is little access to effective treatment. Currently there is no cure for HIV infection, although there are many drugs that significantly decrease the effects of the virus. With access to antiretroviral (ARV) therapy, many people can continue to live a productive life with little adverse impact from the HIV virus. Often people are treated with multiple ARVs, which further enhances their chances of success. There is no vaccine in current use to prevent transmission of HIV.

Prevention of HIV infection is accomplished by avoiding activities that are associated with high transmission (intravenous drug abuse, anal intercourse) and refraining from sexual contact with men who are at high risk of being infected (intravenous drug users, bisexual men, men with a history of multiple sexual partners). Latex condoms for men and female condoms used appropriately prevent the transmission of HIV during sex.

If you acquire any sexually transmitted infection, it is prudent to undergo testing for HIV. If you are in a high-risk group, you should also be tested, particularly if you anticipate becoming pregnant. As many as one-third of all infected women will transmit the infection to their babies, either during pregnancy or delivery. Women with HIV who breast-feed their infants can also transmit the virus to them. Testing is performed on a blood sample. Most healthcare centers will provide HIV testing confidentially. Either your doctor or a healthcare provider at the testing site should counsel patients before and after the test. The blood test for HIV does not register as positive immediately after infection with the virus. Therefore, it is advisable to take a second test approximately six months after the initial screening. You should require HIV testing for any new sexual partner, even if you expect to use condoms consistently. OraQuick, a rapid over-the-counter saliva test for HIV, was approved by the FDA in July of 2012. It does not take the place of laboratory testing for HIV, but should help identify people who otherwise might not get tested.

If you test positive, all current and past sexual partners must be notified and tested. Further sexual activity must be undertaken only with the use of latex condoms (or female condoms) and with the informed consent of your partner. Other contraceptives should be used with condoms to prevent pregnancy. HIV-positive individuals should never donate blood or plasma or register as an organ donor. All health-care providers must be informed of your HIV-positive status, including your dentist. Objects that may be contaminated with blood (tooth-brushes, razors, and nail clippers) should not be shared with others. If you acquire HIV, it is important for you to seek a physician with experience in caring for HIV-positive patients. You should also consult with a therapist or join a support group to help you cope.

For more information on HIV and AIDS, visit: www.avert.org/women-hiv-aids.htm.

Can you get hepatitis through sex?

You bet! Most people think of hepatitis as a disease acquired through food. Indeed, some types of hepatitis are contracted in this manner. Hepatitis type B (and less frequently Hepatitis type C), however, can be transmitted through body fluids such as blood, semen, vaginal secretions, and saliva. It can therefore be transmitted through sexual intercourse. It can also be transmitted through contact with the blood of an infected individual or by sharing needles with drug abusers.

Hepatitis B is a virus that infects the liver, causing fatigue, nausea, abdominal pain, and jaundice (yellowish pigmentation of the skin). In most cases, the body forms antibodies that attack the virus, and the infec-tion is resolved. However, some individuals develop a chronic form of the disease (chronic hepatitis) and are contagious to those who come in contact with their body fluids. Some people infected with the virus never get sick but remain contagious carriers of the virus. Pregnant women can transmit the virus to their unborn children, who may develop hepatitis or become a carrier. People who have chronic hepatitis or are carriers have an increased risk of dying from liver failure or liver cancer. Diagnosis of hepatitis is made through a blood test. Testing can detect whether you have ever had hepatitis and if you can transmit the virus to others. No treatment can eradicate the virus, but a vaccine can prevent you from getting it. Babies are now routinely vaccinated against hepatitis B. Adults who were not vaccinated previously should consider doing so if you:

- Are single and sexually active
- Have multiple sex partners
- Live with someone who has hepatitis or is a carrier
- Have contracted other sexually transmitted infections
- Inject illegal drugs
- Work in the healthcare field
- Work in any field that increases your risk of contact with body fluids
- Have chronic liver or kidney disease
- Are under sixty years of age with diabetes
- Have a disease that requires you to receive blood products

A woman who is pregnant should be tested. If she tests positive, other tests can be performed to ensure that liver function is normal. At birth, her baby can be given hepatitis B immune globulin (antibodies) to fight the virus. The baby will also be vaccinated. This regimen is 95 percent effective at preventing infection of the newborn.

The risk of contracting hepatitis through sex is decreased with the use of latex condoms. The best preventive measure, though, is hepatitis B vaccination.

Hepatitis C is transmitted primarily by exposure to blood containing the hepatitis C virus. Transmission rarely occurs from exposure to other infected body fluids, such as semen. If you're in a long-term, monogamous relationship with a partner who has hepatitis C, your risk of contracting hepatitis C is thought to be low. For these monogamous couples, the Centers for Disease Control and Prevention (CDC) doesn't recommend routine condom use to prevent transmission. However, couples should avoid sharing razors, toothbrushes, and nail clippers. The risk of transmission is higher if you have multiple short-term sexual relationships with partners who have hepatitis C. Your risk of contracting hepatitis C also increases significantly if you have HIV. Under these circumstances, the CDC recommends routine condom use to reduce your risk of transmission. At this time, there is no vaccine for hepatitis C.

If I get a sexually transmitted infection, should I be tested for others?

Sexually transmitted infections (STIs) often coexist. If you have one infection, there is a possibility that other STIs have been transmitted to you, even if they show no signs or symptoms. If your doctor diagnoses an STI, he or she will often swab your cervical and vaginal secretions and order blood work to screen for other sexually transmitted infections. You should also consider screening for STIs if you have been involved in one or more of these high-risk behaviors:

- Sexual activity with more than one partner
- Sexual activity without using condoms
- Sexual contact with a person who has developed an STI

Why can't the gynecologist cure my infection?

Cindy walks into Dr. Donatelli's office for the third time in the past two months. As Dr. Donatelli walks into the room, Cindy looks at her with disgust. "I think I'm going to have to change doctors!"

"Why would you do that?" asks Dr. Donatelli. "Have I done something wrong?"

"No," Cindy begins, "but you haven't gotten rid of my genital warts."

"I understand your frustration, Cindy," Dr. Donatelli responds. "Actually, we have gotten rid of all of the warts that have appeared. The problem is that there is no way that we can permanently get rid of the virus from the skin in your genital area. We can use a cream that will boost your immune system in that area, but ultimately, your body will have to clear the virus itself. I know it's frustrating, but if we stick with it, you will get to a point where no more warts appear."

"Okay, I'll hang in there, but I won't be happy about it."

Cindy expresses a common frustration that people have with viral STIs. Sexually transmitted infections like chlamydia and gonorrhea are curable with antibiotics because they are caused by bacteria that the medication kills. There is no cure, however, for sexually transmitted viruses such as herpes, HPV, HIV, and hepatitis. The immune system mounts a defense against the virus that may clear it or reduce its activity, but often the virus remains and springs up later. Medications can help reduce the activity of the virus, but none can rid the body of the virus.

Dealing with a chronic infection is frustrating and depressing. Advances in genetic technology and pharmacology should eventually provide us with the cure for these infections. Work is also under way to develop more vaccines for the prevention of sexually transmitted viruses (as Gardisil does for certain strains of HPV). Try to maintain a positive outlook. Help is on the way!

What can I do to avoid getting a sexually transmitted infection?

After reading this chapter, you're probably considering a major change in lifestyle, perhaps enlisting as a novice at the nearest convent. That may be a little too drastic of a solution, although abstinence has merit. The only sure way to avoid STIs is to avoid sex. Ideally, you should proceed with sexual intimacy only when you have a long-standing mutually monogamous relationship. At least you should try to limit the number of your sexual partners. Ask a potential sexual partner about his past and any signs of possible infection (sores, warts, discharge). If there is any question of a current or prior STI, he should be examined, ideally by a urologist. Abstain from sex until he has been evaluated, and be adamant about this. If his history includes prior sex partners, strongly consider HIV testing. He should also be screened for herpes type 2 virus. If the herpes test is positive, he can begin daily Valtrex to significantly reduce the risk of asymptomatic transmission. Consider examining a potential sex partner before intercourse (you can combine this with placing a condom on the penis). Look for warts, blisters, and ulcerations. Always use condoms! When using a male condom, use the latex type. Natural "skin" condoms do not offer adequate protection against STIs. An alternative is the female condom, but it is not as well tested for STI prevention. (Refer to chapter 3 for more information on condoms.)

Most STIs have the potential of being spread through oral sex, although the rate is significantly lower compared with vaginal or anal intercourse. Consider incorporating these suggestions into your sexual activities:

- Use a latex barrier from start to finish during oral sex.
- Use a non-lubricated or a flavored condom on a penis or sex toy. Condoms with spermicide can numb the mouth and don't taste very good.
- Don't use food products like whipped cream or chocolate sauce with a condom or dental dam because they may be oil-based, and oil-based products break down latex.
- For oral sex on a woman or for oral-anal stimulation, use a dental dam, plastic food wrap, or a condom cut lengthwise.

Your risk of acquiring an STI during oral sex is increased in the following situations:

- You have gum disease, cuts, or sores
- You've had recent dental work that bruised any tissue in your mouth
- You have vigorously brushed or flossed
- You have had a recent oral or genital piercing (avoid any type of oral sexual contact for six weeks)

If any of these apply, consider postponing oral sexual contact to reduce your risk.

How do I cope emotionally when I discover that I have a sexually transmitted infection?

Society has promoted the concept that sexually transmitted infections should be worn like a scarlet letter. This attitude implies that one must be flagrantly promiscuous and devoid of morality to contract such an infection. This certainly is not true. Because viruses such as herpes and HPV are not yet curable, their prevalence in the general population is very high. You can contract these even with limited sexual encounters. Unfortunately, the prevailing attitude may make you feel embarrassed and ashamed when diagnosed with a sexually transmitted infection. You may feel angry at yourself or the partner that gave you the infection—or even at the entire male population. While working through these issues, keep in mind the following points:

Blaming yourself is not constructive. In many cases, there is nothing you could have done to prevent catching the virus. Obsessing about the past won't help you develop a positive approach to dealing with your infection.

Openly discuss your situation with your partner. If he was not honest with you regarding a history of herpes or HPV, you have every right to feel angry and betrayed. You should question whether it is wise to continue a relationship with a man who cannot be honest, even when your health is at stake. However, keep in mind that sexually transmitted infections can be asymptomatic, and your partner may have been unaware that he was infected. He may have acquired the infection months or even years prior to transmitting it to you. Likewise, you may have acquired the infection before your relationship with him. If both of you are honest and unaware of the origin of the infection, assigning blame only serves to destroy your relationship.

If a marriage or other mutually monogamous relationship has existed for many years and a sexually transmitted infection appears, you should suspect that extramarital sex has occurred. If this is a possibility, confront your husband. Extramarital affairs often reflect serious problems within a relationship. You should definitely consider couples counseling.

If you are in a new relationship and have a history of herpes or HPV, you must discuss this with your partner prior to sexual intimacy. You need to communicate openly with him. If he loves you, this should not be an insurmountable obstacle to deepening your relationship. Make sure he understands the facts about your condition, and help clear up any misconceptions he may harbor about it. A joint visit to your gynecologist may help.

If you are having trouble coping, consider enrolling in a support group. Ask your doctor and call surrounding hospitals to see if there is a support group in your area. There may also be a listing in the phone directory in the "guide to human services" section. Your county medical society may also be able to direct you to a group. At support groups, you will find other women who share your feelings and are struggling with the same issues. Sometimes comfort is gained in discovering that you are not alone. Group members can share approaches that have enabled them to deal with the infection and emotional distress. There are also online support groups and social networks for people with chronic sexually transmitted infections:

www.supportgroups.com

www.stdmatch.net

www.hsvsingles.com

www.datingwithherpes.org

Abstaining from sex during times of active infection doesn't mean you can't share intimate moments with your partner. Spending quiet time talking, kissing, and cuddling can enable you to show affection even during bouts of active infection.

6

WHY CAN'T I GET PREGNANT?

I've been trying to get pregnant for six months. Does this mean I have a problem?

Sandy is upset. She and Scott have been trying to get pregnant for the last six months and nothing has happened. Abby and Liz, her roommates from college, seemed to get pregnant as soon as they tried, but Sandy went off the pill six months ago and still isn't pregnant. There must be something wrong with her, right?

Sandy shouldn't jump to conclusions. Women sometimes get so consumed with preventing pregnancy that they assume it will occur the first month they stop using contraception. In reality, you only have a 25 percent chance of conceiving in any single cycle. Most gynecologists do not suspect an infertility problem until a couple has tried to conceive for one year without success. You should wait at least that long before seeking an infertility evaluation. If you want to increase your chances of success, you can time intercourse to happen just before you ovulate.

Of course, everything is relative. One year seems like an eternity as you're approaching age forty and hearing the tick-tock of that infernal biological clock. In your later reproductive years, after age thirty-five, starting an evaluation after six months of timed intercourse is reasonable. An earlier investigation is also warranted if there is a history of factors that are known to cause infertility such as endometriosis, pelvic infection, or irregular menstrual cycles.

When is the best time in my cycle for conception?

If your sex life is flourishing, you'll be tempted to answer, "All the time!" However enjoyable that may be, successful conception is limited to a specific point in your cycle. The greatest chances of success occur two to three days before ovulation through twenty-four hours after ovulation. The section on natural family planning in chapter 3 shows how to determine your day of ovulation. You can use this information to enhance your chances of conception as well as to prevent it. Try to have sexual intercourse every other day beginning two to four days prior to anticipated ovulation. It is best not to have intercourse every day unless this is your normal sexual practice, as this may decrease your partner's sperm count. Sexual intercourse every other day is sufficient for achieving pregnancy. He should also refrain from masturbation for several days prior to your first scheduled sexual encounter.

Do I need to see an infertility specialist?

It is a whole year now, and Sandy is still not pregnant. It doesn't help that she told her friends that she was trying. Now she constantly hears her friends asking whether she is pregnant. Her mother is also nagging. If Sandy has to hear, "When are you going to give me a cute little grandchild to look after?" one more time, she's going to scream.

Sandy has tried to conceive for a year without success. What does she do now? That depends on the background and philosophy of her gynecologist. Many have the qualifications and interest to start an infertility evaluation. The initial tests are fairly basic and can be performed competently by a general gynecologist. She may feel more comfortable remaining with a doctor she knows rather than starting with a new, unfamiliar one. Also, a gynecologist's fees are generally lower than those of an infertility specialist. However, the evaluation may proceed more expeditiously with a specialist. If the initial tests do not find an obvious source for her problem, she would do best to consult a specialist. She should ask her gynecologist if the tests will have to be repeated if she is referred to a specialist. If so, she is better off seeing an infertility specialist from the start.

What is a BBT chart?

The BBT (basal body temperature) chart reflects your ovarian function. Immediately upon awakening each day, record your temperature on a special chart provided by your doctor. To keep a precise record, this must be done before you begin any other activity. You can purchase a basal body thermometer (also referred to as a basal thermometer) at your local pharmacy or online. There is often a slight dip in your temperature on the day of ovulation. After ovulation, your ovary produces progesterone that induces a temperature rise of half to one degree. By analyzing the chart, your doctor can determine if you have ovulated and the day of ovulation. The doctor also can use your BBT chart when planning the timing of certain tests.

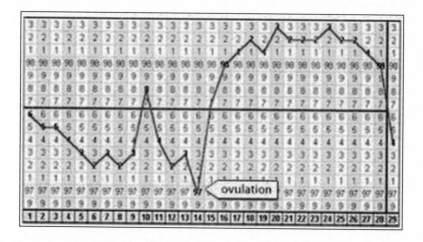

How can the gynecologist tell if I have a problem?

Sandy strolls into Dr. Kramer's office. She's in a good mood. She's convinced that Dr. Kramer will be able to solve her infertility problem today. She feels fine and assumes that there can't be very much wrong. After all, she's been seeing the gynecologist every year since she was sixteen and her exams are always normal.

Dr. Kramer enters the room. "Hi, Sandy, how are things going?"

"I feel fine, Dr. Kramer, but I haven't been able to get pregnant for the last year. I made this appointment so you can tell me why I can't get pregnant and hopefully fix it."

Dr. Kramer sighs. "I'm afraid it's not that easy, Sandy. There may be a few things we can tell by your exam today, but if you're serious about looking into your infertility problem, I'll bring you and your husband into the office so that we can discuss what might be involved."

It is a common misconception that a routine pelvic examination will provide your doctor with enough information to determine if you have an infertility problem. Unfortunately, most infertility problems require specialized testing. The evaluation can be expensive and time-consuming. Some procedures may be uncomfortable (that's what doctors say to avoid the word *painful*). Many tests have to be scheduled at specific times in your cycle. The evaluation often disrupts your daily routines and doesn't exactly enhance the romance of your marriage. About now you're saying, "Gee, you could be a little bit more upbeat about this." We apologize. However, it is important to realize that an infertility evaluation is not to be taken lightly. A strong sense of commitment is needed to launch into a potentially long-term, emotionally draining process. With this in mind, let's identify the various sources of infertility. We will describe each problem, the tests required for its detection, and the treatment. You may want to refer to the illustration of the female reproductive system on page 38.

Problems with Ovulation Ovulatory dysfunction accounts for up to 40 percent of infertility in women. If your ovary doesn't release an egg, you won't conceive. In other words, having eggs in your ovaries does not guarantee that you will ovulate. The sperm can fertilize an egg only after it has been released from the ovary. The eggs reside in small fluid-filled structures in the ovaries referred to as follicles. Signals, called gonadotropins, are sent from the pituitary gland (a small gland located at the base of the brain) to stimulate the follicles in the ovary. Normally, each month one of these follicles reaches maturation and ovulates, thereby releasing the egg. The secretion of gonadotropins from the pituitary must be precisely timed, and anything that interferes with this will result in a failure to ovulate (called anovulation).

Stress or anxiety may temporarily prevent ovulation. Excessive or inadequate weight may also play a role. Numerous medical disorders can have an effect on gonadotropin secretion. The problem may reside within the ovary. The ovary may be congenitally abnormal, may have become resistant to gonadotropins, or may have undergone the effects of early menopause. Many women have no apparent reason for their failure to ovulate.

Your BBT chart and a progesterone level obtained during the second half of your cycle can determine whether ovulation has occurred. If your BBT chart does not show a rise in temperature and your progesterone level is low, you have not ovulated. A rise in temperature and an elevated progesterone level indicates successful ovulation. Sometimes the progesterone level and BBT chart suggests ovulation, but the ovary still doesn't release an egg, a problem that can be detected by performing ultrasound scans when you are in the middle of your cycle. After the diagnosis of anovulation is established, your doctor will order blood work. This helps rule out certain medical disorders, such as thyroid disease, that interfere with ovulation.

To stimulate the release of gonadotropins from the pituitary to induce ovulation, doctors usually first prescribe clomiphene citrate (Clomid or Serophene). Clomiphene induces ovulation in 80 percent of anovulatory women, and 40 percent of those patients conceive (higher if additional causes of infertility are excluded). Overall pregnancy success rates for clomiphene are 16–18 percent per cycle. Clomiphene does not increase the risk of miscarriage and birth defects. The incidence of twins is increased to 5 percent with clomiphene. Multiple births beyond twins are rare. Potential side effects include hot flashes, abdominal bloating, breast tenderness, mood alteration, nausea, headache, and visual changes. Usually these conditions are transient, and most women tolerate clomiphene well. In some cases, the effect of clomiphene on cervical mucus (making it too thick) or the lining of the uterus (making it too thin) may actually impair fertility.

Patients who do not respond to clomiphene are typically treated with gonadotropins, prescription drugs that are similar to the signals normally secreted by the pituitary gland. Injected into the body, they directly stimulate the ovary, inducing follicular maturation. Approximately 60 percent of women who fail to ovulate will do so after receiving gonadotropins. Since these medications are expensive and have the potential for significant complications, it is critical to rule out other causes of infertility prior to using them. Women need to be monitored closely while using gonadotropins, which should be administered under the supervision of an infertility specialist. Side effects and complications include:

- Anywhere from 15–35 percent of women who become pregnant after gonadotropins have a miscarriage. The rate is dependent on age. Since many women receiving gonadotropins will be over thirty-five, their miscarriage rate will be higher than the general population.
- In 5–10 percent of treatment cycles, women develop detectable ovarian enlargement. Multiple follicles (cysts with eggs) make the ovaries larger and tenderer.
- There is a risk of ovarian hyperstimulation syndrome (OHSS), which in rare cases can be life threatening. However, when a woman is closely monitored for side effects, she has less than 1 percent risk of developing severe OHSS.
- Ovarian stimulation increases the likelihood of a multiple pregnancy (twins, triplets, or more). This may at first seem exciting, but a multiple pregnancy is considered high risk for both a mother and her fetuses.
- Other side effects including headache and abdominal pain.

Problems of the Luteal Phase Infertility is not always caused by a failure to ovulate. If the second half of the cycle (known as the luteal phase) is either shortened or inadequate, infertility can result. Three to twenty percent of patients who are infertile and 5–60 percent of patients who experience recurrent pregnancy loss are diagnosed with this condition. You can see the wide range of estimates for how often this affects women's fertility. That is partly because many normal women who are fertile also demonstrate an inadequate luteal phase, making it hard to know whether this is truly the cause of infertility in a woman who is not conceiving.

In this condition, the follicle remaining after ovulation, referred to as the corpus luteum, fails to produce sufficient progesterone. Progesterone prepares the endometrium for implantation of the embryo and supports the early pregnancy. The pregnancy will be unsuccessful if progesterone production is inadequate. The BBT chart suggests a luteal phase disorder if the temperature rise following ovulation is abbreviated. A low progesterone level in the mid-luteal phase also indicates a luteal deficiency. Because progesterone secretion is pulsatile, multiple progesterone levels may be required for this to be of value. Multiple pelvic ultrasound exams can be used to follow follicular development. Ultrasound has also been used in the luteal phase to detect an endometrium that is not responding properly to progesterone, although this has not proven to be particularly useful. An endometrial biopsy may also be obtained to detect luteal phase abnormalities. After inserting a speculum, the doctor introduces a biopsy instrument through the cervix to obtain an endometrial sample. A pathologist interprets the specimen to see if the endometrium has been properly prepared by progesterone. Endometrial biopsy was once considered the "gold standard" for detecting luteal dysfunction, but many infertility experts feel that it lacks accuracy and precision and no longer use it. Occasionally, there is a secondary cause for luteal phase deficiency such as hyperprolactinemia (excess secretion of the hormone prolactin from the pituitary gland) or hypothyroidism (an underactive thyroid gland).

Luteal phase deficiencies are treated in several ways. Hyperprolactinemia and hypothyroidism are treated with medications that specifically address those issues (bromocriptine and levothyroxine respectively). Women without hyperprolactinemia or hypothyroidism (the more common scenario) are treated with supplemental progesterone during the luteal phase. Progesterone is usually given vaginally either by suppository or gel (Crinone). The vaginal route is preferred over both the oral and intramuscular forms of progesterone because of superior endometrial progesterone concentrations. Progesterone will be continued through the first eight to ten weeks of the pregnancy. After that time, the placenta takes over the role of progesterone production from the corpus luteum. The progesterone is not associated with an increased risk of birth defects. If there is evidence of poor follicular development, clomiphene or even gonadotropins (see previous question) will be used to stimulate follicular maturation, thereby producing higher progesterone levels.

Tubal Problems Once the egg is released from the ovary, it must travel down the fallopian tube for fertilization and eventual implantation in the uterus (see the illustration on page 143). If the fallopian tubes are closed or scar tissue (adhesions) is interposed between the ovaries and the tubes, this is not possible. Conditions that may contribute to tubal blockage or adhesions include severe pelvic infections, IUD use (rarely), endometriosis, prior pelvic surgery, tubal pregnancies, and appendicitis.

The hysterosalpingogram (HSG) is a radiologic test used to see whether the tubes are blocked. It is scheduled in the first half of the cycle, at least several days after menstruation has ceased. After inserting a speculum, the doctor places a small catheter into the cervix and injects a contrast dye into the uterus and tubes. X-rays are taken. If the tubes are patent (open), dye emerges from the tubes. If they are obstructed, the doctor notes the location of the blockage. The HSG also provides information regarding uterine abnormalities, such as polyps, fibroids, or an unusually shaped uterus. A sonohysterosalpingogram and sonohysterogram are similar procedures utilizing pelvic ultrasound. Laparoscopy (inserting a telescope into the abdomen under anesthesia) is also employed if the results of the HSG are not clear.

Intrauterine disorders are evaluated by hysteroscopy. The doctor inserts a telescopic instrument through the cervix, allowing him or her to see inside the uterus. Intrauterine fibroids, polyps, and adhesions can be removed through the hysteroscope. Some uterine malformations can also be corrected. (Refer to chapter 9 for more detailed information on uterine disorders and hysteroscopy.)

There are several methods utilized for correcting tubal blockage. If most of the tube is healthy, your doctor may elect to remove the obstructed portion and reattach the remaining sections of tube. This is

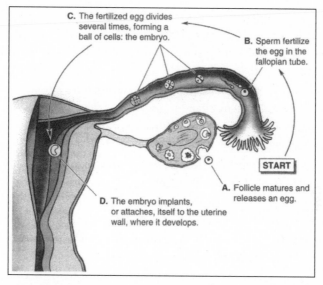

C. The fertilized egg divides several times, forming a ball of cells: the embryo.

B. Sperm fertilize the egg in the fallopian tube.

START

A. Follicle matures and releases an egg.

D. The embryo implants, or attaches, itself to the uterine wall, where it develops.

a surgical procedure referred to as tubal reanastomosis. If the blockage is located at the cornua (where the tube joins the uterus), the doctor may choose to reimplant the tube through an opening created in the uterus. Blockage at the end of the tube (the fimbria) is repaired by releasing the adhesions that encase the tube or by creating a new opening. In some circumstances, a semiflexible wire called a stent can be passed through a tubal obstruction using the hysteroscope.

If your tubes are beyond salvage, you still have the option of in vitro fertilization (IVF). In this procedure, your eggs are removed from the ovaries with a needle that is directed by ultrasonic guidance. The eggs are fertilized with sperm in a laboratory. The fertilized egg divides several times, forming a ball of cells called the embryo, which is placed directly into the uterus through the vagina. Depending on your age, your chances of pregnancy range from 10–70 percent. GIFT (gamete intrafallopian transfer) and ZIFT (zygote intrafallopian transfer) are variations of IVF that involve transferring eggs directly into a healthy portion of tube. Your doctor may also go straight to IVF without attempting tubal surgery if there are additional causes for your infertility such as a partner with a low sperm count. IVF is expensive, although its cost has been decreasing as more centers develop IVF capabilities. Before choosing a center for IVF, investigate the cost and the success rate of the facility. As the cost of IVF has decreased and the success rate increased, more doctors and patients are choosing IVF over surgery for tubes that are blocked.

Cervical Problems Sperm must pass through the cervix to fertilize the egg. Cervical mucus changes prior to ovulation, becoming abundant, watery, thin, and clear. The quality of the mucus may affect the sperm's ability to enter the uterus.

Doctors previously evaluated the cervical mucus by performing a postcoital test (PCT). Immediately prior to ovulation, the woman was asked to have intercourse and then to undergo an examination. The doctor would then examine the quality of the mucus and sperm. Most experts feel that this test is subjective, rarely changes management, and does not accurately predict a woman's ability to conceive. For these reasons, PCT is no longer a routine part of the infertility evaluation. Sperm are assessed for their number, shape, and ability to move through a semen analysis (see below). If your doctor has reason to suspect a cervical problem, he or she may bypass the cervix using intrauterine insemination. The sperm are separated from the seminal fluid and introduced directly into the intrauterine cavity, using a small plastic catheter. Infertility specialists will also use assisted reproductive technology such as IVF. Very poor sperm quality (very low numbers or motility) can be circumvented by directly injecting the sperm into the egg (a process known as Intracytoplasmic Sperm Injection, or ICSI) during an IVF cycle.

What about my husband? Should he be checked?

Dr. Kramer has spent the better part of an hour expounding on the multitude of tests required for the evaluation of female infertility. Sandy is a little upset that she might have to undergo invasive procedures to solve their infertility problem. Scott just sits in silence, eternally thankful that he is not a woman.

Finally Sandy has had enough. "It doesn't seem fair that I have to go through all of this. Our infertility may have nothing to do with me.

Why doesn't somebody look at Scott? It might be his fault that we can't get pregnant."

"You're right," comments Dr. Kramer. "He doesn't completely escape. Scott should undergo a semen analysis."

Upon hearing his name, Scott emerges from his daydreaming. "What's a semen analysis?"

Dr. Kramer explains, "After abstaining from sex for several days, you will provide a semen specimen by masturbation. It must be collected in a clean container and brought to the laboratory within one hour. The semen is examined to determine how many sperm it contains, whether they move, and whether their shape is normal. The semen is also checked for signs of infection."

Male sources for infertility are less common than those found in women. However, abnormalities can be produced by any of the following conditions:

- Past history of mumps, sexually transmitted diseases, surgery near the reproductive organs, or testicular injury
- Use of certain drugs, including some antibiotics, chemotherapy drugs, marijuana, tobacco, and alcohol
- Exposure to radiation
- Excessive heat caused by tight underwear, hot tubs, baths, and saunas
- Varicose veins in the scrotum
- Genetic abnormalities
- Hormonal disorders such as thyroid disease or decreased testosterone production
- Infection
- Structural malformations of the sex organs
- Retrograde ejaculation, in which semen is released backward into the bladder instead of exiting through the penis

Male infertility is usually evaluated and treated by a urologist. You may also be able to locate a physician in your area who specializes in male infertility. Poor sperm quality can also be circumvented through intrauterine insemination and IVF with ICSI (see above).

Why does the doctor want to perform a laparoscopy?

If no source for infertility is found on initial testing, your doctor may want to perform a laparoscopy. Adhesions and endometriosis (refer to chapter 8) are two causes of infertility that cannot be accurately diagnosed by scans and must be examined directly through laparoscopy (a telescope introduced into the abdomen under anesthesia). Endometriosis may be discovered through this procedure, and pelvic adhesions are easily discernible. If a hysterosalpingogram was not previously performed or the results were not clear, dye is injected to exclude the possibility that the fallopian tubes are blocked. Adhesions and endometriosis are treated by employing laparoscopic techniques. Because the cost of IVF has decreased, and the availability has increased, fewer laparoscopies are performed now than in past years. Most of the causes of infertility treated laparoscopically (endometriosis, adhesions, blocked tubes) are circumvented using IVF.

What is artificial insemination?

Occasionally, conception is enhanced by artificially placing sperm in direct proximity to the cervix or uterine cavity. Intrauterine insemination (IUI), where sperm is placed directly into the uterus with a catheter, is the most common form of artificial insemination. Artificial insemination is used when your partner's sperm count is low or if sperm quality is compromised. It is also used when the semen is normal but cannot be properly deposited in the vagina because of retrograde or premature ejaculation. Women with unreceptive cervical mucus, as noted earlier in this chapter, are also good candidates for artificial insemination. Artificial insemination allows the sperm to skip the cervical mucus entirely. Doctors also sometimes suggest artificial insemination when they cannot determine the reason for a couple's infertility.

Your doctor will use ovulation kits, ultrasound, or blood tests to make sure you are ovulating when you undergo artificial insemination. Your partner will be asked to produce a sample of semen after abstaining from sex for two to five days. The sperm will be "washed" in a laboratory which removes chemicals in the semen that may cause discomfort for the woman. The process of "washing" sperm enhances the chance of fertilization. A centrifuge is then used to collect the best sperm. The sperm are placed in a thin tube called a catheter and introduced through the vagina and cervix into the uterus. There may be a small amount of cramping during the procedure, but usually it is a relatively painless procedure. You may be asked to lie down for fifteen to forty-five minutes. After that, you can resume your normal activities.

Artificial insemination will not work for everyone. It is reasonable to try this for three to six cycles. If there is no success, then it is probably best to move on to more advanced forms of assisted reproduction such as IVF. Artificial insemination can also be undertaken with donated sperm. This is referred to as AID, artificial insemination of donor sperm. It is critical for donor semen to be screened to exclude sexually transmittable diseases. Donors should be questioned with respect to family history, genetic disorders, and any past exposure to drugs or chemicals that might increase the risk of birth defects. Your doctor can provide you with details regarding the screening process used for AID specimens.

When am I too old to get pregnant?

Many women think that if they exercise, eat healthy, and take care of themselves properly, then they should be able to have a baby at any age before menopause. However, reproductive health and general health are not the same thing and fertility does decrease with age no matter how well you take care of yourself. Technically, as long as you are having regular menstrual periods, there is the possibility of pregnancy. Unfortunately, fertility progressively decreases after age thirty-five while the chances of losing a pregnancy through miscarriage increases. Older eggs result in declining fertility, miscarriage, and babies with chromosomal abnormalities such as Down syndrome. For thirty-five-year-olds, the rate of pregnancies ending in live births is half that for women in their twenties. By age forty-five, it is down 95 percent. In addition, complications of pregnancy such as gestational diabetes and hypertension progressively increase with advancing age.

The initial approach for patients thirty-five and older will often include an assessment of their ovarian reserves. This may include the following:

- *Day 3 estradiol level*: Lower levels along with a normal FSH result in a higher pregnancy rate with fertility treatments. High day 3 estradiol levels are indicative of advanced ovarian age and a poorer response to fertility treatments.

- *Day 3 FSH (Follicle Stimulating Hormone) level*: This shows how much of this pituitary hormone is necessary to stimulate follicular development. Higher levels indicate that your follicles are more resistant to stimulation, decreasing the chances of successful IVF.

- *Day 3 counting of small follicles (pre antral follicle count)*: This gives an accurate read on how many eggs are left in your ovaries and gives your doctor a sense of how many eggs he or she can retrieve in an IVF cycle. When more eggs are retrieved, there is a greater likelihood of success.

- *Anti-mullerian hormone levels (AMH)*: Blood levels of this hormone reflect the number of eggs remaining in your ovaries (your ovarian reserve). Women with higher levels tend to have a better response to ovarian stimulation, producing more eggs that can be retrieved.

Assisted reproductive technologies such as IVF can help older women achieve pregnancy. An older woman who wants to attempt pregnancy using her own eggs can reduce the risks associated with older eggs by attempting pregnancy using IVF with preimplantation genetic diagnosis (PGD). PGD can screen out most of the chromosomal abnormalities which may occur in older eggs. PGD increases the chance for pregnancy by 15–20 percent and decreases the risk of miscarriage by 50 percent or more. The risk for delivering a baby with Down syndrome can almost be eliminated.

Another option for older women is to use eggs donated from a younger woman, which increases the pregnancy rate and decreases the risk of both miscarriage and chromosomal abnormalities.

Are there natural approaches that increase fertility?

Any woman who is actively trying to conceive should start limiting her caffeine intake, stop smoking, and eliminate alcohol. She should try to normalize her weight. Excessively thin or obese women tend to have a lower fertility rate. While a reasonable amount of exercise is desirable, she should avoid excessive exercise (we're talking about marathon runner or triathlon amounts of exercising). Inordinately low body fat associated with excessive exercise creates ovulatory disorders. Malabsorption disorders such as gluten intolerance, also known as celiac disease or intolerance to wheat, should be identified and treated. Vaginal lubricants, which can kill sperm, should be eliminated. Melatonin, sometimes used for sleep disorders, also appears to play a role in reproduction and high doses should be avoided. Iron deficiency increases infertility. Women with infertility can have their iron and ferritin (the protein that stores iron) checked and iron replacement given if necessary. Thyroid function should also be checked and corrected as necessary. High-protein diets have been shown to adversely affect fertility in rodent studies. While recognizing that humans and mice are quite different, it seems reasonable to not overdo the protein if you are having an infertility issue. Men may want to limit their soy food intake since there is an inverse relationship between soy food consumption and sperm count.

Many supplements have been recommended within the complementary and alternative community (CAM). The following table, developed by Dr. Marilyn Glenville (www.marilynglenville.com), is a reasonable example of vitamins, minerals, and amino acids often recommended for fertility. Many of these have benefit in theory but few have been evaluated through well-designed studies:

Nutrients	You	Your Partner
Folic acid	400mcg	400mcg
Zinc	30mg	30mg
Selenium	100mcg	100mcg
Fish oil	1000mg	1000mg
Vitamin B6	up to 50mg	up to 50mg
Vitamin B12	up to 50mcg	up to 50mcg
Vitamin E	300-400 IU	300-400 IU
Vitamin C	1000mg	1000mg
Vitamin A	up to 2300 IU	-
Manganese	5mg	5mg
L-arginine	-	300mg
L-carnitine	-	100mg
L-Taurine	-	100mg

Dr. Mark Moyad, Director of Preventive and Alternative Medicine in the Department of Urology at the University of Michigan Medical Center, proposes that the following supplements have reasonable evidence for their efficacy in improving male-related infertility: CoQ10 (200–300 mg/day), Fish Oil (1–2 gm/day), L-carnitine (2–3 gm/day), Omega-3 Fatty Acids, and Vitamin C (1000 mg/day).

Herbs often recommended for men include Astragulus, maca, Tribulus, and saw palmetto. Herbs that may hurt sperm production include St. John's wort, echinacea, and Ginkgo Biloba.

Herbs recommended for women include Chaste Tree Berry (Vitex), red clover blossom, dong quai, evening primrose oil, false unicorn root, red raspberry leaf, licorice, damiana leaves, black cohosh, wild yam, and hachimijiogan. Flaxseed oil and other products providing essential fatty acids have also been recommended. Most of these herbs have not been tested in well-designed, randomized, placebo-controlled studies. Chaste Tree Berry, antioxidants, and a product called FertilityBlend (a product combining certain vitamins, minerals, and herbs, available at www.fertilityblend.com) have at least some reasonable studies to recommend them. Many herbs can have significant adverse effects. They should not be used without first consulting your doctor and should not be used with any other fertility treatments prescribed by your doctor. Many traditional doctors have little or no experience in working with herbal products, so you should seek out a physician specializing in complementary and alternative approaches if you choose this path.

Myo-Inositol, a dietary vitamin belonging to the B complex, has been shown in controlled studies to improve ovarian function and ovulation induction in some types of patients with oligomenorrhea (few periods) or amenorrhea (no periods). It is available under the brand name Pregitude, where it is combined with folic acid.

Other alternative approaches include:

- Reflexology: A well-designed study found no benefit.
- Acupuncture: There are at least some studies demonstrating an increase in ovulation induction with acupuncture.
- Mind-body techniques: Studies done in this arena have been mixed. Certainly anything that improves psychological, emotional, and spiritual well-being is of at least some benefit overall, especially in couples undergoing infertility, which can be extremely stressful.
- Homeopathy: There is no data available assessing the effectiveness or lack of effectiveness in infertility patients.

I hear that infertility drugs cause ovarian cancer. Is that true?

Several small studies in the 1990s indicated an increased risk of getting ovarian cancer with previous use of infertility medications, but flaws with the design of those studies made their results questionable. More recent studies are mixed with at least one large, well-designed study not finding an association of ovarian cancer with fertility drugs (clomiphene or gonadotropins) and another finding an increased risk for "borderline ovarian tumors" (a type of ovarian tumor that exhibits some characteristics of cancer, but is far less aggressive and usually is treated successfully).

Although it seems reasonable that drugs that induce ovulation might increase the risk of developing ovarian cancer, since oral contraceptives, which inhibit ovulation, decrease the risk, you must remember that these drugs are used for relatively short periods of time. If there is a small risk, it may be offset if you successfully achieve pregnancy, which confers a degree of protection against ovarian cancer.

At this point, clomiphene and gonadotropins should be used when necessary to induce ovulation.

Why do I feel as if I'm riding an emotional roller coaster?

Sandy is frantic. She received her HCG injection twenty-four hours earlier and now she and Scott are supposed to have sex, but of course he is nowhere to be found. After several attempts, he finally answers his cell phone.

"What's up?" he asks.

"What do you mean 'what's up'? You're supposed to be home so that we can have sex. I'm ovulating now. What's all that noise? Where are you?"

"Oh, I forgot. Some of us from the office went out to The Golden Goose after work for a few drinks. We just got a big account and we're celebrating."

Sandy can't believe what she's hearing. "I can't believe you don't remember. You knew I got my HCG injection yesterday. If we don't have sex today, we will have missed another cycle."

"It's always another cycle with you," Scott shouts over the noise in the bar. "How many times are we going to try this, Sandy? This whole infertility thing has ruined our sex life. It used to be spontaneous and fun. Now it's just all about making a baby."

Sandy is on the verge of tears. "I thought you wanted to have a baby?"

"I do," Scott responds. "It's just that I've had enough of this. Injecting your wife's butt is not exactly sexy. I used to look at you as my hot wife. Now I look at you as a science experiment. Then last month you had that

complication from the injections and you were in pain and bloated and miserable. I couldn't get near you."

Sandy is taken aback. *This must be the alcohol talking. This does not sound like her husband.* *"I'm the one who has to go through all of this. Aren't you being just a little selfish? All I'm asking is that you be available for us to have sex when it's the right time."*

Scott relents. *"Okay, okay, I'm coming home, but I don't know how much longer I can persist with these infertility treatments. One minute your hopes are up and you're as high as a kite and the next you're totally depressed. Maybe it's time for us to look into adoption."*

"We can talk about that later. Just get home so we can give it another try."

Infertility can play havoc with your emotions. Discovering that you have an infertility problem can elicit feelings of anger, denial, guilt, grief, and isolation. You assume that pregnancy will occur naturally. When it doesn't, your self-esteem can be shattered. Additional pressure may come from friends and family: "Your sister Judy just had her third baby. When are you going to start?" Avoiding contact with siblings and friends who have already conceived may lead to social isolation.

The infertility evaluation itself is laden with emotional upheaval. Many tests and procedures require scheduled intercourse, which zaps the romance out of marriage. Hopeful anticipation accompanies each attempt at conception. This is soon replaced with frustration and despair if the attempt is not successful. Counseling or therapy with a psychologist may help if you are having trouble coping. You can ask if there is a support group available in your area. If you have trouble finding a support group, contact the national office of RESOLVE (www.resolve.org). Taking periodic breaks from all the testing for one to three months may also help you cope with the stress.

Throughout the evaluation, your doctor must give you a clear assessment of your chances of success. As long as there is a reasonable chance of becoming pregnant, you should persist. Most women who persevere through the infertility evaluation will achieve a successful pregnancy. However, there may come a time when it becomes clear that success is unlikely. At that point, you must try to accept that you may never become pregnant. You can then start investigating alternatives such as adoption.

For more information and help with infertility issues, visit:

The American Society of Reproductive Medicine (ASRM): www.reproductivefacts.org

The American Fertility Association: www.theafa.org

Fertile Hope: www.fertilehope.org

Resolve: www.resolve.org

The Society for Assisted Reproductive Technology (SART): www.sart.org

Infertility Resources: www.ihr.com

WHEN SOMETHING GOES WRONG: COMPLICATIONS OF EARLY PREGNANCY

Stephanie is ecstatic! She found her soul mate in Robbie. They had a storybook wedding in Antigua, and after trying for two years, she has finally conceived. The whole world just has to know! She is so excited that she posts it on Facebook. But her joy doesn't last, at least not this time. Three months into the pregnancy she begins bleeding. Her doctors reassure her that this is not uncommon, but it doesn't stop and she has a miscarriage.

Perhaps the only thing worse than not being able to get pregnant is conceiving, only to lose your pregnancy. Stephanie is left with a thousand questions: What did I do wrong? What is wrong with me? Why did this happen? Am I ever going to have a successful pregnancy? This chapter addresses Stephanie's questions and others that arise when there are complications early in a pregnancy.

I missed my period and have a positive pregnancy test. Now I'm bleeding. Am I having a miscarriage?

This seems to be a good time to panic, right? Not necessarily. It is common to have light bleeding early in a normal pregnancy. If the bleeding is light, your odds of maintaining the pregnancy are good. If the bleeding is heavy, your chances of success are diminished. When you pass tissue other than blood or clots from the vagina, miscarriage is inevitable.

You should schedule an appointment with your gynecologist at the first sign of bleeding. The doctor will determine your B-HCG (beta human chorionic gonadotropin) level. B-HCG is a hormone produced by the placenta. The amount of this hormone rises steadily through the first ten weeks of the pregnancy. The value doubles approximately every two days. By comparing sequential values of B-HCG, the doctor can assess the health of the early pregnancy. Even when the B-HCG does not double every two days, a good quality pregnancy may still develop. However, a B-HCG level that fails to rise significantly over time will predict an unsuccessful pregnancy. As long as it rises significantly, there is hope of keeping the pregnancy. The doctor may also want to measure a progesterone level, and if it is low, prescribe supplemental progesterone to support the pregnancy. A very low progesterone level suggests a pregnancy that may be growing poorly and will ultimately fail. Low B-HCG and progesterone levels may also reflect a pregnancy that is growing in the fallopian tube (ectopic pregnancy).

Once the B-HCG reaches a certain level, your doctor will order a pelvic ultrasound scan, which should demonstrate a pregnancy sac containing an embryo. At this point, or shortly thereafter, a heartbeat should be detectable. If these are not seen, the pregnancy is not viable. As the embryo grows, consecutive studies can be done. If growth ceases or the heartbeat stops, the pregnancy has ended.

What needs to be done if I'm having a miscarriage?

Once it is determined that pregnancy loss is inevitable, the doctor often recommends a D&E (dilation and evacuation) or gives you misoprostol, which helps the uterus expel the nonviable pregnancy tissue. If the pregnancy is very early, this may not be necessary. The uterus spontaneously expels the nonviable pregnancy completely. After the first few weeks, this is less likely. Your chances of developing prolonged, heavy bleeding are substantial, and it's better to use additional medical or surgical approaches. Misoprostol helps your uterus expel the tissue by dilating the cervix and inducing contractions. With this approach, you will have bleeding that can last anywhere from several hours to several weeks, with the heaviest bleeding lasting three to four days. The most common side effects from misoprostol are gastrointestinal, especially diarrhea. D&E is the surgical procedure used to remove the nonviable pregnancy tissue. After sedation or anesthesia, a suction instrument is placed through the vagina and into the uterus. The tissue is evacuated from the uterus, which then allows it to return to normal. Miscarriage beyond fourteen weeks may necessitate an extended D&E or labor-inducing procedure (refer to page 79).

Why did I have a miscarriage?

Stephanie is still very upset from her miscarriage. She has accepted that there wasn't anything she could have done differently that would've made a difference in her pregnancy loss, but she is still left with questions: Why did I have this miscarriage? What went wrong? Is it likely to happen again?

This is one of life's mysterious questions. Often your doctor will not be able to identify the cause of your loss. The mechanisms involved in a developing pregnancy are intricate. Following fertilization, the egg must divide repeatedly and produce perfect duplication of chromosomes (the structures containing your genetic blueprints). A ball of cells forms and implants itself on the inside wall of the uterus before developing into the placenta and embryo. The placenta must evolve successfully to provide nutrients to the embryo. The cells of the embryo must develop into tissues, and tissues into organs. The complexity of this series of events is almost incomprehensible. If any of these processes fail, the pregnancy will end. Miscarriage is nature's way of eliminating abnormal pregnancies.

Miscarriages are very common. Twenty percent of all conceptions result in miscarriage. This is important to understand. The tendency is to feel guilty about having one. "Is it something I took (a drink or a medication)? Is it something I did?" Such possible causes are unlikely. Women often feel they are at fault for losing the pregnancy or defective in some way. But in general, the woman is not responsible for the miscarriage.

How long should I wait after a miscarriage before trying again?

Stephanie decides that she wants to get pregnant again immediately in order to prove to herself that she and Robbie can have a successful pregnancy. Does this make sense? Is this the right way to move forward?

This depends on her emotional state. Some women will want to try again as soon as possible, whereas others need more time for grieving. She should wait at least two menstrual cycles before attempting to conceive again. This permits ample time for her reproductive organs to recover and reestablish a normal ovulatory cycle. She may increase her risk of subsequent miscarriage if she attempts to conceive sooner. Waiting also allows for a period of observation in case she develops a complication from the miscarriage, such as erratic bleeding or infection. Finally, it provides her doctor with a better opportunity for dating the pregnancy. If she conceives prior to regaining regular periods, it is harder to establish her estimated date of confinement, or due date.

I had two miscarriages. Is there something wrong with me?

We have already said that it is unlikely for there to be anything wrong with Stephanie or her husband after having one miscarriage. But what about two or three successive miscarriages? Does that increase the risk of there being a specific problem with either Stephanie or Robbie?

Two or three (the American Society for Reproductive Medicine uses two; classically it was three) successive miscarriages is classified as recurrent pregnancy loss (RPL). Approximately 3–5 percent of couples suffer from RPL. RPL warrants further investigation. Even after investigation, the source of the recurrent pregnancy loss may not be evident. Approximately 50 percent of the time a source is found.

Chromosomal aberrations are associated with miscarriage 30–50 percent (varies with age) of the time. Chromosomes are the structures that contain genes, the material encoded with the information that determines a person's constitution. Every cell in the body has an identical set of chromosomes. If there is a failure in the duplication or distribution of the chromosomes during the development of the baby, a miscarriage will occur.

Most chromosomal problems are isolated to a specific pregnancy and do not result in repeated pregnancy loss. However, if you or your husband carries a chromosomal irregularity (3 percent incidence), it may cause recurrent pregnancy loss. This condition can be detected through genetic analysis of chromosomes obtained from cells in the bloodstream (both of you provide a blood specimen). If a chromosomal disturbance is the cause, a genetic counselor can aid you in determining your future chances of success and also advise you about genetic studies that might be required during a future pregnancy.

Another potential cause for pregnancy loss is progesterone deficiency caused by a luteal phase disorder (see chapter 6). Progesterone prepares the endometrium for implantation of the embryo and subsequently is required for sustaining the pregnancy. Blood progesterone levels can be measured early in the pregnancy and supplemented if low. Unfortunately, most medical research has shown this not to be effective at preventing miscarriage.

The medical community has often blamed infection as a cause for recurrent pregnancy loss. While certain infections may cause a single pregnancy loss (toxoplasmosis, rubella, cytomegalovirus, herpes), they are not a cause of recurrent pregnancy loss. Bacterial vaginosis, an imbalance in the bacteria of your vagina (see chapter 5), has been associated with pregnancy loss between four to six months and preterm delivery. Tests on your vaginal secretions can easily detect bacterial vaginosis and appropriate antibiotics given if it is found.

Abnormalities in the contour or shape of the uterine cavity can produce recurrent pregnancy loss. Some of these may be congenital, meaning that the woman was born with the abnormality. Fibroids— benign, smooth muscle tumors that develop in the wall of the uterus and project into the uterine cavity—can interfere with pregnancy, resulting in miscarriage (see chapter 9). Scar tissue from prior surgery or infections may also cause pregnancy loss. Uterine abnormalities are diagnosed through a hysterosalpingogram or other similar tests (see chapter 6) or hysteroscopy and are corrected through surgery. Often the surgery can be performed through the hysteroscope, a telescopic instrument introduced through the vagina into the uterus. An "incompetent" cervix can prematurely dilate, leading to pregnancy loss in the second trimester (middle of the pregnancy). An incompetent cervix can be treated with placement of a circlage (a special stitch placed around the cervix to keep it closed) at approximately twelve weeks into the pregnancy.

Certain medical disorders may increase the risk of miscarriage. These include systemic lupus erythematosus (an autoimmune disorder), hyperprolactinemia (over secretion of the hormone prolactin), thyroid disease, chronic kidney disease, congenital heart disease, and diabetes. A thorough medical history and physical exam, in conjunction with screening blood work, will detect these problems. Often conception can be attempted once these conditions are treated or stabilized.

Disorders of the immune system may result in recurrent pregnancy loss. It is natural for the body to treat the baby as something foreign. Normally, the immune system has a mechanism that prevents the body from rejecting the baby, but this may malfunction. In another immune disorder, the body makes antibodies that cause clotting in placental blood vessels. This disorder is treated with low doses of blood thinners (aspirin and heparin).

Also, factors under a woman's control may be responsible for recurrent miscarriages. Smoking, heavy alcohol consumption, excessive caffeine, obesity, and illicit drug use all increase the risk of pregnancy loss. Eliminating these habits is critical to sustaining a healthy pregnancy. Exposure to high doses of radiation or toxic chemicals has also been implicated in causing miscarriage.

Recurrent pregnancy loss can be psychologically devastating. From the moment of conception, you begin to prepare yourself mentally and emotionally for pregnancy and childbirth. Failure of the pregnancy can bring grief, guilt, and anger. Feelings of hopelessness and loss may persist long after the miscarriage, only to be compounded when another miscarriage occurs. Only 50–60 percent of affected couples ever discover the cause for their recurrent loss. Anger at the medical community for not solving this problem is an understandable reaction. If you are having difficulty coping, contact a support group or psychologist. You may also find the book *A Silent Sorrow: Pregnancy Loss* by Ingrid Kohn valuable in dealing with these difficult emotions. Finally, take heart in the fact that 75 percent of women with recurrent loss that has no identifiable cause will ultimately have a successful pregnancy with no treatment necessary.

For additional help in obtaining support, visit:

www.resolve.org

www.nationalshare.org

What is a tubal pregnancy?

Fertilization of the egg occurs in the fallopian tube. The fertilized egg divides several times, forming a ball of cells called the embryo. Usually the embryo becomes implanted in the uterus. However, if the fertilized egg cannot reach the uterus, it implants itself in the wall of the tube and begins to grow. (See the illustration below.) This is referred to as a tubal pregnancy. It is the most common form of ectopic pregnancy, meaning one that is not located in the uterus. Other rare forms of ectopic pregnancy include ovarian pregnancy (implanted on the surface of the ovary) and abdominal pregnancy (implanted elsewhere in the abdomen). Tubal pregnancies occur in approximately one out of every fifty pregnancies.

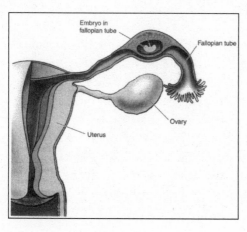

Conditions that may obstruct the fallopian tube increase the risk of developing a tubal pregnancy. Pelvic inflammatory disease, endometriosis, and pelvic surgery can produce scar tissue, which then interferes with passage of the fertilized egg to the uterus. A history of infertility or prior tubal pregnancies heightens the risk of this as well. In many cases, the cause of the tubal pregnancy cannot be identified. Sometimes this indicates a congenital defect in the structure or function of the tube.

Tubal pregnancies are very dangerous. Because the fallopian tube is narrow and cannot expand, the pregnancy eventually bursts through the wall of the tube, resulting in heavy internal bleeding. If left untreated, this condition ultimately results in shock, followed by death. Fortunately, symptoms such as pain or abnormal vaginal bleeding raise suspicion and allow the doctor to intervene. Other symptoms include shoulder pain (caused by blood gathering under the diaphragm) and dizziness or faintness caused by blood loss. Tubal pregnancies are never successful. Once this problem is diagnosed, treatment to minimize complications should begin.

Angela's Story

Angela misses her period and has a positive pregnancy test. She makes a doctor's appointment, unaware of any problems. A few weeks later she starts to feel a "pulling" pain on her left side. She calls her doctors, who reassure her that this is not uncommon and that she can expect that type of pain as the uterus starts to grow. A few days later, the pain seems to intensify and she starts to bleed a little. Worried that she might be having a miscarriage, Angela calls the office. Dr. Thompson, the on-call gynecologist, tells her to go to the emergency room for further testing.

As she waits in the emergency room, the pain worsens and she starts to feel faint. Dr. Patel, the emergency room physician, examines Angela and orders a blood pregnancy test and pelvic ultrasound. The blood pregnancy test returns at a level where one would expect to see a pregnancy inside the uterus on her ultrasound, but no such pregnancy is found. Instead, there is a bulge in the area of her left tube and free fluid in the pelvis, suggesting a ruptured tubal pregnancy. While Dr. Thompson is notified, arrangements are made for emergency surgery.

Dr. Thompson informs Angela and her husband Louis of the findings on ultrasound and the need for surgery. At this point Angela speaks up, saying, "Dr. Billings is my gynecologist. He told me that he would be available whenever there was a problem. I won't undergo surgery with anyone else." Somewhat taken aback, Dr. Thompson reiterates the need for immediate surgery given the fact that Angela is losing blood. Angela is about to object when she loses consciousness and starts seizing from excessive blood loss. Dr. Thompson gives Louis a stern look and he instantly agrees to surgery. With surgery and blood replacement, Angela survives.

If you are pregnant and develop pain or bleeding, ask your gynecologist for a pelvic ultrasound! It is better to be cautious and not take the chance of missing a tubal pregnancy.

I am pregnant and have pain. Do I have a tubal pregnancy?

Have we scared you out of your wits? Thanks to us, every time you get a pain early in pregnancy, you'll be convinced that you have a tubal pregnancy. Actually, many common sources of pain characterize early pregnancy, and most of them are not serious. As the uterus begins to grow, it may cause crampy pain or discomfort. The stretching of the ligaments, the structures that attach the uterus to the pelvic walls, also causes discomfort. Usually these types of pain are transient. Cramping and bleeding that occur together are far more likely to represent a threat of a miscarriage than a tubal pregnancy. Pain confined to one side raises more concern. Even then, it may not signify a tubal pregnancy. It is fairly common to develop an ovarian cyst early in pregnancy that can cause pain. This cyst derives from the corpus luteum, a normal follicular structure in the ovary. It will resolve spontaneously and requires no treatment.

If you have pelvic pain or bleeding early in pregnancy, don't panic. Call your doctor and ask to be evaluated. If the doctor is concerned after reviewing your history and performing an exam, he or she will obtain an ultrasound scan and check the level of serum B-HCG, the hormone produced by the placenta (see page 156). If the pregnancy is located inside the uterus and no tubal abnormalities are found, no further evaluation is necessary. If the pregnancy cannot be seen in the uterus and the B-HCG level indicates that it should be visible, an ectopic pregnancy must be suspected. If your history includes heavy bleeding or passage of tissue, miscarriage is more likely than an ectopic pregnancy. Sometimes an ultrasound clearly shows that the pregnancy is located in the tube. If the doctor is uncertain about the status of your pregnancy, you'll be scheduled for laparoscopy. By inserting this telescopic instrument through an incision near your navel, the doctor can look at the tubes to confirm the tubal pregnancy and then either remove the tube (salpingectomy) or remove the pregnancy from the tube (salpingostomy).

Is surgery always necessary to treat a tubal pregnancy?

In the past, most tubal pregnancies were treated surgically. If the tube has ruptured, surgery is required to stop the bleeding. Copious amounts of free blood may be seen on your ultrasound scan or blood loss may be detected through a low blood count, low blood pressure, or high pulse rate. These are all signs of an unstable patient who requires surgery. If your doctor is not certain that you have a tubal pregnancy, laparoscopic surgery may be performed to confirm it.

Ultrasound, used in conjunction with serial B-HCG measurements, can often diagnose an early tubal pregnancy prior to its rupture. In this scenario, the tubal pregnancy will be treated with a medication called methotrexate, which arrests the pregnancy development and allows the body to absorb the tissue. Methotrexate cannot be used to treat women who have significant liver, kidney, or peptic ulcer disease.

It should only be used in women who are willing to be closely monitored. Sometimes a second dose of methotrexate is required for resolution of the tubal pregnancy. Occasionally, the tubal pregnancy will rupture despite the methotrexate. Therefore, women must follow up with the doctor if their pain worsens or they become faint.

Can I get pregnant again after a tubal pregnancy?

Because you have two tubes and ovaries, your chances of achieving a subsequent pregnancy are good. There is approximately a 50 percent chance that you will have an intrauterine pregnancy. If you conceive, there is a 10–20 percent chance that you will experience another tubal pregnancy. Therefore, your doctor will want to monitor you carefully.

After two tubal pregnancies, your odds of future success diminish significantly. Only 30 percent of such women will conceive, and the odds of having another tubal pregnancy are high. In vitro fertilization (see chapter 6) should be considered in this situation.

8

ENDOMETRIOSIS:
THE GREAT MASQUERADER

I was told I have endometriosis. What is that?

At first Joan wasn't too concerned when her menstrual cramps worsened. After all, she always had cramps with her periods. Aleve or Advil would take away her discomfort and the cramping never really interfered with her everyday life. Now, however, it seems different. The cramps have worsened over the last year or two and now start even before her period. The cramps last longer and are more disruptive. Sometimes the Advil helps, but other times she is sidelined with pain. Over spring break, she sees her gynecologist, Dr. Seaver.

Dr. Seaver enters the exam room. "Hi Joan, how's it going? Your mother tells me that you're doing well at Penn State. What brings you in today?"

"I don't know," Joan begins. "It might be nothing, but my period cramps seem to be starting earlier and are more severe than they ever were before."

"Well, it may be nothing, but we'll look into it and see what we can do to help you," responds Dr. Seaver. He proceeds to examine Joan. Her exam appears to be normal. He obtains a sample from her cervix to rule out uterine infection, and orders a pelvic ultrasound. The tests come back normal and Dr. Seaver gives Joan a call. "Joan, it's Dr. Seaver. Your scan and tests for infection were all negative. There probably isn't anything serious going on, but given the fact that you are sexually active, we will start birth control pills, which tend to make your periods lighter and less crampy. You can still take Advil or Aleve as necessary. Also, make sure you

continue to use condoms. Remember, the birth control pill does not protect you against STIs."

Several months later Joan returns to Dr. Seaver's office. "Dr. Seaver, my cramps haven't decreased with the birth control pill. They're as bad as ever. What can we do about this?"

Dr. Seaver responds, "I'm afraid that you might have endometriosis. If I remember correctly, your mother was also treated for that condition, and it tends to run in families."

Endometriosis is the bane of every gynecologist's existence. You've heard the expression *a thorn in your side*. Well, this is more like a spear. Okay, maybe we're getting overly dramatic. Nevertheless, it can be an extremely difficult problem for patients and their doctors.

Inside the uterus is a glandular lining referred to as the endometrium. When this tissue is located outside of the uterus, the condition is referred to as endometriosis. There are a number of theories explaining how it gets outside. The most common hypothesis is that pieces of endometrial tissue flow back out of the fallopian tubes during the menstrual flow and become implanted on the surfaces of the other organs in the pelvis, such as the uterus, ovaries, bladder, and bowel. (See the illustration below.) Each month during the menstrual flow, the endometrial implants bleed, causing inflammation and pain. Ultimately, scar tissue forms in affected areas. Blood from ovarian endometriosis may accumulate inside the ovary, producing a benign (noncancerous) cystic growth of the ovary, referred to as an endometrioma.

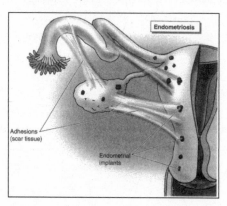

If I have painful periods, does it mean that I have endometriosis?

A common misimpression is that everyone with painful periods has endometriosis. Many women with painful periods, or dysmenorrhea, have no definable disease (see chapter 1). Conversely, there may be no symptoms and a woman may have severe and extensive endometriosis. Pain may be recent in origin and progressively worsening, while some women go undiagnosed despite having severe pain from the onset of their first menstrual cycle. Pain from endometriosis typically starts a day or two before the menstrual flow begins, but may start after bleeding begins or simply cause pain mid-cycle with ovulation. The probability of having endometriosis increases if there is a family history of the disorder.

What other symptoms characterize endometriosis?

Endometriosis can produce a multitude of different symptoms, depending on its location. That is why we call it the *"great masquerader."* Painful periods are the most common symptom. However, it can also cause chronic pelvic pain that is not related to the menstrual cycle. Disturbances of menstruation may also occur, and infertility is often seen in conjunction with endometriosis. Painful intercourse, occurring with deep penetration, is another fairly common symptom. Endometriosis associated with the bowel can result in painful defecation, changes in bowel function, and rectal bleeding. Urinary frequency, urinary urgency, or blood in the urine may occur if the bladder is involved.

Well, by now you should be convinced that you have endometriosis. The fact that it can produce quite an array of symptoms is problematic. We have encountered many women throughout the years who have read or been told about symptoms of endometriosis and are now convinced that they must have it. In reality, most of them don't. Many of the same symptoms more commonly signal other medical disorders.

How is endometriosis diagnosed and treated?

Joan is taken aback by Dr. Seaver's call. "Endometri . . . what?"

"Endometriosis," Dr. Seaver reiterates. "It is a condition where bits of the inside lining of the uterus are implanted on the outside of your pelvic organs."

"How do you know I have that?" asks Joan.

"Well, I don't know for sure. But your history suggests that you might have the condition. Most women with functional menstrual cramps will improve with birth control pills, but you didn't. The fact that it runs in your family also makes me suspicious. I recommend that we perform a laparoscopy."

"What's a laparoscopy?" Joan asks.

"I will insert a telescope-like instrument into your abdomen under anesthesia. We can see endometriosis through the laparoscope and often treat it at the same time. Some doctors will make the diagnosis just based on history, or findings on an exam, but that isn't really a definitive way to diagnose the condition." Joan isn't thrilled about the prospect of surgery. Hoping for a different solution, she asks, "Aren't there medications that we can use for this?"

"There are numerous approaches to endometriosis," Dr. Seaver begins, "but most of the medications used to treat endometriosis have significant side effects. It is my preference to first make sure that we're dealing with endometriosis through laparoscopy." He then proceeds to educate her on the many approaches to endometriosis. Some involve medications, usually of a hormonal nature, that reduce the endometrial implants. Surgical techniques are used to remove the abnormal tissue and adhesions.

Surgery Since endometriosis is usually diagnosed via laparoscopy, surgery is often done at the time of diagnosis, using laparoscopic techniques. A telescopic instrument is placed through a tiny incision near the navel. Other small incisions are made through which instruments are inserted to perform the surgery. Endometrial implants are destroyed or resected and scar tissue is removed.

Laparoscopic surgery is not always appropriate. If there is deep involvement of the bowel, ureters, or bladder, your doctor may feel that it is safer to operate through a larger incision (laparotomy). This may be more appropriate if pelvic adhesions are extensive.

Often surgical and drug treatments are combined. The most common approach is laparoscopic surgery followed by treatment with a medication called a GnRH agonist.

GnRH Agonists Because this group of medications has relatively few side effects, they are generally used as the first line of nonsurgical treatment for endometriosis. By placing a woman in a pseudomenopausal state (a state that mimics menopause), GnRH agonists turn off the signals that stimulate ovarian hormone production. Menstruation ceases, and the endometrial implants regress.

GnRH agonists are available in the form of injections (Lupron), implants placed under the skin (Zoladex), or as a nasal spray (Synarel). They are effective but also very expensive, which limits their use for individuals without prescription plan coverage. Common side effects include hot flashes, sweats, vaginal dryness, mood change, and headaches. More recently, low doses of hormones have been added back during treatment which has reduced the most disabling side effects (hot flashes and night sweats). Treatment is continued for six to nine months. Over this time, there may be a small decrease in bone density related to the low estrogen levels. This problem seems to disappear when the treatment is finished.

Danazol A steroid closely related to androgens ("male hormones"), danazol (Danocrine) decreases estrogen and progesterone production, thereby eliminating the hormonal stimulation causing the growth of the endometrial implants. In addition to stopping menstruation, the drug has many side effects, including weight gain, decreased breast size, acne, oily skin, deepening of the voice, and increased facial hair. Other side effects include hot flashes, night sweats, and vaginal dryness.

After hearing this, you probably wonder who in their right mind would use danazol. Although most women will experience at least some of these side effects, only about 10 percent find them sufficiently disturbing to discontinue the medication. The usual length of treatment is six months.

Oral Contraceptives The birth control pills have been used to treat endometriosis for decades, although they are less effective than GnRH agonists or danazol. Endometrial implants are less active during use of birth control pills, particularly when the pills are taken continuously without a break for menstruation.

Progesterone Progesterone alone, without estrogen, can also be used to treat endometriosis. The most common progesterone used for this purpose has been medroxyprogesterone (Provera), administered either orally or injected in the form of Depo-Provera. Like continuous birth control pills, progesterone stops menstruation and renders the endometrial implants inactive. Overall, progesterone use has fewer side effects than taking combination birth control pills, although erratic bleeding is more common. Weight gain and mood change are also somewhat more likely to occur with Provera than with birth control pills. Because it delays ovulation, Depo-Provera is not recommended for women who have fertility problems. Other progestins have also been used for the treatment of endometriosis including "natural" progesterone (Prometrium). Prometrium is not as potent as the synthetic progestins, so when it is used to treat endometriosis, it must be used in doses that are higher than those used in hormone replacement therapy. Natural progesterone creams are not absorbed into the bloodstream in sufficient quantities to impact endometriosis. Mirena, a progesterone-releasing IUD, has also shown efficacy in the treatment of endometriosis.

Aromatase Inhibitors Aromatase inhibitors (AIs), drugs more commonly used to decrease estrogen production in breast cancer patients, have been used in refractory cases of endometriosis and have been shown to provide relief in 90 percent of patients. Unfortunately, the pain usually returns immediately after cessation of therapy. AIs also increase ovarian cyst production in premenopausal women. Combining an oral contraceptive or progestin with AI treatment can reduce the likelihood of cyst formation.

Mefipristone (RU-486) Mefipristone is an anti-progestin agent more commonly used in pregnancy termination. However, it has been shown to reduce pelvic pain in patients with endometriosis by inhibiting ovulation and disrupting endometrial integrity (considered experimental at this time).

Pentoxifylline Pentoxifylline is another experimental drug that theoretically might provide benefit to endometriosis patients. It decreases the production of inflammatory factors called cytokines and inhibits the activation of immune cells. Therefore it would seem to have the potential for decreasing pain from endometriosis and improving fertility. Randomized trials have shown a trend toward improving pregnancy rates and a trend toward decreasing pain scores, but the results do not achieve statistical significance. More studies are needed to address immune-modulators such as Pentoxifylline before they can be recommended in the treatment of endometriosis.

Complementary and Alternative (CAM) Approaches One theory of endometriosis proposes that it is an autoimmune condition. If the immune system is compromised with food intolerance, then theoretically removing that food can have an effect on the disease. Various dietary recommendations have been made including the elimination of wheat (gluten), sugar, meat, and dairy. In this theory, decreasing foods that are high in hormones and inflammatory fats, such as red meat, while increasing fruits and vegetables would be helpful. However, there are no scientific studies to support this approach. In one case-controlled study, diets high in fat and low in fruit were actually associated with a lower risk of endometriosis, contradicting the common sense approach mentioned above. Supplementation with Omega-3 fatty acids and anti-oxidant vitamins such as A, C, and E has also been recommended. At least two reasonable studies suggest that Chinese herbal medicine can be effective at reducing the pain from endometriosis. In one study it was found to work more effectively than danazol (see above) and in another it was as effective as gestrinone, an anti-progestin used outside of the United States to treat endometriosis. Chinese herbal medicine is often combined with acupuncture in the treatment of endometriosis.

Vaginal childbirth appears to decrease the recurrence of endometriosis compared with women who have not given birth or women who have delivered by cesarean section.

After hearing the options, Joan agrees with Dr. Seaver that laparoscopy is necessary. During the laparoscopy, Dr. Seaver sees multiple endometrial implants, but little in the way of adhesions. He uses a laser to vaporize the visible endometrial implants at the time of laparoscopy. After the surgery, he gives Joan Depo-Provera injections every three months for continuous suppression of further endometriosis and contraception. With regular administration of the Depo-Provera, Joan no longer has menstrual periods and remains pain-free.

If I have endometriosis, does that mean I can't get pregnant?

After graduation, Joan marries her college sweetheart, Bubba. (I know. Really? But it's better than his real name, Bartholomew. What were his parents thinking?) Joan wants to start a family right away, so she stops her Depo-Provera. After approximately four to five months her menstrual cycle resumes, but one year later she is still not pregnant. She begins to wonder if this is related to the endometriosis.

There is an increased chance of infertility with endometriosis. Adhesions formed from endometriosis may obstruct the fallopian tube or encase the ovaries, thereby preventing the egg from reaching the tube. Tubal scarring can hinder the egg's movement down the tube, preventing it from reaching the uterus. Even when no adhesions are present, infertility may occur. The mechanism that causes infertility when no adhesions exist is not clearly understood. In some women with mild endometriosis, the levels of certain chemicals called cytokines (released in response to inflammation) are increased in the abdominal cavity, and these hormone-like proteins may have a negative effect on reproductive processes.

You can find solace in knowing that most women with endometriosis and infertility will succeed in conceiving after treatment. The method of treatment depends on the severity of endometriosis. The American Society for Reproductive Medicine has developed a classification system based on the extent of the problem, the size of the endometrial implants, and the severity of adhesions. Approximately 75 percent of patients with mild endometriosis and 60 percent of those with moderate disease conceive after treatment. Patients with severe disease have a significantly lower pregnancy rate. If all else fails, in vitro fertilization may still provide an opportunity for a successful pregnancy (see chapter 6).

Dr. Seaver reassures Joan, reminding her that it may take a year or two for women to get pregnant even if they do not have a problem such as endometriosis. If she were in her mid-thirties, he might refer her to an infertility specialist, but she is only twenty-five, so he encourages her to be patient. Six months later she is pregnant with Bubba Jr.

Will endometriosis come back?

Unfortunately, endometriosis often reappears, even after treatment. This is extremely disconcerting after you have undergone extensive treatment to eradicate it. Symptoms may recur within months of treatment or a number of years later. Persistence is the name of the game. If one method of treatment is unsuccessful, another should be tried. You might consider consulting an infertility specialist if the endometriosis recurs, since he or she will usually have greater expertise in dealing with this disorder. If you suspect that you have endometriosis, your best bet is to start your family sooner rather than later. If infertility has been a problem, the best window of opportunity for successful conception immediately follows treatment. Chronic pelvic pain is often associated with recurrent disease, and working with a physician who specializes in pain control can be beneficial if one is available in your area.

Dealing with a recurrent or chronic disease is demoralizing. Seek emotional support through psychological consultation or support groups. Contact the national headquarters of the Endometriosis Association to find a support group in your area at www.endometriosisassn.org.

My doctor said I'll eventually need a hysterectomy because of my endometriosis. Is that necessary?

If your primary problem is pelvic pain and childbearing is not an issue, the doctor may recommend removal of the uterus, fallopian tubes, and ovaries. Obviously, this is a very aggressive step. It is based on the rationale that endometriosis is least likely to recur if the reproductive organs are removed. Other options include conservative surgery or drug treatment. However, if you have severe symptoms that have not responded well to conservative treatment, this more aggressive approach may be appropriate.

What happens to my endometriosis after menopause?

Yeah! We finally get to say something reassuring about this disorder. Endometriosis regresses with menopause. Menopause occurs when the ovaries stop producing estrogen. Since the endometrial implants depend on estrogen, the condition improves after menopause. However, adhesions produced by the disease will not disappear. Severe pain from the scar tissue requires surgery. If the adhesions are particularly extensive, removal of the uterus, fallopian tubes, and ovaries is a reasonable solution to the problem.

As you enter menopause, keep in mind that hormone replacement therapy must be undertaken carefully if you have a history of endometriosis. Progesterone must be given to counteract the estrogen. Cyclical regimens (those that create periodic menstrual flow) should be avoided.

For more help with endometriosis, visit the Endometriosis Association at www.endometriosisassn.org.

9

DISORDERS OF THE UTERUS

What are fibroids?

Fibroids of the uterus are very common. They occur in up to 40 percent of black women and 20 percent of white women. So what is a fibroid? It's a tumor composed of smooth muscle that originates in the wall of the uterus. (See the illustration on page 177.) Fibroids vary considerably in size. They may be indiscernibly tiny or larger than a grapefruit. They can remain small throughout adulthood or grow rather quickly over a few months. Because of this variation, a gynecologist may want to examine a woman more frequently if fibroids are present—at least every six months—even if the fibroids are not causing problems.

Doctors really don't know what causes fibroids to develop. We do know that their growth accelerates in the presence of estrogen. Conditions associated with high estrogen levels, such as pregnancy, increase the growth of fibroids. Conditions with decreased estrogen levels, such as menopause, decrease their growth. There is a genetic

> ### A Funny Tidbit
>
> *Dr. Thornton was taking a history from Viola, a forty-three-year-old woman. He asked her whether she had any past gynecologic problems. Viola answered, "I used to have problems with fireballs in my Eucharist." It took Dr. Thornton a moment, but he quickly surmised that Viola really meant "fibroids in my uterus."*

predisposition for fibroids. If your mother or sisters have fibroids, your chance of developing them is increased.

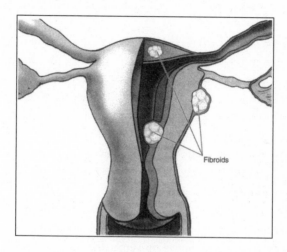

Will my fibroids turn into cancer?

When you hear the word *tumor*, thoughts of cancer jump into your mind. Stop worrying! Fibroids are benign tumors. They can transform into a rare type of cancer called a sarcoma, but the incidence of this is very low—less than 1 percent. Thus fibroids should not be removed simply because of a concern that they could become malignant (cancerous).

What problems do fibroids cause?

Actually, most fibroids never cause problems. However, numerous difficulties may be encountered. As Elizabeth Barrett Browning said, "Let me count the ways."

1. *Prolonged or heavy bleeding*: Fibroids growing into the cavity of the uterus characteristically cause heavy and prolonged periods. Occasionally, they cause bleeding between periods. The abnormal bleeding can cause anemia.

2. *Pain*: Depending on their size and position, fibroids can cause pain or pressure in the lower abdomen or back. They may also trigger pain during intercourse, particularly with deep penetration.

3. *Difficulties with urination*: Large fibroids may cause frequency and urgency of urination if they put pressure on the bladder. Occasionally, fibroids grow in a way that obstructs the urethra, thereby creating difficulty with emptying your bladder. Very large fibroids can obstruct the ureters (the tubes carrying urine from the kidneys to the bladder). The obstruction usually causes no symptoms but nevertheless is important to address, since over time it can cause damage to the kidneys.

4. *Difficulties with bowel movements*: Pressure on the rectum can cause rectal spasms, pain with bowel movements, or difficulty with completing bowel movements.

5. *Problems with pregnancy*: Most often fibroids do not interfere with pregnancy. However, they may cause infertility or repeated miscarriages. Because of increased hormone levels during pregnancy, they tend to increase substantially in size. In doing so, a fibroid may outgrow its blood supply and degenerate, causing pain. Medication can relieve it.

When do fibroids need treatment?

Just because you have fibroids doesn't mean you have to do anything about them. Fibroids may never cause you problems. They may grow slowly or not at all. Examinations performed at six-month intervals are sufficient. However, if you are having any of the problems mentioned in the previous list, further evaluation and treatment may be necessary. If you have heavy bleeding during your period, you should see a doctor. If the bleeding is heavy enough to cause anemia, you should also consider a more aggressive approach. Remember that pelvic pain, urinary difficulties, and problems with defecation are often incorrectly attributed to fibroids and may be caused by other conditions. If you have one or more of these problems, obtain a thorough evaluation before pursuing treatment of the fibroids.

Treating fibroids prior to conception is not usually recommended. Most pregnancies progress uneventfully despite their presence. The unlikely chance that you *may* have a problem with them does not justify aggressive treatment of the fibroids. However, if you experience recurrent problems that your doctor attributes to the fibroids, treatment may be indicated.

Historically, physicians automatically removed large fibroids (greater than the size of a grapefruit), even if asymptomatic. At that size, there is a greater risk that a fibroid will obstruct the ureters. It is also unlikely that your doctor will be able to check your ovaries successfully during an examination if you have very large fibroids. This attitude began to change with the advent of pelvic ultrasound scans which can be used to monitor the status of your ovaries and ureters. Doctors were more willing to observe fibroids with periodic ultrasound without intervening. With the advent of laparoscopic myomectomy (removing fibroids from the uterus and repairing the uterus through tiny incisions under telescopic visualization), attitudes have once again changed. If you have a rapidly growing fibroid(s) and are not close to menopause (when the fibroid is likely to stop growing), it is reasonable for your gynecologist to remove the fibroid(s) through this minimally invasive surgical procedure.

Sometimes it is assumed that a rapidly growing fibroid needs aggressive treatment because it may be developing into a type of cancer called a sarcoma. However, even rapidly growing fibroids are not typically cancerous. There is concern if fibroids grow rapidly in menopause. Fibroids usually shrink during that time. Rapidly growing fibroids after menopause indicates the need for a hysterectomy.

If you and your doctor conclude that treatment of your fibroids is indicated, you must review the range of options available. They are discussed under the next two questions.

Can fibroids be treated with medications?

There are medications that can lessen some of the adverse effects related to fibroids. Oral contraceptives, oral progestins, the progesterone-releasing IUD Mirena, and tranexamic acid (Lysteda) have all been used to decrease excess bleeding associated with fibroids. Nonsteroidal anti-inflammatory drugs (NSAIDs) like naproxen sodium (Aleve), ibuprofen (Advil, Motrin), and acetaminophen (Tylenol) can be used to reduce pain or discomfort associated with fibroids.

The most common drugs used to treat fibroids are GnRH agonists (see chapter 8). These medications shut off your ovarian hormone production creating a state of false menopause. By reducing hormone levels, they make fibroids shrink, often by as much as 50 percent. That's the good news. The bad news is that the fibroids will resume their previous size when the medication is discontinued. Maximum shrinkage occurs within three months of treatment. GnRH agonists (Lupron, Synarel) are often used before surgery to reduce the size of fibroids, thereby making the surgical procedure easier. You may ask, "Why can't I just stay on this medication?" Unfortunately, prolonged use of GnRH agonists produces a decrease in bone density. You would also develop symptoms similar to those of menopause: hot flashes, night sweats, and vaginal dryness. Doctors will often add back small amounts of hormones to diminish the bone loss and alleviate the menopausal symptoms. While this has achieved some success, the long-term treatment of fibroids with GnRH agonists is impractical for all but those who are close to natural menopause, when the fibroids will shrink spontaneously. In addition, GnRH agonists are expensive, which limits prolonged therapy.

There are several other drugs that have been shown to both shrink fibroids and reduce bleeding from fibroids. Mifepristone (also known as RU-486) is an anti-progestin drug that is more commonly used in high doses for pregnancy termination. At very low doses, it has been shown to be very effective in treating fibroids. Ulipristol, a drug used in higher doses for emergency contraception (Ella), is a drug that modulates progesterone receptors and has also been shown to reduce fibroid size and bleeding. Finally, aromatase inhibitors such as anastrozole (Arimidex), drugs more commonly used in the treatment and prevention of breast cancer, have also been shown to effectively treat fibroids. None of these drugs are currently approved for the treatment of fibroids, but they may be available in research studies. It is anticipated that eventually one or more of these medications will be approved for the treatment of fibroids once we have a better idea of the long-term ramifications of using them in this way.

What type of surgery is used to remove fibroids?

If you and your doctor determine that surgery is necessary, fibroids can be treated through a variety of techniques. Each is described here, together with a discussion of each one's potential advantages and disadvantages.

Abdominal or Vaginal Hysterectomy In the past, hysterectomy (removal of the uterus) was the most common treatment for fibroids. Hysterectomy is only an option if you no longer wish to bear children, as it is the most aggressive approach to fibroids. During an abdominal hysterectomy, a uterus with large fibroids is removed through an incision made through the abdomen. During a vaginal hysterectomy, a uterus with smaller fibroids is removed without the necessity of an abdominal incision. If the hysterectomy can be safely performed vaginally, recovery will be quicker.

Advantages

- Hysterectomy is the most thorough way of removing fibroids. More conservative methods of treatment involve the chance that more fibroids will develop and cause problems in the future, possibly requiring additional surgery.
- Removing the uterus prevents the development of other uterine problems, including endometrial and cervical cancer.

- It is easier to provide hormone replacement therapy (discussed in chapter 13) in menopause without the uterus in place. If you have had a hysterectomy, you can take estrogen alone for hormone replacement. Many of the potential risks, such as breast cancer, associated with hormone replacement therapy are significantly reduced if you do not have to add progesterone to the hormone regimen.

Disadvantages

- Hysterectomy is a major operation. Although most hysterectomies proceed without complication, chances of experiencing a complication are greater than they would be with less invasive surgical procedures.
- Compared with laparoscopic and hysteroscopic procedures, length of stay in the hospital will be greater. The recovery period after hospitalization will also be substantially longer.

Abdominal Myomectomy An incision is made through the abdominal wall. An incision is then made into the wall of the uterus and the fibroid(s) is removed. The defect in the wall of the uterus is then repaired. As with a laparoscopic myomectomy (see below), the uterus remains in place, thereby maintaining the potential for future pregnancies. However, delivery by cesarean section may be necessary after a myomectomy.

Advantages

- The primary advantage of myomectomy is preservation of the uterus and the ability to have children.
- For some women, removal of the uterus is emotionally traumatic, and this procedure keeps it in place.
- Although it is debatable, leaving the uterus in place may help maintain pelvic support and sexual responsiveness.

- Surgery through a larger open incision is easier for the surgeon and requires less expertise than laparoscopic myomectomy. Depending on the size, location, and number of fibroids, surgery through an open incision can be faster and safer.

Disadvantages

- If the myomectomy is performed through a large incision on the abdomen, hospitalization and recovery will be prolonged.
- The time required for this surgery and the blood loss associated with it may exceed those of hysterectomy.
- Adhesions may form along the incisions made in the wall of the uterus, thereby causing infertility or pelvic pain.
- Preservation of the uterus means that other fibroids may develop in the future. If they do, the risk of requiring future surgery is 20–40 percent. Future fibroids may also increase the chances of bleeding abnormally when taking hormone replacement during menopause.

Laparoscopic Techniques Depending on the size, number, and location of the fibroids and expertise of the doctor, many fibroids can be treated through laparoscopic surgery. Only tiny incisions are made on the abdomen, and the doctor views the surgery through a telescopic instrument hooked up to a monitor. Single-incision laparoscopy and robotic surgery are additional variations of this type of surgery. The laparoscopic technique chosen depends on your doctor's familiarity and comfort level with the available equipment. Sometimes GnRH agonists are used prior to surgery to reduce the size of your fibroids. Myolysis is a procedure performed during laparoscopy in which the fibroids are either treated with electrical energy through needles or frozen with probes. Often this will help shrink fibroids and prevent them from growing in the future. As laparoscopic instruments have improved, many doctors now are comfortable with performing myomectomy and hysterectomy procedures laparoscopically.

Advantage

- Laparoscopy requires a much shorter hospitalization and recovery than surgery performed through larger abdominal incisions. Laparoscopy is often performed as outpatient surgery.

Disadvantages

- Advanced laparoscopic surgery requires special skills and equipment that are not universally available.
- Laparoscopic myolysis appears to control the fibroid, but it is still present and therefore has potential to cause problems down the road.

Hysteroscopic Techniques In hysteroscopy, the gynecologist introduces a telescopic instrument through the cervix into the uterine cavity. If most of the fibroid is located within the cavity, it can be removed through this procedure. If most of the fibroid is not located within the cavity, bleeding issues can still be controlled by performing an endometrial ablation, a procedure that destroys the inside lining of the uterus. There are a variety of different techniques used for endometrial ablation, but they all are 80–90 percent effective at controlling heavy bleeding. More recently, some doctors have used cryomyolysis (freezing the fibroid with a probe) through the hysteroscope.

Advantage

- Hysteroscopy can be performed at an outpatient facility, and the patient recuperates quickly (there are no incisions or sutures).

Disadvantages

- Hysteroscopy requires advanced skills and equipment.
- It can only remove fibroids that project well into the cavity of the uterus.
- If the entire fibroid cannot be removed through this procedure, there is an increased chance of having future problems.
- Large fibroids (greater than 3 to 5 cm) often cannot be removed through hysteroscopic techniques without increasing risks from the procedure.

Are there any other nonsurgical treatments for fibroids?

Uterine artery embolization is a procedure in which an interventional radiologist threads a catheter into the uterine artery. He or she then injects particles to block the blood flow to the fibroid, which causes the fibroid to shrink. This procedure allows patients to avoid the risks associated with surgery. Complications are unusual and include bruising or bleeding from the entry site of the catheter, allergic reaction to dye used during the procedure, and uterine infection. Postprocedure pain and fever can usually be treated with acetaminophen (Tylenol) or NSAIDs (Advil, Motrin, Aleve). More severe pain can be treated with narcotics. Most women do well and can return to normal activities within seven to ten days. Not all patients are candidates for this procedure. The radiologist will have you obtain a pelvic MRI before the procedure to assess the size, number, and location of your fibroids. He or she will then determine if you are a candidate for the procedure.

MRI-guided focused ultrasound is a newcomer in the treatment of fibroids. During this procedure, a high-intensity ultrasound beam is used to heat and destroy the fibroid. Since this is a newer development in the treatment of fibroids, it may not be available in your geographical location. There isn't much known about the long-term impact of using this technique.

Individualizing Treatment

Let us look at three different women to demonstrate the impact of age on the treatment of fibroids. In each case, the patient has multiple fibroids causing heavy menstrual periods and symptoms of fullness in the pelvic region.

Kathy is a twenty-nine-year-old woman who would like to have children in the future. Obviously, hysterectomy is not an option. The medications listed above can be used to alleviate her symptoms until she is ready to conceive (preferably sooner rather than later). If more definitive treatment is necessary, Kathy would be a good candidate for either laparoscopic or hysteroscopic myomectomy. At this time, it is not recommended that women undergo uterine artery embolization or MRI-focused ultrasound treatment if they plan on having future pregnancies.

Isabelle is a forty-one-year-old woman who has completed childbearing. Since Isabelle no longer wants children, hysterectomy is a reasonable option. Often a hysterectomy is easier to perform and less risky than undergoing multiple myomectomies, especially if the hysterectomy can be performed laparoscopically or vaginally. Uterine artery embolization and MRI-focused ultrasound are two additional reasonable options. Medical management can be considered, but these options are usually only a temporary solution and Isabelle is probably ten years away from menopause.

Martha is a fifty-two-year-old woman, a perfect candidate for medical management since menopause should be right around the corner. The medical management can be discontinued after menopause. In all likelihood, the fibroids will shrink after menopause and cease to be a problem.

Can fibroids grow back?

If a total hysterectomy is performed (entire uterus removed), you will not redevelop fibroids. If your uterus remains, there is a possibility that additional fibroids will appear. The chance of this recurrence may be as high as 40 percent. The further you are from menopause (the younger you are), the more likely this will happen. However, remember that most fibroids do not cause problems. Most women who redevelop fibroids will not require treatment.

If a particular fibroid is completely removed, as during a myomectomy, that fibroid cannot reappear, but others may develop. If only a part of the fibroid is removed, there may be regrowth of the remaining portion. Fibroids that shrink during GnRH agonist treatment will return to their pretreatment size when therapy is discontinued.

Where do polyps come from?

Uterine polyps originate from the surface lining of the uterine cavity and cervical canal. Cervical polyps can often be detected on routine examination. They tend to be small and can usually be removed in the office. Endometrial polyps are usually hidden from view inside the uterus. Often they will cause abnormal bleeding that leads to their detection.

Can polyps turn into cancer?

Most endometrial and cervical polyps are benign. However, cancer can develop within polyps. All polyps that are removed should be sent to a pathologist, who will examine them under a microscope to rule out the presence of cancer.

How are polyps removed?

Small cervical polyps are generally removed in the office. Your doctor may administer a local anesthetic to the cervix, although most of the time this is not necessary. The polyp is attached to the cervix by a stalk. Your doctor snips the stalk with a biopsy instrument or scissors, thereby removing the polyp. You may feel a pinch when this is done, but significant pain from the procedure is uncommon.

Endometrial polyps aren't quite as easy to approach because they are located inside the uterus where they cannot be seen during examination. Most are discovered during surgery performed to determine the cause of abnormal bleeding. Any of the following conditions constitutes abnormal bleeding:

- Prolonged bleeding (duration of greater than one week)
- Exceptionally heavy bleeding
- Bleeding between periods
- Postmenopausal bleeding

Historically, the standard procedure for evaluating abnormal bleeding was a D&C (dilation and curettage). The doctor performed a D&C by dilating the cervix and placing a scraping instrument into the uterus. A sampling of the endometrium was removed and studied under a microscope. Although this was very good at diagnosing endometrial cancer, it was very mediocre for removing polyps. Even special instruments that were designed to help remove polyps commonly failed to do so.

Today, gynecologists evaluate abnormal bleeding with pelvic ultrasound and hysteroscopy. A pelvic ultrasound can reveal a significant abnormality within the uterus. During hysteroscopy, the doctor inserts a telescopic instrument through the vagina and cervix into the uterine cavity and removes the polyp(s). This procedure is performed as outpatient surgery. Recovery is usually quick. Varying degrees of cramping and bleeding may ensue for a short time after the procedure, but serious complications are uncommon and most women can return to normal activities within a day or two.

My doctor said my heavy bleeding is from adenomyosis. Is that the same as endometriosis?

Patients often confuse adenomyosis and endometriosis. Endometriosis, which is discussed in chapter 8, is a condition in which endometrial tissue is located outside the uterus. Although it may be associated with abnormal bleeding, it does not usually cause heavy periods. In adeno-myosis, endometrial tissue grows into the muscular wall of the uterus (the myometrium). Adenomyosis is not a cancerous condition. It most often becomes apparent in a woman's thirties or forties and manifests itself as heavy or prolonged periods.

How can the gynecologist tell if I have adenomyosis?

It can be difficult to diagnose adenomyosis. Your doctor may suspect the presence of adenomyosis if your uterus feels symmetrically enlarged and boggy; fibroids, in contrast, cause the uterus to feel irregular in shape. Heavy and crampy periods are a defining characteristic of adeno-myosis. No test or procedure reliably diagnoses this condition. Certain radiologic studies (pelvic MRI, ultrasound) or hysteroscopy may suggest that this condition exists. Most often it is diagnosed by excluding other causes of heavy periods. If your periods are not improved through hormonal regulation and no polyps or fibroids have been discovered, you probably have adenomyosis.

How is adenomyosis treated?

Adenomyosis may not require any treatment. If your periods are somewhat heavy but still tolerable, you don't have to do anything. However, you should drink more fluids during your period and take an iron supplement. Over-the-counter medications such as ibuprofen (Advil, Motrin) and naproxen sodium (Aleve) may help relieve cramp-ing. Progressively heavier periods or prolonged periods require fur-ther investigation to rule out polyps, fibroids, and cancer as causes. This may include an endometrial biopsy, D&C, pelvic ultrasound, or hysteroscopy. Hormonal regulation of heavy periods can be attempted, although it is not likely to succeed if you have severe adenomyosis. The progesterone-releasing IUD Mirena has been used with some success. Lysteda (tranexamic acid), a nonhormonal prescription medication can also be used for heavy monthly periods. Lysteda should not be used at the same time as oral contraceptives or in women at risk for the development of blood clots.

The most successful conservative procedure used in the treatment of adenomyosis is hysteroscopic endometrial ablation. A variety of modalities have been used to destroy the endometrium including cautery, laser, freezing, microwave, and scalding. All techniques have their advantages and disadvantages and all are approximately 80–90 percent successful at eliminating or decreasing menstrual bleeding. In many cases, periods are eliminated altogether and in other cases, a woman continues to have periods, but they are lighter. Women who cease menstruation after an ablation are not menopausal. The endometrial ablation does nothing to destroy ovarian function, so it has no direct adverse impact on female hormone production. The 10–15 percent of women who fail to respond to endometrial ablation usually have deeply penetrating adenomyosis. Hysterectomy is a reasonable choice for women with severe adenomyosis that is unresponsive to conservative approaches. Hysterectomy in these cases can often be performed laparoscopically or vaginally. Uterine artery embolization (see above) has also been employed to treat adenomyosis, but with less success than when it is used to treat fibroids.

I'm sixty years old, and now I'm bleeding. Does that mean I have cancer?

Most women realize that it is not normal to have vaginal bleeding during menopause. If you have not bled for years and start to bleed, it is natural to feel anxious. Try to remain calm. Most postmenopausal bleeding does not indicate cancer. Often benign growths such as polyps of the cervix or endometrium will bleed (see page 188). Without estrogen replacement, the lining of the vagina and uterus becomes thin and can bleed. Another cause of bleeding after menopause is endometrial hyperplasia, a condition represented by an excess number and crowding of the glands in the lining of the uterus. Certain types of hyperplasia are considered precancerous. When discovered, hyperplasia can often be reversed by administering progesterone.

It is not unusual for women on hormone replacement therapy to have bleeding (refer to chapter 13). If you are taking hormone replacement, ask your doctor what to expect in terms of vaginal bleeding.

Certainly postmenopausal bleeding should be investigated because it may be a sign of cancer. Other signs of endometrial cancers such as pelvic pain, a mass or swelling in the pelvis or lower abdomen, and weight loss don't usually present until later when the cancer has already advanced.

What is endometrial cancer?

Cancer of the inside lining of the uterine cavity, or endometrium, is referred to as endometrial cancer. The cancer begins inside the uterus and gradually extends into the myometrium, or muscular wall of the uterus. It is also not uncommon for it to extend downward into the cervix. In its more advanced stages, the cancer spreads elsewhere in the pelvis or into the vagina. If the cancer cells spread into the lymphatic drainage of the pelvis or the blood stream, they can invade other parts of the body, particularly the lymph nodes, lungs, liver, and bones. Fortunately, most endometrial cancers cause abnormal bleeding that prompts the doctor to investigate and discover the cancer while it is still early.

Doctors sometimes divide endometrial cancer into two types. Type 1 is more common and generally emerges in women with excess estrogen (see below). Type 1 cancers are usually not very aggressive and spread slowly. Type 2 cancers are more likely to grow outside of the uterus and have a poor outlook. Type 2 cancers include serous carcinomas, clear cell carcinomas, and poorly differentiated (grade 3) carcinomas (cells that look very bizarre and aggressive under the microscope).

Uterine sarcomas are cancers that develop from muscular and other supporting tissues of the uterus (as opposed to the glandular lining).

These are usually aggressive cancers that spread fairly quickly beyond the uterus.

In this chapter, we focus primarily on type 1 endometrial cancer, which accounts for the vast majority of uterine cancers. Type 2 endometrial cancers and uterine sarcomas are generally treated very aggressively because of their poor prognosis.

How did I get endometrial cancer?

Nobody completely understands why women get endometrial cancer. Estrogen stimulates endometrial growth, whereas progesterone decreases it. Conditions that produce excess estrogen, unbalanced by progesterone, increase the risk of getting endometrial cancer. They include the following:

- *Obesity*: Fat cells in the body convert other hormones in the body to estrogen.
- *Women with infrequent periods*: During the months that periods are missed, the ovaries are still producing estrogen. However, no progesterone is produced during those months to oppose the effects of the estrogen on your endometrium.
- *Women who have an early onset of periods (menarche) or a late cessation of periods (menopause)*: The average age of onset is eleven and the average age of cessation is fifty-one.
- *Women with polycystic ovarian disease*: Women who have this condition infrequently ovulate and develop multiple small cysts in their ovaries.

There is sometimes a genetic, or familial, predisposition to endometrial cancer. If you have a close family member who has had endometrial cancer, your risk of developing it is increased. Your risk is also greater if you have had cancer of the breast, ovary, or colon, especially if you have HNPCC (hereditary nonpolyposis colon cancer) syndrome, also known as Lynch syndrome.

Women who use tamoxifen, a hormonal medication used to prevent and treat breast cancer, are also at increased risk for endometrial cancer.

Oral contraceptives, pregnancy, and breast-feeding lower your risk for endometrial cancer. Additional factors that may lower your risk include increased physical activity and a diet that is low in saturated fat and high in fruits and vegetables.

How is endometrial cancer diagnosed?

If you have abnormal bleeding past the age of thirty-five (some doctors use age forty as a cutoff), it must be investigated. Prolonged periods, bleeding between periods, and very erratic bleeding constitute abnormal bleeding prior to menopause. If you are in menopause and have *any* bleeding (presuming you are not on hormone replacement), it is abnormal. Do not wait to see if it will recur. Early detection of cancer is the mainstay of success.

Investigation of the bleeding might include pelvic ultrasound or MRI, endometrial biopsy, D&C, or hysteroscopy (see earlier sections of this chapter). Complications from these procedures are uncommon. If you have abnormal bleeding, the need to obtain more information outweighs the risk of undergoing any of these procedures. The least invasive of the procedures is a pelvic ultrasound, but it does not provide your doctor with a tissue specimen for analysis. An endometrial biopsy can be performed in the office and is an effective tool for diagnosing cancer. A D&C provides a greater amount of tissue than the endometrial biopsy, but is usually performed in the operating room under anesthesia. Hysteroscopy provides the most thorough evaluation of the uterine cavity and enables your doctor to remove other benign causes of abnormal bleeding, such as fibroids and polyps. Hysteroscopy is also usually performed in the operating room under anesthesia, although some gynecologists perform it in the office.

The most important take-home message is that you shouldn't defer investigation of the bleeding. It may not represent cancer. However, if cancer is discovered, early diagnosis greatly increases the likelihood of successful treatment.

Why didn't this show up on my Pap smear?

There are many misconceptions regarding the Pap smear. The most prevalent is that Pap smears screen women for all types of gynecologic cancer. The standard Pap smear is obtained from the cervix and can detect only cervical cancer. Cancer of the endometrium begins inside the uterus and is therefore not usually detected on a Pap smear. Occasionally, malignant cells from inside the uterus drop down the cervical canal and are discovered on a Pap smear, but that is unusual. Abnormal bleeding must be investigated, even if your Pap smear is normal.

Do I need a hysterectomy to treat endometrial cancer?

Surgery is the mainstay of treating endometrial cancer. If it is determined that surgery would be too risky, you can be treated with radiation. If you are healthy enough to undergo surgery, your doctor will recommend a hysterectomy with removal of both fallopian tubes and both ovaries. The doctor may also want to remove lymph nodes in the pelvis or abdomen to help determine if the cancer has spread beyond the uterus. Your physician may be willing to perform a vaginal hysterectomy or a complete laparoscopic hysterectomy. These are usually reserved for early, low-grade cancers. If the cancer is more advanced, the surgery may be performed through an open abdominal incision that allows your surgeon the best opportunity to assess the extent of your cancer and remove it successfully.

I'm scared. What will happen if I don't do anything?

Our mouths drop open whenever we hear a patient ask this question. You will die from endometrial cancer if it is not treated. Nobody can predict how long you will live without treatment, but it is likely that you will die within a few years, and maybe sooner.

Generally this question stems from fear, not a genuine desire to avoid treatment. The word *cancer* evokes apprehension in even the bravest of individuals. You may mistakenly assume that death is inevitable if you have cancer. However, most women with endometrial cancer are diagnosed early. With appropriate treatment, the vast majority survive their cancer. You may also be scared of surgery, particularly if you have never undergone an operation. Discuss these concerns with your doctor. Serious complications from the surgery are uncommon. There is no doubt that the benefit from surgery far outweighs the unlikely possibility of experiencing a complication.

I had a hysterectomy for endometrial cancer, and now my doctor says I need radiation therapy. Is that really necessary?

Many women will need only surgery for the treatment of endometrial cancer. However, in the following situations, additional therapy may be required:

- The cancer is assigned a high grade. High-grade cancers look particularly bizarre under the microscope. They are more likely to behave aggressively.
- The cancer penetrates deeply into the wall of the uterus. The chance of cancer cells existing outside the uterus is increased in this situation.
- The lymph nodes test positive for cancer.
- There is evidence of cancer spreading to other organs.
- The uterine cancer is a variety other than type 1 endometrial cancer.

Additional therapy in these situations can include radiation, chemotherapy, or both. Each case is unique and reviewed by specialists (gynecologic oncologist, pathologist, medical oncologist, and radiation oncologist) in order to decide whether the benefit of additional therapy outweighs the risks.

Complications associated with radiation include bowel difficulties (bleeding, spasms, colitis, constipation, or diarrhea) and bladder problems (increased frequency and urgency of urination, burning, or bleeding) that can persist after the treatment. Before submitting to the radiation, you will consult an oncologist who specializes in radiation therapy (radiation oncologist). Radiation can also be used to treat endometrial cancer that has spread to a specific site outside of the pelvis.

Chemotherapy is discussed in chapter 10, so we won't expound on it at this point other than to say that it may be recommended if your doctor thinks there is a reasonable probability of cancer cells extending beyond the pelvis.

Hormonal therapy in the form of high-dose progesterone or an aromatase inhibitor (more commonly used for breast cancer, see page 264) can also be used if there is evidence of cancer in distant organs (or a high probability that it will spread there). This treatment will not cure the cancer, but it may hold it in remission or slow its spread.

When considering radiation or chemotherapy, inquire about the frequency and severity of side effects from the treatment. If your survival rate is increased by 15–20 percent or more with the addition of radiation or chemotherapy, it is probably in your best interest to proceed with it. If survival is boosted only 5 percent, it may not be warranted.

Three Women . . . Same Cancer . . . Different Outcomes

We start with three women: Martha, Gloria, and Bonnie. All three women are two years beyond menopause and notice several days of light vaginal bleeding.

Martha

Martha wakes up her husband. "Al, wake up. I'm bleeding!"

"Where?" asks Al.

"From my vagina," Martha explains.

"I thought you were all done with that," Al replies.

"I was!" exclaims Martha. "You don't think this could be a period after all this time, do you?"

"Do I look like a doctor?" replies Al, clearly annoyed. "Call Dr. Sussman in the morning."

Martha calls her gynecologist, Dr. Sussman, the following day. "Is this abnormal? Does this mean I have cancer?"

"Martha, try to calm down," Dr. Sussman begins in a reassuring tone. "There isn't anything that we'll be able to tell over the phone. You'll have to come into the office. I can examine you and will probably order a pelvic ultrasound. Since your bleeding occurred more than one year after menopause, it is not normal. However, this does not mean that it is related to cancer. Postmenopausal bleeding is more likely to be from something benign like a polyp. Let's just take it one step at a time."

Martha is examined by Dr. Sussman, who finds no source for her bleeding at the time of her pelvic exam. Since the pelvic exam cannot evaluate the inside of the uterus, he orders an ultrasound study, which does show thickening of the endometrium (uterine lining). In the operating room, under sedation, he places a hysteroscope inside the uterus. He sees abnormal endometrial tissue, which is biopsied. The pathology report reveals this to be a grade 1 or well-differentiated (cancer cells that do not look particularly bizarre or aggressive under the microscope) endometrial cancer. He obtains an MRI scan that suggests her cancer is superficial with little invasion into the muscular wall of the uterus.

Dr. Sussman calls Martha the next day. "Martha, it turns out that you do have cancer, but you are very fortunate. It may not seem that way to you, but your cancer is not aggressive and at this early stage, I can treat you with surgery alone. We should be able to perform a laparoscopic hysterectomy. You will only be in the hospital a day or two and should recover very quickly."

Endometrial cancer is often diagnosed while it is still early and confined to the uterus. Women usually bleed while the cancer is still in its early stages. Contacting Dr. Sussman with her first bleeding episode has enabled Martha to be treated with surgery alone and she should have a 90–95 percent chance that her cancer will never recur.

Gloria

Gloria is a little surprised when she notices bleeding two years after menopause, but the bleeding is very light and she feels fine, so she ignores it. She doesn't tell her husband Carl. After all, why bother him with something minor? Six months later she bleeds again, this time heavier. Gloria makes an appointment to see her gynecologist, Dr. Jackson.

"Good morning, Gloria. How are you doing?" Dr. Jackson inquires while entering the room.

"Well, I feel a little silly," Gloria starts, "but I have some bleeding and I just want to make sure that it's okay. I'm sure it's nothing, but I guess it's better to see you and be sure."

"No, you're not being silly at all," responds Dr. Jackson. "Your bleeding is abnormal and needs to be investigated. When did you first notice this bleeding?"

"I had some bleeding about six months ago," confesses Gloria, "but I didn't make too much of it since it was very light and stopped after a few days."

"Well, it won't help to scold you at this point," Dr. Jackson begins, "but you really should've brought this to my attention six months ago. I'm not too busy today, so why don't we do an endometrial biopsy while we have you here in the office."

Dr. Jackson examines Gloria and performs an endometrial biopsy, which demonstrates a moderately differentiated (grade 2) endometrial cancer. Ultrasound shows this to be rather large and an MRI examination demonstrates extension deep into the wall of the uterus. Dr. Jackson performs a hysterectomy on Gloria, but also samples lymph nodes from the pelvic and peri-aortic (around the aorta) region since her cancer is rather large, moderately differentiated (grade 2), and has significant extension into the wall of the uterus. The pathology report indicates that there is no involvement of the lymph nodes, but the cancer has extended from the endometrial lining down into the cervix.

Because of the cervical involvement, large size, and deep penetration into the wall of the uterus, Dr. Jackson refers her to a radiation oncologist for additional treatment. Gloria will receive pelvic radiation, which has the possibility of altering her bowel or bladder function. However, with the surgery and radiation she has a 70 percent chance that her cancer will not recur.

Bonnie

Bonnie is an anxious woman. However, unlike some anxious patients who run to the doctor every time they get a symptom, Bonnie deals with her anxiety by ignoring symptoms. It was easy to ignore her first episode of bleeding, which was very light and only lasted a few days. She never really had much in the way of menopausal symptoms, so she convinced herself that her ovaries were still functioning. Over the next two years she bleeds for a few days every three to six months, convincing herself every time that this is a normal menopausal bleeding pattern. Like many anxious patients, Bonnie skips her GYN appointments and sees her gynecologist, Dr. Truman, every few years at best. Finally, she develops heavy bleeding that continues for three weeks. When it looks like it won't stop, she finally makes an appointment to see Dr. Truman.

Dr. Truman greets Bonnie. "Hi, Bonnie. Long time, no see."

"Yeah, I've been very busy," responds Bonnie.

Dr. Truman tries to contain herself, but in the end can't keep from responding sarcastically. "Too busy? It's been three years since you have been here. There must've been some time in there you could have seen me. So what's going on? I know you don't like coming here so by the time I see you, all hell's broken loose."

"Please don't yell at me," Bonnie pleads. "I'm nervous enough already. I've been bleeding for three weeks now."

Dr. Truman is unconvinced. "Tell me when you first started to bleed."

"About two and a half to three years ago probably," confesses Bonnie, "but I just thought that it was normal for menopause. Maybe I was just telling myself that because I didn't want to face the problem."

"Yeah, that sounds like the Bonnie I know. Let me take a look and see if there's anything obvious on your exam. Since you've been bleeding for three weeks already, I'm going to call over to the ultrasound department and see if they can squeeze you in for a study. After that we'll probably have to get a sample of tissue from inside the uterus."

Bonnie's ultrasound study reveals a large uterine mass. Because of the heavy bleeding, Dr. Truman admits Bonnie to the hospital where she performs a D&C and acquires an MRI study. The D&C reveals a grade 3 or poorly differentiated (cells that look bizarre and aggressive under the microscope) endometrial cancer and the MRI study suggests that it may have penetrated beyond the wall of the uterus. A hysterectomy with pelvic and peri-aortic lymph node sampling is performed. It is obvious at surgery that the cancer has perforated the outer surface of the uterus and the pathology report reveals several positive lymph nodes. Fortunately, there does not appear to be any invasion of adjacent organs such as the bowel or bladder.

Bonnie is referred to a radiation oncologist and medical oncologist. It is decided that she will have pelvic radiation followed by chemotherapy. Unfortunately, even with treatment, she has a 50 percent chance of her cancer recurring.

Lessons Learned from Martha, Gloria, and Bonnie

- Investigate any bleeding that occurs more than one year after menopause. There is no way to be sure whether Gloria and Bonnie worsened their prognosis by delaying evaluation, but there is a reasonable likelihood that earlier diagnosis would have reduced the chances of them needing radiation or chemotherapy.
- "Feeling fine" does not exclude the presence of cancer. In fact, most people have no symptoms from early cancer. Symptoms such as pain, fatigue, and weight loss usually present later. We are very lucky that endometrial cancer often presents early with abnormal bleeding.
- Woman can have heavy bleeding from a benign process such as a polyp and only light bleeding with cancer.
- You cannot let anxiety or fear of cancer delay evaluation when you exhibit an abnormal symptom. First, there is always a greater likelihood that your symptom is unrelated to cancer. Secondly, if it is related to cancer, you increase your chances of being treated successfully through early evaluation. If you find that anxiety interferes with your ability to function at home or work and leads you to make irrational decisions, then you should consider evaluation by a therapist or physician for treatment.

Can I use hormone replacement after treatment for endometrial cancer?

Most doctors will not allow you to take estrogen after being treated for endometrial cancer. There is a concern that any remaining cancer cells will be stimulated by the estrogen and increase the chances of a recurrence. Recently, doctors have been less strict regarding that recommendation. If your cancer was detected very early, your risk of recurrence is very low (5 percent). This small risk must be weighed against the benefits you will receive from the estrogen. You also must consider the timing of your treatment. Most endometrial cancers that recur will do so in the first five years after treatment. Recurrence after ten years is rare. Many gynecologic oncologists feel that hormone replacement is permissible if your cancer was not advanced when it was discovered and if you have been free of disease for ten years (some use five).

How often should I see the doctor after my treatment for endometrial cancer?

Initially you will be seen frequently, possibly as often as every three to four months. Your doctor will examine your pelvic region to feel for a mass that could represent a recurrence. He or she also will obtain frequent Pap smears from your vagina, which is one of the more common sites for recurrence. If your cancer was more advanced, follow-up may also include periodic pelvic, abdominal, and chest imaging (CT scans, chest X-ray, PET scan), and a CA-125 blood test (a tumor marker). The frequency of your visits can be decreased after two years, but most physicians will recommend that you still be seen every six months.

For more facts about endometrial cancer, contact these organizations:

The National Cancer Institute: www.cancer.gov/cancertopics/types/endometrial

The American Cancer Society: www.cancer.org/cancer/endometrialcancer/index

The Mayo Clinic: www.mayoclinic.com/health/endometrial-cancer/DS00306

My Pap smear is abnormal. Does that mean I have cancer?

You have been taught that Pap smears are used to detect cervical cancer. Therefore, you automatically assume that an abnormal Pap smear represents cancer. Actually, most abnormal Pap smears reflect cervical conditions that are not life-threatening. Your Pap smear may become atypical because of any of the following conditions that do not indicate cancer:

- Cervicitis (infection or inflammation of the cervix)
- Irritation of the cervix from intercourse, a tampon, an IUD, or another agent
- Changes that occur as cells repair the cervix
- Changes due to inadequate estrogen levels, for example, menopause

Your doctor may want you to return to the office to be examined or to obtain cultures if the Pap smear suggests the presence of an infection. An infection may require specific treatment with an antibiotic or antifungal medication (see chapter 5). Often no infection can be identified although cervicitis is present. If the cervicitis persistently causes abnormal Pap smears, it can be treated with either cryotherapy (a freezing technique) or laser. Other changes usually reverse themselves spontaneously without specific treatment. Changes due to inadequate estrogen can be reversed with vaginal estrogen therapy.

If my Pap smear is abnormal, why isn't the doctor doing something about it?

Nancy is very worried. Linda, the nurse practitioner at Dr. Irving's office, calls and tells her that her Pap smear came back a little abnormal. What the heck does that mean? *she wonders.* She's never had an abnormal Pap smear before. This must mean that she's going to get cancer. Right? *Linda says that Dr. Irving tested it for a virus called HPV and since that test was negative, nothing special needs to be done.* It doesn't sound reasonable.

After all, if the test reveals something abnormal, shouldn't he be doing something about it right away?

Actually, minor abnormalities of the Pap smear often take care of themselves. If the Pap smear appears slightly atypical but does not show precancerous or cancerous changes, it is often given the designation ASCUS (atypical squamous cells of undetermined significance). Depending on your age, your doctor may have the laboratory test ASCUS smears for the presence of high-risk HPV viruses (not currently recommended for women under age twenty-five). We now understand that all cervical cancer is induced by high-risk HPV. Therefore, if your Pap smear tests negative for HPV, it is reasonable to continue with routine screening without intervention. Most of the time ASCUS smears unrelated to HPV will resolve spontaneously.

What cervical conditions are precancerous?

The next degree of abnormality beyond ASCUS is low-grade squamous intraepithelial lesion (LSIL). In the past, this was also referred to as CIN 1 or mild dysplasia. LSIL most typically develops from acquiring a high-risk HPV virus, which is sexually transmitted. Having multiple sexual partners increases your risk of acquiring HPV. Condoms lower the risk of acquiring HPV but do not eliminate it. Two vaccines are now present (Gardasil and Cervarix) that protect against the transmission of HPV types 16 and 18, which are responsible for 80 percent of cervical cancer. The Gardasil vaccine also protects against types 6 and 11, which are instrumental in the development of genital warts. The vaccines are now recommended for both sexes between the ages of eleven and twenty-six. Insurance companies will usually cover the vaccine within that age range. However, it is not unreasonable to offer the vaccine to women or men over the age of twenty-six if they are single and sexually active. The risk of developing cervical atypia from HPV is increased in smokers.

In the past it was common for doctors to treat low-grade cervical abnormalities because it was assumed that they would ultimately

It's So Confusing!

The terminology for atypical Pap smears seems to change every ten years. Thirty years ago abnormalities were classified as mild, moderate, or severe dysplasia. Twenty years ago this switched to CIN I, CIN II, and CIN III. Currently we classify these abnormalities as low-grade or high-grade SIL. It seems that the only thing you can be sure of is that given enough time, the terminology will change again.

progress to more significant abnormalities. However, we now understand that most cases of LSIL will not progress, especially in young women (teens and twenties). Younger women usually develop an immune response that clears the virus in six months to two years. Once the virus clears, the LSIL often resolves. Therefore, doctors rarely intervene to treat LSIL, presuming that the diagnosis is confirmed with colposcopically directed biopsies (see below). Older women are less likely to clear the high-risk HPV virus. However, most cervical cancer develops while the cervix is undergoing a transformation that occurs in the earlier reproductive years. Therefore, you may have less chance of clearing the HPV virus if you are older, but the HPV virus may also be less likely to cause a cervical abnormality.

Less commonly, a woman develops a high-grade squamous intraepithelial lesion (HSIL). In the past this was referred to as moderate/severe dysplasia, or CIN 2/CIN 3. Approximately 20 percent of HSIL will progress to cervical cancer. The risk is particularly high if you harbor HPV types 16 or 18. Most doctors will proceed with treatment if you are diagnosed with HSIL.

How do you diagnose LSIL and HSIL?

LSIL or HSIL are initially indicated through your Pap smear. If the Pap smear suggests either of these, a colposcopy is usually performed (current guidelines allow for annual Pap smear follow-up in women under twenty-five without colposcopy, initiating colposcopy only if the condition persists). This procedure is performed in the office. Your doctor inserts a speculum into the vagina and examines the cervix through an optical instrument that magnifies images of the cervix. Dilute acetic acid (sounds bad—it's just vinegar) is applied to the cervix. You may feel a slight burning when the acetic acid is applied, but usually this is tolerated well. SIL of the cervix has a characteristic appearance when visualized through the colposcope. The doctor will take biopsies of any suspicious areas. You will feel a pinch when a cervical biopsy is taken. The doctor may also perform endocervical curettage, in which a small scraping instrument is used in the cervical canal to obtain tissue that cannot be seen with the colposcope. This helps the doctor make sure there is no abnormality beyond the field of vision provided by the colposcope. The biopsies are sent to a laboratory for microscopic evaluation.

How do you treat LSIL and HSIL?

LSIL is usually observed with serial Pap smears (with or without HPV testing) without intervention. HSIL will be generally treated in one of the following ways:

- Observation—HSIL does not always progress, and may regress to normal in young women. A minority of physicians would continue to observe HSIL in a patient under the age of thirty, hoping for this regression. This requires an extremely compliant patient and frequent (every six months) observation intervals with Pap smears and colposcopy.

- Cautery—The SIL is destroyed by electrosurgical techniques that apply heat.

- Cryotherapy—The SIL is treated through the application of freezing agents to the cervix.

- LEEP procedure—An electrosurgical loop "scoops" the SIL out of the cervix. This may be followed by application of an electrosurgical ball that cauterizes the cervix.

- Laser surgery—A high-energy beam vaporizes the SIL.
- Cervical conization—If there is a suggestion that there may be SIL or cancer in the cervical canal, a cervical conization may be recommended. A cervical conization removes a cone of tissue from the cervix. The cone may be removed using a scalpel, laser, or LEEP loop.

The method chosen by your doctor may vary depending on the degree of your SIL, and your doctor's suspicion regarding the possibility of CIS (carcinoma in situ, cervical cancer that is still confined to the glands lining the cervical canal) or invasive cancer. The most common modalities used today are laser and LEEP procedures. In cases of persistent HSIL, CIS, or early invasive cancer, hysterectomy is often recommended.

Why is my doctor treating my SIL differently than someone I know who has the same thing?

Debbie is having lunch with Aunt Martha. The two have been close ever since Debbie was a child. Debbie lost her mother in a car accident when she was twelve and Aunt Martha is like a second mother. Even though Debbie has grown into an independent young woman, she and Aunt Martha have remained close.

"I got my results from Dr. Suswick's office today," begins Debbie. "He says that I have a low-grade cervical problem. He assures me that it is nothing overly serious and that we can just follow it. Dr. Suswick says that most of the time it regresses back to normal in women my age."

"I don't know about that!" exclaims Martha. "I had the same thing when I was your age and they had to remove part of my cervix to fix it. You'd better get a second opinion. It doesn't sound right to me that they would just watch a problem like that."

Aunt Martha has Debbie worried. Her aunt is not one to get excited over minor problems. Debbie calls Dr. Suswick's office back. "Can you have Dr. Susswick give me a call?" she asks the receptionist.

"Can I tell Dr. Sussman why you are calling?" inquires the receptionist.

"Yes, he told me that I have a cervical problem and that we only need to watch it. But my Aunt Martha had the same thing and she had to have part of her cervix removed. I want to know why Dr. Susswick isn't doing the same thing for me."

We hear this all the time. How come you are not treating me like my sister, or my aunt, or my friend? From our discussion above you must reach two conclusions. First, there are varying degrees of cervical abnormalities. Some require no treatment while others are likely to progress into cervical cancer. Try not to compare your situation to someone else's that may not be exactly the same. Second, there are many treatment modalities used that successfully treat cervical SIL. Remember, different doesn't mean better. Therefore, it is not uncommon for two doctors to treat the same condition using different yet equally successful methods.

Will SIL come back again after treatment?

Unless a hysterectomy is performed, there is a chance of redeveloping SIL. Initial treatment eradicates the SIL but it doesn't remove the cervix or the presence of HPV. It is important that you undergo regular Pap smears (usually every six months) following treatment for SIL. If a Pap smear indicates recurrent SIL, it will again be approached as outlined above. If childbearing is not a concern, one might consider hysterectomy (particularly with HSIL). If your body clears the high-risk HPV virus that induced your cervical problem, then you have a good chance of not getting a recurrence.

If the SIL can recur, why don't you just do a hysterectomy?

Treating cervical SIL via hysterectomy is like killing an insect with a sledgehammer: it's usually more than you need. Many women will never have recurrence of SIL. Submitting a woman to a major operation when a minor procedure may solve the problem is not justifiable. If it is obvious that there will be a problem with compliance after treatment (the patient is unwilling or unable to submit to regular fol-low-up Pap smears), hysterectomy is indicated. It is also reasonable if you continue to persist or recur with HSIL or CIS. Otherwise, it is in your best interest to use one of the conservative modalities (ex. Laser, LEEP, or cone biopsy) to treat the SIL. They are performed either in the office or as an outpatient in the operating room and have fewer complications than hysterectomy.

What's the difference between cervical SIL and cervical cancer?

Many women assume that SIL is an early form of cervical cancer. Women tell us that they have a family history of cervical cancer. Upon further questioning, it becomes apparent that their relative had SIL. SIL of the cervix is not cancer. It is potentially (as in not necessarily) precancerous (could develop into cancer). This is an important distinc-tion. SIL can be treated with conservative approaches (as described above), while cervical cancer mandates an aggressive approach.

How will I know if I have cervical cancer?

You probably won't know! There are no symptoms associated with early cervical cancer. That is why it is critical for you to regularly visit your gynecologist for Pap smears and HPV testing. There are approximately twelve thousand new cases of invasive cervical cancer each year. This number is dramatically lower than prior decades' because of Pap smear screening. Regular Pap smears and HPV testing will almost always detect cervical abnormalities prior to the development of invasive cer-vical cancer. Most commonly, cervical cancer is detected in women who have not been evaluated by a gynecologist for many years. Sexual activity with multiple partners increases your risk for cervical cancer by increasing your risk for HPV infection. Smoking also increases your risk. Cervical cancer may occur at any age but is most commonly seen between ages thirty-five to fifty.

The earliest sign of cervical cancer is abnormal bleeding (particularly between your periods, with intercourse, or in menopause). Don't panic! The vast majority of abnormal bleeding is not from cancer. Nevertheless, it needs to be evaluated. Advanced cervical cancer may cause difficulty with urination from obstructing the urinary tract. The tumor may also impede drainage of fluid from your legs, causing them to swell. Once again, these symptoms are much more likely to be related to other causes, but should be evaluated by a physician.

How do you diagnose and treat cervical cancer?

When your Pap smear indicates the possibility of cancer, your doctor will biopsy any area on the cervix that looks abnormal, either on direct vision or with colposcopy (see above). If there is nothing that appears distinctly abnormal, he or she will probably perform a cervical cone biopsy (removing a cone of tissue from your cervix in the operating room). If cancer is confirmed, additional imaging studies (ultrasound, CT, MRI, PET) will be done to evaluate the extent of the cancer. Your doctor may also do special procedures to look into the bladder or rectum if imaging studies indicate involvement of those organs. Cervical cancer is staged according

Avoid Cervical Cancer!

Dr. Thornton has only seen three cases of invasive cervical cancer in thirty years. In one case, a woman had not seen a gynecologist for ten years. The second woman had not seen a gynecologist in twenty years. The third woman had an abnormal Pap smear obtained by an older gynecologist who was not trained in colposcopy. He performed a few random cervical biopsies and missed her cancer.

Almost all women who regularly go for Pap smears and HPV testing will have their cervical problem detected before it has developed into invasive cancer. Do not skip your routine annual GYN appointment!

to how far it has invaded. Stage I cervical cancer has invaded only minimally and is confined to the cervix. As the cancer spreads beyond the cervix, the stage increases. In stage IV, it has spread to the bladder, rectum, or other parts of the body. Very minimally invasive cervical cancer (microinvasion) is sometimes treated with a cervical cone biopsy in women who are trying to retain their uterus for childbearing. Most early cervical cancer is approached surgically with a hysterectomy. The uterus and its adjacent tissues are removed. Pelvic lymph nodes and the upper part of the vagina may also be excised. If the ovaries are normal, they do not need to be removed (although it is often recommended if you are beyond menopause). More advanced cervical cancer is often treated with radiation. Initially, cervical cancer spreads locally, so pelvic radiation is very effective. Complications from pelvic radiation include voiding difficulties (bladder spasms, burning with urination, frequent and urgent urination), and bowel problems (rectal spasms, diarrhea). As radiation therapy has become more sophisticated, these complications have become less frequent. Medications are available to help ease these symptoms should they occur.

Cervical cancer that has spread to distant areas of the body is treated with chemotherapy. Unfortunately successful treatment at this point is limited.

Will HPV Testing Replace Pap Smears?

We now know that certain strains of high-risk HPV are the cause of cervical cancer. If you test negative for these high-risk strains of HPV, you should not be at risk for cervical cancer. Clinical studies seem to indicate that HPV testing is a better predictor for cervical cancer than Pap smears. If further clinical trials concur with this assessment, we may see a recommendation down the road for HPV testing alone as the primary screening tool for cervical cancer. Pap smears or other additional studies would only be performed if high-risk HPV is present.

Currently, screening recommendations for cervical cancer include both Pap smears and HPV (see page 15 in chapter 1), but don't be surprised if in the future Pap smears are deemed unnecessary for patients who test negative for HPV.

What are my chances of surviving cervical cancer?

Early cervical cancer has an excellent prognosis. With stage I disease (confined to the cervix), you have an 85–90 percent chance of surviving. Your chances decrease as the stage of cancer increases. Survival with advanced disease that has spread to other parts of the body is very low (5–10 percent).

The take-home message here is visit your gynecologist regularly. A complete examination should be performed annually, and Pap smears should be obtained after age twenty. HPV testing should be included in women over thirty every three to five years (more frequently in women who have had prior cervical abnormalities). Advanced cervical cancer is exceptionally rare in women who comply with regular exams.

For more information on cervical cancer, visit:

The National Cancer Institute: www.cancer.gov/cancertopics/types/cervical

The American Cancer Society: www.cancer.org/Cancer/CervicalCancer/index

10

DISORDERS OF THE OVARY

I was told I have a cyst. What is that?

Any fluid-filled structure seen in the ovary is referred to as an ovarian cyst. Your doctor may discover an ovarian cyst when he or she examines you, or it may be detected by a radiologic scan (ultrasound, CT, MRI). Radiologists often call any fluid-filled structure in the ovary a cyst, but in premenopausal women this term should be reserved for structures greater than 2 cm. The follicle containing the egg to be released at ovulation is a cystic structure. It increases up to 2 cm (slightly less than 1 inch) before ovulation. Because follicles are normally seen in the ovary, they should not be referred to as cysts. Postmenopausal women no longer develop follicles, so any fluid-filled structure in the postmenopausal ovary is abnormal (but not necessarily dangerous; see below).

The most common cysts seen in the premenopausal ovary are "functional" cysts. Sometimes a follicle doesn't rupture in the middle of your cycle. It continues to increase in size, evolving into a follicular cyst. Sometimes the follicle does rupture, and blood collects in the corpus luteum (the follicular structure after ovulation). This is referred to as a corpus luteal, or hemorrhagic, cyst. Follicular and luteal cysts are "functional" because they relate to the normal function of the ovary. They comprise 90 percent of all premenopausal and perimenopausal ovarian cysts. Functional cysts resolve spontaneously. Your doctor may place you on oral contraceptives to suppress ovarian function. Some physicians believe this decreases the amount of time it takes for resolution of a functional cyst, although studies do not back up that assertion.

Polycystic ovaries represent a variation of functional cysts. In this condition, there are an excess number of unruptured follicular cysts within the ovaries. This abnormality is associated with infrequent ovulation that may cause infertility. Infrequent periods, obesity, and masculine traits (such as increased facial hair) may also develop. Polycystic ovary syndrome is also associated with features of a metabolic syndrome that include type 2 diabetes, hypertension (high blood pressure), and dyslipidemia (abnormal levels of cholesterol and triglycerides). For additional information, go to the Polycystic Ovarian Syndrome Association at www.PCOsupport.org.

Another type of ovarian cyst is an endometrioma. Before menopause, little bits of endometrium can reflux out of your fallopian tubes and land on the surface of your ovaries and other pelvic organs. If the capsule of the ovary envelops these "endometrial implants," then each month they bleed and the blood cannot escape from the ovary. This produces a cyst filled with old blood, sometimes referred to as a "chocolate cyst" because the contents look like chocolate syrup. Associated with this, there may be other symptoms related to endometriosis such as pelvic pain or infertility. After menopause, endometriomas tend to shrink, but often they do not disappear. More recently, it has been shown that there is an increased association of endometriosis with certain specific types of ovarian cancer. However, most cystic tumors found in the presence of endometriosis will be benign. See chapter 8 for more information on endometriosis.

There are many types of benign cystic tumors that can evolve from ovarian tissue. Cystadenomas are cystic tumors that emerge from the cells that cover the surface of the ovary. Dermoid cysts are particularly unique. They may contain many types of tissue within the cyst including skin, hair, and teeth. (Yes, they look as disgusting as they sound!) Because most benign tumors are removed (see below), it is not known how many of them would become cancerous if not treated.

Malignant tumors of the ovary may also be cystic. The most common of these are referred to as cystadenocarcinomas. Fortunately, malignant (cancerous) tumors comprise a small minority of ovarian cysts. Ninety-five percent of all ovarian tumors in women under the age of forty-five are benign. The chances of a cyst being malignant increases with age, although the majority of cysts are benign even after menopause.

Why do I have pain from my ovarian cyst?

An enlarged cystic ovary may twist and turn, causing intermittent, sharp pain. If the ovary is enlarged sufficiently to press on other pelvic structures, it may be felt as a dull, continuous pain. You may also feel pain with intercourse, particularly on deep penetration. A very large cyst may be first noticed as abdominal swelling.

Occasionally, a cystic ovary undergoes continuous twisting until it cuts off its blood supply. This is called ovarian torsion. You develop profound, unrelenting pain with ovarian torsion. We're talking about the kind of pain that brings you to the emergency room any time, day or night. Ovarian torsion is treated through surgery. Most doctors approach ovarian torsion using laparoscopic techniques (surgery using a telescopic instrument and small incisions). Historically, doctors removed the ovary if there was torsion. More recently, physicians are untwisting the ovary. In a premenopausal woman, particularly a woman who wants to have more children, the ovary is untwisted and preserved, as long as the torsion has not destroyed the blood supply to the ovary. Ovarian torsion is less common in menopausal women, but when it does occur, the ovary will usually be removed.

Rupture of an ovarian cyst also produces sharp pain. The pain then decreases in intensity but may persist as a continuous "achy" feeling in the pelvis. The diagnosis is suspected when an ultrasound examination demonstrates "free" fluid in the pelvis. This represents the contents of the cyst lying free in the pelvis. If there is continuous bleeding from the ruptured cyst (demonstrated by repeatedly checking your blood count), surgery is required. However, most of the time ruptured cysts can be observed without treatment. Most ruptured cysts occur in premenopausal women, are functional in nature, and will resolve spontaneously. Your pain usually resolves quickly (anywhere from hours to several days). Any ruptured cystic structure in a postmenopausal woman must be further investigated to exclude cancer.

Did She Really Rupture a Cyst?

Kristen wakes up with a severe pain. She has noticed a similar type pain in the past when she ovulates, but this is much worse. When she can't take it anymore, she wakes up her mother.

"Mom! I have this terrible pain and can't go back to sleep. I think you need to take me to the emergency room."

"Are you having any other symptoms?" asks her mother anxiously. "You weren't sick yesterday, were you?"

"No, I felt fine yesterday," answers Kristen, "but I can't stand this pain anymore. Take me to the emergency room."

After a few hours in the waiting room, Kristen is finally seen by the emergency room physician, Dr. Andrews, who examines her. Kristen has a little bit of tenderness in the right lower abdomen, but nothing else is overly impressive. Dr. Andrews orders blood work, a urinalysis, a CT scan, and a pelvic ultrasound. Nothing is overly remarkable, other than a small amount of free fluid in the pelvis. Kristen is told that she ruptured an ovarian cyst. She is assured that everything will be fine, but she should follow up with her gynecologist within the next week.

So, did Kristen really rupture an ovarian cyst? The answer is maybe. Unfortunately, when no other source for lower abdominal or pelvic pain is found in a young woman, she is almost always told that she has ruptured an ovarian cyst. Once the cyst ruptures, often it is no longer visible as a distinct entity in the ovary on imaging studies. The little bit of free fluid found on Kristen's ultrasound scan is consistent with a recently ruptured ovarian cyst, but small amounts of free fluid can be seen in the pelvis of normal women. Kristen's scenario is fairly common; many women will recurrently suffer from periodic intense pain, presumably from rupturing ovarian cysts. If symptoms develop before a cyst ruptures, then it will be apparent on pelvic ultrasound, but many times there are no symptoms until a cyst actually ruptures. One way to deal with this dilemma is to suppress the ovary with moderately high doses of hormonal contraceptives.

Do I need surgery if I have a cyst?

Most ovarian cysts do not require surgery. In the premenopausal or perimenopausal patient, the majority of cysts are functional (see above) and will resolve spontaneously over one to three months. You need surgery for your cyst in the following situations:

1. Your cyst does not resolve after several months, particularly if you have been placed on oral contraceptives.
2. Your cyst is exceptionally large. Functional cysts are usually under 10 cm. If your cyst is larger than 10 cm, surgery may be recommended.
3. You are menopausal. After menopause your ovaries no longer function. Therefore, functional cysts are not possible after menopause. If your cyst is small and has benign characteristics on an ultrasound scan, your doctor may be willing to follow it conservatively. You must meet the following criteria for conservative management:

   - Your cyst should be no larger than 5 cm.
   - Your cyst must be purely cystic (fluid-filled). There can't be any solid areas within the cyst.
   - The walls of the cyst must not be thick.
   - There must not be thick septations (walls going through the cyst).
   - You must not have other evidence of cancer on your scan such as ascites (free fluid in the abdomen), enlarged lymph nodes, or other tumor masses.
   - You must have a normal CA-125 test, a blood test that screens for ovarian cancer.
   - You must be willing to undergo frequent ultrasound scans (initially every three to six months).

All menopausal cysts that do not meet these criteria should be removed. Some doctors feel that all menopausal cysts should be removed if you are otherwise healthy (at low risk for undergoing surgery), but gradually doctors are willing to be more conservative. Very few postmenopausal cysts with a benign appearance will ever develop into cancer.

4. Your symptoms are severe. If the pain you have cannot be adequately controlled, surgical intervention may be justified.
5. You develop ovarian torsion (see above).
6. Your cyst causes internal bleeding that does not spontaneously abate.

What type of surgery is done for ovarian cysts?

Historically, ovarian cysts were removed by laparotomy, which requires a larger incision in the abdomen. Today, laparoscopic approaches for ovarian surgery are commonly used. A telescopic instrument is inserted through a small (1 cm or less) incision near your navel. Operative instruments are introduced through secondary incisions (also small) and either the cyst is removed from the ovary (ovarian cystectomy) or the entire ovary is removed (oophorectomy). Laparoscopic surgery for an ovarian cyst is only appropriate if the cyst is benign. The contents of a cyst may spill into the abdomen during laparoscopic removal, which is not ideal if the cyst is malignant. Rarely, an ovarian cyst appears benign on imaging studies, such as ultrasound, but looks suspicious at the time of laparoscopy. When this happens, the laparoscope is removed and your surgery will be performed through a laparotomy. The ovary will be removed intact, and more extensive surgery is performed if the ovary is found to be malignant on frozen section examination by a pathologist. Laparotomy for a suspicious ovary may be rescheduled so that a gyneco-logic oncologist (a GYN doctor who specializes in cancer) is present for the procedure.

How does the doctor know that my cyst is not cancerous?

There is no way of knowing for sure. This can be very upsetting. Many women overreact when informed of an ovarian cyst. You may assume that it is malignant and have yourself dead and buried. In reality, it is far more likely that the cyst is benign, particularly if you are premenopausal.

If the ultrasound criteria mentioned above indicate that the cyst is benign, and your CA-125 test is normal, then you have at least a 95 percent chance that your cyst is not malignant. If you are premenopausal, wait to see if the cyst will resolve.

The doctor says I have an ovarian tumor. Does that mean I have cancer?

Gladys is hysterical. She has just returned home after her routine annual visit with her gynecologist, Dr. Simpson. He has informed her that she has an ovarian tumor and will need surgery. She immediately calls her best friend, Erica, on the phone.

"I'm going to die!" exclaims Gladys, sobbing into the phone.

"Calm down, what are you talking about? I saw you yesterday and you were fine."

"I just got back from my gynecologist. Dr. Simpson says I have an ovarian tumor. He says it's the size of a grapefruit. How can that be? I get my exam every year and it's always been fine," says Gladys, wondering how this could happen.

"Aren't you having any pain?" asks Erica. "I can't believe that you could have something that big without pain."

"I haven't noticed anything. You know me—if I get anything at all I run to the doctor right away."

"Does this mean you have cancer? Maybe you should be going to a hospital that specializes in cancer," Erica suggests.

"Dr. Simpson says that this probably isn't cancer, but I was pretty upset so he may have just been trying to calm me down. He says he will do surgery with a cancer specialist. Why would he bring in a cancer specialist if it's not cancer? I'm so confused."

"Well, let's hope for the best," Erica says, trying to sound reassuring. "I'll be with you the whole time."

"I know you will," responds Gladys, thankful that she has such a good friend.

Words like *tumor* and *neoplasm* are tossed around cavalierly by health professionals. Without further definition, they are likely to be misinterpreted by patients. A tumor, or neoplasm, is an abnormal mass of tissue that grows more rapidly than normal. It may be noncancerous (benign) or cancerous (malignant). The words *tumor* and *neoplasm* are usually used for ovarian growths that appear to have a solid component. Fluid-filled ovarian masses that do not appear to be functional cysts (see above) are referred to as cystic tumors or neoplasms.

The majority of ovarian tumors are benign. The incidence of ovarian cancer increases with age, but even after menopause more ovarian tumors are benign than malignant. Certain ultrasound characteristics help your doctor decide if the tumor is likely to be cancerous. The CA-125 and HE4 tumor markers, measured through blood work, are also helpful. However, until the tumor is removed surgically, there is no way of being sure that your tumor is benign. When possible, a gynecologic oncologist (gynecologist who specializes in cancer) should be consulted for tumors that may be malignant. He or she should be available at the time of surgery (see below).

Does ovarian cancer run in families?

Most ovarian cancer is sporadic, occuring without the patient having a family history of ovarian cancer. However, there are familial genetic syndromes that can increase a woman's chance of developing breast, ovarian, endometrial, and colon cancer. The most common of these familial syndromes is Hereditary Breast and Ovarian Cancer Syndrome, related to a BRCA1 or BRCA2 mutation.

In the general population, ovarian cancer occurs in approximately one out of every seventy to eighty women. It occurs more frequently in white women than black women and is most common between the ages of fifty and seventy-five. Your chances of developing ovarian cancer are increased if you have a history of infertility. It is also higher if you have not had children. Your chances are decreased with childbearing and usage of birth control pills. Tubal ligation may also have a protective effect.

If there is one relative in your family who has had ovarian cancer, your risk is increased, but no more than 3–5 percent. If there are multiple relatives (particularly first degree relatives such as your mother and sisters), your risk is increased substantially. In this situation there is a reasonable likelihood of hereditary breast and ovarian cancer syndrome and your risk of developing ovarian cancer may be as high as 25–50 percent. Genetic testing should be strongly considered under these circumstances (first testing the family members who have actually had ovarian cancer). With a BRCA1 or BRCA2 mutation, most gynecologists and oncologists will recommend prophylactic removal of the ovaries between ages thirty-five and forty. Early detection of ovarian cancer is difficult, even with screening. Your ovarian hormones can be replaced until you are closer to the age of natural menopause.

Are there screening tests for ovarian cancer?

Screening tests for ovarian cancer include pelvic ultrasound and a blood test called CA-125. Routine pelvic exams will detect some ovarian cancers, although early detection by pelvic exam is uncommon. Your Pap smear does not screen for ovarian cancer. It is valuable for the detection of cervical cancer, but does nothing to detect ovarian problems.

A pelvic ultrasound scan is good at detecting ovarian cysts and growths. So why aren't we getting pelvic scans every year? First, the scans are relatively expensive, ranging from five hundred to a thousand dollars per scan. That is a large amount of healthcare dollars to detect a disease that occurs in only 1.3 percent of women. We perform mammography annually in women after forty years of age, but breast cancer develops in more than 10 percent of women. Even if we had unlimited finances, there are other problems. Ovarian cancer can progress rapidly. For early detection, we would have to screen women every six months. Also, ovarian cancer tends to spread to other areas in the abdomen fairly early in its course. Although screening will detect some cancers still confined to the ovary (which have a good prognosis), many will have already spread. It is therefore debatable how many lives can be saved with ultrasound screening. Finally, the ultrasound scan cannot precisely determine if your ovarian growth is cancerous. Many benign ovarian cysts and tumors detected by the scan would be removed for every one that actually is malignant.

There are also problems using the CA-125 blood test. Not all ovarian cancers increase the CA-125 level. No more than 50 percent of early ovarian cancers will have an elevated CA-125. On top of that, many benign conditions raise the CA-125 level (fibroids, endometriosis, pelvic infection, pregnancy). False positive elevations create anxiety and may lead to unnecessary surgical procedures. The noncancerous conditions that raise CA-125 usually occur before menopause. It is not recommended to screen premenopausal women with the CA-125 test because of this high false positive rate. It is more reliable when used after menopause.

There are other individual tumor markers such as HE4 and tests looking at multiple markers such as ROMA and OVA1 that can be used by your gynecologist to help him or her decide if an ovarian mass is malignant. While these markers are not recommended for general screening, they may help gynecologists decide which patients with a pelvic tumor might require the services of a gynecologic oncologist.

So where does this leave us? Opinions vary among gynecologists as to the value of screening for ovarian cancer. It is probably not cost effective. However, if you are the one who develops the cancer, there will be little solace gained by someone telling you that screening wasn't cost effective. Studies are continually under way to decide if screening can substantially decrease the death rate from ovarian cancer. So far, the results have been mixed. If you have a positive family history of ovarian cancer, consider screening with ultrasound and CA-125 every six to twelve months. If there is a strong family history, consult your doctor regarding the possibility of genetic testing, or if this is not feasible, ask whether you should have your ovaries removed.

What symptoms will I have if I develop ovarian cancer?

Unfortunately, you probably won't have any symptoms while your cancer is early. Ovarian cancer tends to be asymptomatic until your abdomen begins to swell. By that time, your cancer has often spread into the abdomen. Abdominal swelling is either from free fluid in your abdomen, called ascites, or the tumor itself, which at this point is very large. Early ovarian cancers may cause pelvic pain or painful intercourse in similar fashion to ovarian cysts. Occasionally, the cancer will alter ovarian hormone secretion and cause abnormal bleeding. Advanced ovarian cancer may create indigestion, abdominal cramps, or bloating.

Whatever you do, don't assume you have an ovarian cancer if you have any of the above symptoms. They all are quite common and usually caused by conditions that are totally unrelated to cancer. On the other hand, don't ignore persistent, unusual symptoms. Consult your gynecologist and let him or her decide if further investigation is warranted.

If the tumor is on my ovary, why does the doctor want to perform a hysterectomy?

Okay, you're told there is an ovarian growth that needs to be removed. That makes sense. "But why in the world does he want to remove my uterus, and why does he need to remove the other ovary?" Ovarian cancer can spread to the uterus and may also involve the other ovary. If it is obvious that your tumor is malignant (either by appearance at surgery or a "frozen section"), the uterus and other ovary should be removed. If you still desire childbearing and the cancer appears to be confined to one ovary, the uterus and opposite ovary are sometimes preserved. However, a second operation is usually recommended after you have completed your family to have the uterus and other ovary removed. If you are beyond menopause, your doctor may recommend removal of your uterus and other ovary even if he or she feels that the tumor is benign. Until your tumor is analyzed, you can't be sure that there is no cancer. If the tumor appears benign but is found to be malignant on further evaluation, a second operation would be required. Removal of the uterus and opposite ovary also eliminates them from developing benign or malignant tumors in the future. If both ovaries are removed in a premenopausal woman, hormone replacement can be given in order to prevent premature menopausal symptoms.

Ovarian cancer surgery also entails removal of the omentum. The omentum is a fatty drape that lies over your intestines. It can be safely removed without any repercussions and is a frequent site for metastasis (spread of your cancer cells). Your doctor should also take biopsies throughout the abdomen and sample lymph nodes to see if there has been any spread of the cancer. Your doctor may consult a gynecologic oncologist for this more extensive surgery. If the cancer has spread to involve your bowel, one or more sections of bowel may be resected in order to optimize your chances of survival after the surgery.

The doctor says all of the cancer was removed. Why do I need chemotherapy?

Even when all of the gross tumor (tumor your doctor can see) is removed, there are microscopic cancer cells that remain in the pelvic and abdominal areas. If these are not treated, your cancer will definitely recur. In certain situations, radiation will be used to treat the remaining cancer cells. However, chemotherapy is more effective for most types of ovarian cancer. If there is no evidence of your cancer progressing beyond the ovary, chemotherapy may not be necessary. Unfortunately, only 25 percent of ovarian cancers are confined to the ovary when first diagnosed. Most women with ovarian cancer will need chemotherapy in addition to their surgery.

I know people who had chemotherapy and died anyway, so why should I take chemotherapy?

The success of chemotherapy is predicated upon many factors. Not all types of cancers are sensitive to chemotherapy. Fortunately, most ovarian cancers respond well to chemotherapy. Therefore, you can't compare someone else's situation to your own. Your response to chemotherapy depends on the following factors:

- The extent of your cancer when it is first discovered—if the cancer is limited, your chances of success with chemotherapy are better than if the cancer is widespread.
- The type of ovarian cancer—some varieties of ovarian cancer respond better to chemotherapy than others.
- The grade of your cancer—cancers with a very atypical or bizarre microscopic appearance (higher grade) have a poorer prognosis.
- The success of your surgery—if all of the visible tumor can be resected at surgery, your chances are better than if tumor is left behind.

If your doctor can successfully remove all of the visible cancer at the time of surgery, your chances of surviving at least five years after chemotherapy is 50 percent, referred to as the five-year survival rate. The benefit of chemotherapy in this situation clearly outweighs any risks associated with its use. If the cancer was initially confined to the ovary, your five-year survival can be as high as 90 percent.

As the extent of the cancer increases, your chances of survival decrease. If your cancer cannot be optimally resected at the time of surgery, your chance of surviving to five years is very low (under 10 percent). In this situation, you must weigh the benefit of chemotherapy extending your life against the side effects you will experience with the chemotherapy. Most patients will begin chemotherapy to see if their cancer responds (noted by a decrease in the size of the residual cancer when followed by scans). If the cancer shrinks and the side effects from the chemotherapy are tolerable, it is continued. If there is no response, or the chemotherapy is not tolerated well, it is discontinued.

Chemotherapy is not always recommended with ovarian cancer. If your cancer appears to be very early and confined to the ovary, chemotherapy may not be recommended. Other types of tumors referred to as "borderline" have a good prognosis without chemotherapy. Some types of ovarian cancer are more successfully treated with radiation. Each case of cancer is unique. Openly discuss the pros and cons of recommended treatments so that you can make an informed decision.

Ask your doctor to be honest with you regarding your prognosis. If you have trouble getting information, consult a gynecologic oncologist.

Tensie
An Empowering Story

Tensie and Bob were truly beautiful people. Now that I look back, I can't remember when either one of them said anything bad or judgmental about another person. I don't think that I can say that about anyone else I know. Tensie's brother and his wife had three beautiful daughters. Unfortunately both parents were involved with illicit drugs, progressively descending into the abyss created by their addiction. When it became apparent that they could no longer safely parent the three girls, Tensie and Bob took them in and raised them as their own. The girls were still young when Tensie was first diagnosed with advanced stage ovarian cancer. When diagnosed with ovarian cancer, most women assume it is a death sentence. Indeed, most women aren't diagnosed until stage III, when cancer has already spread into the abdomen. Tensie, however, was not one to dwell on misfortune. She and Bob decided to focus on everything positive that could be done to treat the cancer. It's not that they were unaware of the potential devastation that ovarian cancer can inflict on the body, but obsessing over that couldn't possibly be of any benefit.

Tensie was treated by the gynecologic oncologists at one of our community hospitals. As with most ovarian cancer patients, she underwent surgery and chemotherapy. Her cancer responded well to the treatment, and she remained free of cancer for two years. Unfortunately, the cancer did recur; in fact it recurred numerous times. Each of those times Tensie would undergo a course of chemotherapy that would temporarily place her into remission. Only those who were particularly close to Tensie knew of her treatments. She was not one to advertise her disease. In fact, her ovarian cancer was never a focus during the two to three times we encountered her over the course of each year. Raising the three girls was life affirming, and perhaps life sustaining, for Tensie. She and Bob did an amazing job with the girls who all have grown up to be fine young women. In addition to being a mother, Tensie pursued a very successful executive career at a major corporation.

After eleven years, Tensie did eventually succumb to her ovarian cancer. However, it seems to me that she provides us with a good model of how we should think about this cancer. In the past, the vast majority of women with ovarian cancer died within two years of diagnosis. However, more recently we have encountered many women whose experience with ovarian cancer parallels those who have other chronic diseases. The cancer waxes and wanes, requiring intermittent treatment with surgery, chemotherapy, or both. However, there is a good quality of life for many years after diagnosis. Women shouldn't automatically feel hopeless if they are diagnosed with ovarian cancer. Yes, there will be some cancers that are extremely aggressive and resistant to treatment. Some women will have rapidly progressive disease, leading to an abrupt end of their life. However, more and more women are living rich lives despite their cancer. New advances in the type and delivery of chemotherapy have increased survivorship. Progressively more women will experience a fulfilling life after diagnosis, just as Tensie did. Survivorship will continue to increase as treatments advance, and earlier diagnosis will become available as we refine our ability to detect cancer in its earliest stages.

Will I get sick from chemotherapy?

Side effects from chemotherapy vary depending on what agent is used. The most common side effects from chemotherapy are nausea, vomiting, decreased appetite, change in bowel function, fatigue, and hair loss. Nowadays, patients are premedicated to limit some of the side effects.

Most chemotherapeutic agents suppress your bone marrow. This can lead to anemia, poor blood clotting, and an increased susceptibility to infections. Your blood counts are monitored very closely during chemotherapy, and sometimes special drugs are administered to boost the bone marrow's production of certain blood components.

In addition to those effects mentioned above, each therapeutic drug has its own unique profile of toxicity. Chemotherapy is administered by doctors who specialize in this area, usually either a gynecologic oncologist or medical oncologist. The doctor will review possible side effects from any chemotherapeutic drug that is recommended.

How long will I get chemotherapy?

Duration of chemotherapy ranges from three to six months. It is given in cycles, with most patients receiving three to six cycles. Each cycle is three weeks. You are given the chemotherapeutic agents through an intravenous (IV) catheter either as an outpatient or during a very short hospitalization. The following three weeks allow your body to recover from the effects of the drugs. Throughout the course of therapy, your response to the chemotherapy may be monitored using scans. The CA-125 level (and possibly HE4, a new tumor marker) will also be followed if it was elevated when your cancer was initially diagnosed. Tumor markers should decrease with successful treatment, and they tend to rise again if there is a recurrence.

Sometimes chemotherapy is injected directly into the abdominal cavity through a thin tube or catheter. This process is known as intra-peritoneal (IP) chemotherapy. The advantage of IP chemotherapy is that it bathes the cancer cells directly with the cancer-killing drugs. When IP chemotherapy is chosen, doctors will often place the catheter for IP chemotherapy during the initial surgery. The tube is attached to a port, which makes it easy to deliver the drugs into the abdomen each time treatment is given. Unfortunately, IP chemotherapy can have more severe side effects than standard intravenous chemotherapy, including abdominal pain and infection. Sometimes, IP chemotherapy and IV chemotherapy are combined to maximize survival.

Occasionally, very large cancers, or cancers that appear to have extensive spread within the abdomen, will be treated with chemotherapy for several cycles before surgery (neoadjuvant chemotherapy). The hope in this situation is that the cancer will shrink to a point that makes surgery more successful.

In the past, a second-look operation was often used after your chemotherapy was completed, especially if there was no evidence of persistent cancer. By looking inside a second time, doctors could look for the presence of residual cancer that was not detectable by scans and tumor markers. If residual cancer was found, chemotherapy would be continued for a longer period of time. However, ovarian cancer commonly recurs even when there is no evidence of persistent tumor during second-look surgery, and survival is poor in patients who have chemotherapy continued because of persistent tumors found on second-look. Therefore, it is not clear that substantial benefit is to be gained from second-look surgery. With the advent of newer scans (ex. PET scan) and tumor markers and the lack of a clear survival advantage, initial enthusiasm for second-look procedures has waned.

Can I be cured, or will my cancer come back?

You have a good chance of survival (oncologists don't tend to use the word *cure*) if the cancer is confined to the ovary when it is discovered. Unfortunately, early ovarian cancer is usually asymptomatic. It doesn't take long for tumor cells to slough off the ovary and implant elsewhere in the pelvis and abdomen. Tumor masses evolve from the implants and are often present at the time of initial diagnosis. Most women treated at this stage will eventually have a recurrence of their cancer. However, many will have prolonged disease-free intervals after being treated with surgery and chemotherapy. If you develop a recurrence after a disease-free period, reoperation or additional chemotherapy may be recommended. If the cancer responded well to chemotherapy previously, it may do so again, placing you in remission. Most ovarian cancer will recur within the first five years after initial treatment. If you reach five years without any evidence of recurrence, your long-term prognosis is good.

For more information on ovarian cancer, visit:

National Cancer Institute: www.cancer.gov/cancertopics/types/ovarian

American Cancer Society: www.cancer.org/cancer/ovariancancer/index

11

PROBLEMS OF THE VAGINA AND VULVA

What is that lump by my vagina?

Patients use the word *lump* to describe numerous conditions. Boils, warts, polyps, cysts, tumors, and dropped pelvic organs have all been referred to as lumps at one time or another. Normal genital structures may also be mistaken for lumps. Folds of tissue in the labia or remnants of the hymenal ring, which is located just inside the vagina, often feel lumpy but are perfectly normal.

Raised skin lesions are most likely to be warts or moles. A mole is raised and usually darker than the surrounding skin. If it increases in size or changes in shape or color, it must be removed in case it proves to be a malignant melanoma. This rule applies to any pigmented area in the vulvar region, even if it is not a raised lesion. Genital warts are caused by infection with the HPV virus (see chapter 5). Vulvar cancer may also appear as a raised area on the vulva. Consultation with a physician is imperative if you notice an unusual skin lesion; don't assume it is a mole or wart. For best results, vulvar cancer requires early diagnosis. If your doctor finds a questionable skin lesion, he or she will biopsy it to rule out cancer.

Cysts are quite common in the genital region. If ducts in the glands located near the opening of the vagina become blocked, the gland will fill with fluid and feel like a lump. If it becomes infected, it evolves into a painful abscess and must be drained. If the gland is infected but has not developed into an abscess, your doctor will have you soak it in a warm sitz bath (a basin that fits on your toilet seat—you can buy it in a pharmacy) or tub. He or she may also give you antibiotics. The infection will either clear up without further treatment or develop into an abscess, which is drained under local anesthesia. Vulvar cysts that are not infected do not require any treatment unless they are causing discomfort.

With the exception of vulvar skin cancer, solid tumors are less common. They include fatty tumors, nerve tissue tumors, and blood vessel tumors. These are usually benign but may warrant removal. If a solid growth has been present for many years without changing, it almost inevitably is benign. However, any new or enlarging growths should be removed.

A lump that appears to be arising from within the vagina may be a uterine or vaginal polyp. These are noncancerous growths from the lining of the vagina, cervix, or endometrium. Vaginal polyps and cervical polyps can usually be removed in the office (see chapter 9). If the uterus, bladder, or rectum does not have adequate support, any one of them can descend down the vagina and appear at or beyond the vaginal opening, producing a lump. (For more information on this problem, see chapter 15.)

Why do I keep getting boils?

There are many skin glands in the pubic area. There are two different types of sweat glands and oily (also known as sebaceous) glands. When their ducts become blocked, skin bacteria are trapped in the glands, causing pustules or boils (a big pustule). Shaving your pubic region also increases the likelihood of developing a boil. Surface bacteria are able to penetrate the skin when you shave. If you have already shown a tendency to develop boils in the pubic region, you are much better off using a grooming instrument to shear the hair in this region.

Warning!

MRSA Changes Everything

In the past, most skin infections were easily treated with common antibiotics. Now, however, there are skin bacteria like MRSA (methicillin-resistant Staphylococcus Aureus) that are much harder to treat. Eleanor was a seventy-year-old woman who ignored a boil. She just assumed it would clear up on its own sooner or later. Unfortunately, the infection was caused by MRSA and quickly spread. She was taken to the operating room for drainage and a large amount of dead tissue had to be resected from above her pubic bone all the way into her buttocks. Eleanor nearly died from the MRSA and its toxins, which were shutting down her cardiovascular system, liver, and kidneys. With aggressive surgery, antibiotics, and the intense intervention of a team of specialists, Eleanor survived. Her case demonstrates the importance of following skin infections closely, since minor skin infections can evolve into life-threatening situations. Any skin infection, insect bite, scrape, or cut that does not quickly begin to heal should be seen by a physician. For more on MRSA, visit www.CDC.gov/MRSA.

When a boil occurs, you should soak it in warm water either in a sitz bath or tub. It may resolve by itself or spontaneously drain. If at all possible, see a physician. Skin-related infections are increasingly being caused by bacteria that are resistant to many antibiotics (see above). Some of these bacteria have significant potential for causing tissue damage. A large, unruptured boil must be lanced (surgically drained using a scalpel).

You can try to prevent recurrences by keeping the pubic area clean and dry. Loose-fitting cotton clothing is best. Avoid synthetic fabrics and tight slacks or underwear. Sleep in a loose nightgown or nude. Use a blow-dryer on a cool setting after showering, swimming, or working out. Your doctor may recommend a course of mupirocin (Bactroban), or Phisohex, antibacterial creams to lower your recurrence.

Sometimes boils recur despite preventive measures. Often one will redevelop in the same location as a previous boil and may be caused by an ongoing smoldering infection of your sweat glands (hidradenitis) in that location. Antibiotics usually do not prevent the repeated infections. Surgical removal of the infected sweat glands may be the only cure.

234 • ASK YOUR GYNECOLOGIST

I constantly have burning in my vulva. What can I do?

While waiting for their Starbucks order, Susie glances over to her friend Heidi, who appears to be scratching her crotch.

"What in the world are you doing? Quit that. You're embarrassing me."

"I can't help it. It feels like my vagina is on fire."

"Well, go see a doctor for goodness sake!"

"I have. He keeps telling me that I have yeast infections, but nothing he gives me seems to work."

Welcome to the perplexing world of vulvar disorders. Most women, and many healthcare providers, automatically blame yeast for all vulvar symptoms. While yeast infections are common, there are many other skin conditions that can cause vulvar itching, burning, or pain. *Vulvodynia* is a general term that denotes vulvar pain. It is most commonly used when there is no obvious source for the pain. Hypersensitivity to yeast, allergic and irritant skin reactions, inflammation associated with estrogen deficiency, chronic skin conditions (see below), and trauma from activities such as bicycle and horseback riding should be excluded before one is given the diagnosis of vulvodynia. Often there is no specific source identified for the vulvodynia. It is postulated that the condition results from anything that currently or in the past caused injury or irritation of the nerves that supply sensation to the vulva.

If your vulvar pain is limited to the area between the inner labia at the opening of the vagina (the vestibule), your condition may be referred to as vulvar vestibulitis. You may have one or more painful areas that are tender to touch within the vestibule. Often intercourse is exquisitely painful, precluding penetration of the vagina.

Because the condition is somewhat perplexing and often there is no specific identifiable cause, multiple approaches have been taken to treat vulvodynia:

- *Topical creams and ointments*: These may contain medications that are anti-inflammatory (steroids), anesthetic (lidocaine), or hormonal (estrogen, testosterone). Sometimes topical creams or ointments are specially compounded. These may contain antidepressant or anticonvulsant medication.

- *Pain-blocking medication*: These are medications which in many cases are used for other diagnoses, but often are successful in treating vulvodynia. Medications that can be tried include antidepressants (ex. Amitriptyline, Cymbalta), anti-seizure medications (ex. Tegretol), and two other medications commonly prescribed for nerve pain, gabapentin (Neurontin) and pregabalin (Lyrica).
- *Diet modification*: Some doctors will prescribe a low oxalate diet supplemented with calcium citrate (Citracal). A low oxalate cookbook can be obtained through the Vulvar Pain Foundation (www.thevpfoundation.org). There is not much in the way of legitimate medical research to support this approach, but it can certainly be tried.
- *Pelvic floor muscle therapy*: Often women with this disorder will have excessive tightness or spasm of the pelvic floor muscles. Retraining these muscles, alone through Kegel exercises (see chapter 14) or with the help of a healthcare professional who specializes in this disorder, can be helpful.
- *Nerve blocks*: Physicians who are familiar with the course of the pudendal nerve, which supplies sensation to this area, can employ a series of nerve blocks using anesthetics (with or without steroids). In rare cases, sacral nerve stimulators can be implanted.
- *Surgery*: When your vulvar pain is limited to the vestibule (vestibulitis), your gynecologist can resect the affected area.

Chronic vulvar pain can be very demoralizing. Doctors may tell you that there is nothing abnormal, implying that it is all in your head. You know that there is something wrong but cannot get help. First you must locate a doctor who acknowledges the existence of your problem. If he or she is not well versed in the peculiarities of vulvodynia, ask for a referral to someone who is. Unfortunately, it may be difficult to find an effective treatment. For more information on vulvodynia and support groups, contact these organizations:

The National Vulvodynia Association: www.nva.org
The Vulvar Pain Foundation: www.thevpfoundation.org
The Vulval Pain Society: www.vulvalpainsociety.org

The doctor wants to do a biopsy of the skin on my vulva. Does that mean I have cancer?

Your gynecologist should biopsy any skin abnormality involving the vulva. It is very difficult to accurately assess all of your skin changes based on their appearance. After injecting a local anesthetic in the office, your doctor can remove a small piece of skin for microscopic analysis. Most changes are not cancerous. Inflamed skin is often due to contact dermatitis or vulvar infection. If this is obvious from the skin's appearance, treatment can be given without a biopsy.

There are many chronic skin conditions (ex. lichen sclerosis, squamous cell hyperplasia, and lichen planus) that target the vulvar tissues. Other dermatologic conditions (ex. psoriasis) affect many areas of the body but can also be found in the vulvar region. These often present with a change in color or texture of the skin and their diagnosis confirmed by biopsy. Most of these will present with symptoms of itching or burning and are treated with steroid ointments.

Self-Exam

You may only see your doctor once or twice yearly. With self-examination you can follow skin changes monthly and may be able to detect changes earlier than the doctor. Wash your hands thoroughly and get into a comfortable position that will enable you to view the vulvar region with a hand mirror. You don't have to be a contortionist, although experimentation may be required. Move the mirror as necessary to look at the inner and outer labia, clitoris, vaginal and urethral openings, perineum, and perianal region (see the illustration on page 15). Any skin lesions, such

Precancerous changes in the skin of the vulva are referred to as VIN, vulvar intraepithelial neoplasia. VIN is classified into two types. "Usual-type" VIN is associated with HPV and risk factors that help HPV persist, such as smoking. "Differentiated" VIN is usually not associated with HPV and is more often associated with vulvar skin conditions such as lichen sclerosis (described in chapter 5). VIN is most commonly treated by local excision, laser ablation, or Imiquimod (Aldara, a cream applied three times weekly for twelve to twenty weeks). When *as ulcerations, warts, and moles, should be noted. Pay attention to their size, shape, and color, and bring them to the attention of your doctor. Also note any change in the texture and color of the skin. Special attention should be given to pigmented areas. Don't have an anxiety attack if you discover something unusual. Remember: Most changes are not malignant.*

the disease is widespread, large areas of vulvar skin may be removed and a skin graft is then used to re-cover the vulva. Untreated VIN may progress to vulvar cancer. Fortunately, progression occurs slowly. If you or your doctor regularly examines the vulva, there is a good chance of early detection.

Your doctor may also want to examine the vulva under magnification. Various dyes or acetic acid may be used to enhance the visibility of subtle areas of VIN or cancer. They direct your doctor to tissue that should be biopsied.

How is vulvar cancer treated?

Vulvar cancer develops within the skin covering the labia, clitoris, vestibule, perineum, and perianal areas. Most often it evolves from VIN (see the previous question). Vulvar cancer may emerge as a growth on the vulva but often appears as a change in skin color or texture. Alert your doctor to any change in the appearance of skin in the vulvar region.

When invasive cancer is detected during biopsy, more advanced surgery is necessary. The surgery removes the cancerous tissue along with some of the surrounding normal tissue. In more advanced cases, the entire vulva is removed (radical vulvectomy). Usually, lymph nodes near the groin are also removed. Complete removal of lymph nodes in the groin and upper leg has a significant potential for adverse effects such as lymphedema (swelling in the leg), persistent infections, and poor wound healing. Removing and examining only one or two "sentinel" nodes in the groin and upper leg (the first nodes likely to be involved with cancer) is an effective way to detect whether cancer has spread in women with early stage cancer of the vulva and has fewer adverse side effects. If lymph nodes are cancerous, radiation therapy will be needed to prevent recurrence or spread of the cancer. Doctors may employ chemotherapy for widespread disease.

Early detection of vulvar cancer has an excellent prognosis. Ninety percent of patients with small lesions (defined as less than 2 cm in size) and no enlargement of lymph nodes will survive. This confirms the benefit of self-examination mentioned earlier.

Another form of cancer seen on the vulva is Paget's disease, which is a type of skin cancer. Symptoms include persistent soreness and itching. The skin may appear thick and whitened or have well-demarcated red patches.

Malignant melanoma is a skin cancer that arises in pigmented areas of skin. Many women have a pigmented area or mole present on the vulvar skin. Any change in the size, shape, or color of such an area needs prompt medical attention. Melanomas are treated with radical vulvectomy and removal of lymph nodes.

Can you get vaginal cancer?

Yes, but it is uncommon. The doctor examines the vagina during a pelvic examination. If there is an abnormality, he or she will obtain a Pap smear or biopsy. Precancerous changes are treated conservatively with local surgery or laser vaporization. Treatment of invasive cancer is similar to that used for cervical cancer if it is located in the upper vagina and similar to the treatment for vulvar cancer if it is found in the lower vagina.

Historically, gynecologists performed vaginal Pap smears every three to five years in women who underwent a hysterectomy. Since primary vaginal cancer is rare, gynecologists currently obtain vaginal Pap smears only on women who underwent their hysterectomy for the treatment of cervical or endometrial cancer.

For more information on vulvar or vaginal cancer, visit:

National Cancer Institute: www.cancer.gov/cancertopics/types/vulvar

www.cancer.gov/cancertopics/types/vaginal

American Cancer Society: www.cancer.org/Cancer/VulvarCancer/index

12

PROBLEMS OF THE BREAST

Why do my breasts hurt?

Dr. Spencer enters the exam room to see Trudy for her annual visit.

"Hi, Trudy, how are you today?" begins Dr. Spencer. "Is it hot enough out there for you? There's nothing like Philadelphia in July."

"Yeah, it's terrible out there," responds Trudy. "Of course in here it feels like you're chilling a Chardonnay."

"I know," acknowledges Dr. Spencer. "There's nothing worse than a freezing room when you have to take off all your clothes. Unfortunately, we don't have much control over the temperature in this building. So are there any issues you would like to discuss today?"

"Yes, my left breast has been hurting on the outside," Trudy says as she reaches over to show Dr. Spencer the location of her pain. "There must be something wrong."

Dr. Spencer has Trudy raise her arms over her head as he examines her breasts. There is nothing particularly impressive found on the exam. "Actually, your breast is probably fine. I don't feel anything remarkable. Breast tenderness is very common. More than half of the women coming in today will tell me that they have tenderness in one or both breasts. We get accustomed to thinking that pain must be a reflection of something terribly wrong, but this is not usually the case when it comes to your breasts. You're likely to have an area of fibrocystic change where it is tender, but tenderness in and of itself is not really a sign of breast cancer, which is what most women worry about when they get pain in their breast. We can have you get a diagnostic mammogram on that side and add a breast ultrasound, but more than likely everything will turn out fine."

This may be the most frequently raised question in this entire book! Most women will ask it at one time or another. We are conditioned to assume that tenderness and pain reflect an abnormal condition that warrants further investigation. Women assume that something must be wrong if the breasts hurt. However, pain and tenderness in the breasts (mastalgia) are quite common and only rarely reflect an ominous situation.

The exact cause of breast tenderness is unclear, although it appears to result primarily from an exaggerated response of breast tissue to the female hormones estrogen and progesterone. Normal breast tissue is composed of glands, ducts, fat, and fibrous tissue. The glands may become cystic (enlarged and full of fluid), and nodules of fibrous tissue can form within the breast. When these changes are very pronounced, doctors often label the condition fibrocystic breast disease (FBD). Since this is not really a disease, most physicians now refer to the condition as fibrocystic breasts or fibrocystic breast changes. There are different variations of fibrocystic breasts, depending on microscopic appearance.

You will experience fibrocystic breasts as pain and tenderness associated with an increase in lumpiness. The condition usually worsens premenstrually. This is why you should examine your breasts and have mammograms early in your menstrual cycle. The changes may be localized to a specific area within your breast or involve the entire breast. Fibrocystic changes may be present in one or both breasts. Fibrocystic breast changes may regress along with the breast discomfort after menopause. Hormone replacement therapy will tend to aggravate symptoms related to fibrocystic breasts.

Many approaches have been used to reduce breast tenderness associated with fibrocystic breasts. Reducing nicotine, caffeine (coffee, tea, cola, and chocolate), and salt is often recommended by physicians. Supplemental vitamin E (800 units per day) and evening primrose oil (3,000 mg per day) are also frequently recommended. Most studies that have looked at caffeine reduction have concluded that there is little or no benefit. Likewise, studies looking at vitamin E and primrose oil are mixed, with some showing benefit and others not. However, anecdotal reports suggest that some women find these measures useful. Diindolylmethane (DIM 100–300mg per day) has also been shown to be an effective treatment for breast pain. Over-the-counter analgesics (Tylenol, Motrin, etc.) may provide some relief. Some studies indicate that fibrocystic breasts improve with the use of oral contraceptives. This certainly should be a consideration if you also need contraception. Other hormonal agents used to treat fibrocystic breasts include:

- Tamoxifen (an anti-estrogen used to prevent and treat breast cancer)
- Danazol (see page 170)
- Bromocriptine (also used to suppress lactation)

Each of these has side effects that limit their usefulness, but they should be considered if your discomfort is severe. Weight reduction through a healthy diet can help by decreasing body fat and breast size, and a well-fitting bra that provides good support will help by limiting breast motion.

Do fibrocystic breast changes increase your risk of breast cancer? Most doctors feel that fibrocystic changes in and of themselves do not increase your risk for breast cancer. If the fibrocystic changes are associated with hyperplasia (detected on biopsy), especially atypical hyperplasia, then your risk of breast cancer is increased by two to four times. Clearly fibrocystic breasts are more difficult to examine and are more difficult to interpret with mammography. Self breast exams are often not performed because "I feel lumps all the time and I don't know what I'm feeling." Detecting lumpiness increases your anxiety, and you stop examining yourself. You should try to examine yourself even if you can't interpret what you are feeling. Develop a mental image of your breasts. Describe to yourself the position and size of palpable nodules and ridges. Essentially, you create a topographical map of your breasts. After several months, you will have a good feel for the contours and texture of your breasts. If there is a change, you will be as likely to detect it as your doctor (see page 255 for more information on self-examination).

Are breast implants dangerous?

After getting the kids off to school, Dina and her neighbor Traci retreat to the kitchen for a cup of coffee, a ritual moment of relaxation they have shared since sending the kids off to kindergarten.

"I have some exciting news," Dina begins. "I've decided to get breast implants."

"You've got to be kidding," responds Traci.

"No, really. I've been thinking about this for awhile and I think I'm really going to do it."

"Did Dave put you up to this?" asks Traci, referring to her friend's husband.

"No, this is something that I want to do for myself. After nursing the three kids, my breasts are sagging."

"Your breasts look fine," reassures Traci.

"Sure, when I have my clothes on they look fine. Without clothes they look like a couple of deflated water balloons. I can't stand it when I see them in a mirror. We're not talking about porn star breasts. I just want them to look closer to the way they did before the children."

"Aren't breast implants dangerous?" asks Traci.

"I don't think so," Dina responds. "I have an appointment with a plastic surgeon next week. I'll ask him if they are safe."

Breast implants are used in breast augmentation (enlargement) surgery as well as reconstructive surgery following mastectomy (see below). Implants have an outer shell of silicone (similar in texture to a thick plastic freezer bag). It is filled with either silicone gel or saline (salt water). The implant should be placed under your chest wall muscles through a small incision.

Breast implants containing silicone gel have been placed in women for more than forty years. Liquid silicone from these implants can slowly leak through the outer shell, which may cause local tissue reaction around the implant. There is also concern that the silicone may travel to other areas in the body and cause problems. It was reported that silicone breast implants could induce the development of autoimmune diseases such as systemic lupus and rheumatoid arthritis. Because of these concerns, in 1992 the FDA placed limitations on the use of silicone gel implants.

Since 1992, studies have compared women with and without silicone gel implants. The results do not indicate a greater incidence of connective tissue or autoimmune disease in women with silicone gel implants. These diseases are more frequent in women than men. They are often diagnosed in the third or fourth decade of life, when insertion of implants is common. In 2006, the FDA reapproved the use of silicone gel implants for all women. Many women prefer this type of implant because it has a softer, more natural feel. A cohesive gel implant, also known as a "gummy bear" implant, has been developed to address the problem of leakage. Cohesive gel does not spread if there is a rupture in the outer shell of the implant.

Saline implants are also used for augmentation and breast reconstruction in place of silicone gel implants. Although they have a firm external shell of silicone, this does not seem to be a problem. Saline is totally nontoxic to your body, so there is no concern if the saline implant leaks or ruptures. It is unlikely that saline implants pose a substantial health risk.

The most common complication of breast augmentation is capsular contracture. In this condition, your body forms a hard fibrous capsule around the implant. This produces a firm breast that has lost its soft, natural texture. The breast may also be painful. Fortunately, improved implants and surgical techniques have decreased the frequency of this complication. When contracture is severe, a second operation may be required for correction of the problem, or the implant may have to be removed. Occasionally, decreased nipple sensitivity will occur after breast augmentation. A breast implant may also rupture or deflate. When this happens, it must be replaced to maintain breast symmetry. It also may be more difficult to visualize breast abnormalities with mammography after you have implants.

Can anything be done if my breasts are too large?

Exceptionally large breasts, referred to as macromastia, create numerous problems. They often produce a sense of heaviness and pain, particularly before a menstrual period. Large breasts cause shoulder, neck, and upper back strain with pain in those regions. Chronic skin irritation may develop in the folds under the breasts.

Reduction mammoplasty is a surgical procedure that reduces the volume of breast tissue. It can significantly improve the comfort and quality of life in women with exceptionally large breasts. However, there are drawbacks. Breast reduction involves rather extensive incisions in contrast to breast augmentation. Scar formation along these incision lines can be unsightly. Lactation and breast-feeding may not be possible following breast reduction surgery. There may also be decreased sensitivity of the nipples. Women may experience mammographic abnormalities as a result of the rearranged breast tissue. Nevertheless, the vast majority of women who undergo breast reduction surgery are pleased. The relief obtained appears to outweigh the shortcomings of this procedure.

I have a tender area in my breast. Does that mean I have cancer?

A tender area within the breast is usually a focal area of fibrocystic change. If a lump is palpated in the area, it is probably a cyst. This can be confirmed by ultrasound or aspiration in the office. Breast cancer is not typically associated with focal tenderness. It is more apt to present as a painless, hard lump. Other causes of tenderness include trauma, infectious mastitis, superficial phlebitis, and inflammatory breast cancers. Fibrocystic breasts do not appear inflamed (redness, heat, and swelling) and are not associated with fever. If you develop localized tenderness associated with either fever or inflammation, contact your doctor.

Why does the doctor want to aspirate my breast lump?

Jill is trying to keep herself from getting hysterical. She's in the shower and feels a lump in her right breast. Quickly she checks her left breast but, no, it's not her imagination. She definitely feels something in the right breast that isn't there on the left side. Anxiety gets the better of her. Does this mean she has cancer? It can't be. I'm only thirty-five. On the other hand, Luanne at church got breast cancer in her thirties. Oh my God, I have three children. What will happen to them if I die? Okay now, calm down. This doesn't have to be cancer. Let me call Dr. Pierson.

"Dr. Pierson's office. Can I help you?" asks the receptionist.

"This is Jill Harrington. I'm a patient of Dr. Pierson's. I feel a lump in my breast. When can she see me?" asks Jill, trying not to sound too panicked.

"Jill, this is very common and most of the time it will not turn out to be anything bad like cancer," reassures the receptionist. "But there is no problem with getting you in for something like this. We will add you on today after our regular hours so Dr. Pierson can see you."

"Thanks so much. I'll see you later." Jill tries to remain calm, but there is no way she will feel comfortable until this is resolved.

Later that day Dr. Pierson sees Jill. Jill has a well-defined 2 cm tender lump in the right breast. "Well, I think this is good news, Jill. A well-defined tender lump is usually a cyst. I'm going to send you for a breast ultrasound. Presuming this confirms that it is a cyst, we can either ignore it or aspirate the fluid, which will make it magically disappear and take away the tenderness."

Indeed, the ultrasound confirms the lump to be a cyst which is aspirated, resolving the issue. Jill finally begins to relax.

Most breast lumps are benign cysts. Your doctor may attempt to aspirate the lump to confirm that it is cystic. Once the fluid is aspirated, the lump should disappear. Occasionally, the fluid is sent to a laboratory for analysis. Cells in the fluid are evaluated microscopically for atypical features. Inability to aspirate fluid from the lump suggests that it is solid. Most solid lumps should be biopsied (see below). However, don't assume that the lump is cancerous if your doctor cannot aspirate fluid from it. The lump may represent a conglomeration of fibrocystic tissue, as opposed to an isolated cyst. It may also be a fibroadenoma, which is a benign, solid tumor of the breast. If a lump is confirmed to be a simple cyst on an ultrasound, there is no specific need to aspirate it. However, if the lump is bothersome, aspiration is certainly an easy fix of the problem. "Complicated" cysts (cysts that have particles in them on an ultrasound) are generally aspirated to confirm their benign nature.

What does discharge from the nipple indicate?

Nipple discharge is fairly common and usually not indicative of a severe problem. Almost half of women in their reproductive years can express a few drops of liquid from their breasts. In fact, squeezing the nipple during self breast exams is no longer encouraged by the American Cancer Society (although you should still look for spontaneous discharge and report it to your physician). Let's examine the significance of various types of nipple discharge.

A milky discharge from the nipple is normal during pregnancy. It is also seen for up to one year following the cessation of nursing. It is not commonly seen at other times. Milky discharge from the nipples (may be one or both) is referred to as galactorrhea. Usually, it is from inappropriate secretion of prolactin, the hormone responsible for breast milk production. Most of the time it is white or clear, although it may also appear yellow or green. When the color is yellow or green, consideration must be given to other breast diseases (see below).

Elevated prolactin in association with galactorrhea may be seen in the following situations:

- Use of birth control pills
- Use of certain medications—ask your doctor to check in the PDR (Physicians' Desk Reference) to see if it is listed as a side effect.
- Prolonged and intense suckling
- Conditions that stimulate the nerves of the chest wall (thereby simulating suckling) such as shingles, chest surgery, and upper spinal cord lesions
- Hypothyroidism—a decrease in circulating levels of thyroid hormone indirectly stimulates the secretion of prolactin.
- Central nervous system injuries or tumors that affect the pituitary gland—the pituitary gland is located at the base of the

brain and is responsible for the secretion of many important hormones including prolactin.

- Pituitary tumors—a prolactin secreting tumor can grow in the pituitary gland itself. Although it is a benign tumor, it can have disabling neurologic (affecting the brain), endocrinologic (hormonal), and ophthalmologic (affecting the eyes) consequences.

Your doctor will order a prolactin level if you have galactorrhea. Your doctor may also check your thyroid status. If the prolactin is elevated without explanation, he or she may order a scan to rule out a pituitary tumor. When a pituitary tumor is discovered, it can usually be treated with medication that inhibits prolactin secretion and shrinks the tumor. Bromocriptine (Parlodel) and Cabergoline (Dostinex) are two medications used for this purpose. Occasionally, surgery will be recommended for removal of the tumor.

Nipple discharge may also be purulent (pus), watery (clear), yellow, multicolored, or bloody (pink or red). Purulent discharge can be caused by a bacterial infection and is accompanied by pain, tenderness, redness, and swelling. Breast infection (mastitis) is most common after pregnancy (especially with nursing). Bloody discharge is of greater concern since it may be a sign of cancer. The rare occurrence of a profuse, crystal-clear discharge may also be associated with cancer. Not all bloody discharges are secondary to cancer. In fact, the most likely culprit for a bloody discharge is an intraductal papilloma. An intraductal papilloma is a benign growth located within one of the breast ducts, usually near the nipple. It may produce a discharge that is yellow or bloody. Ductal ectasia is an uncommon disease of the breast that causes nipple discharge. The discharge is usually non-bloody and may be multicolored (green, brown, grey, reddish-brown, yellow, or white). Ductal ectasia may present as thickening and inflammation around the nipple and areola (the darker skin surrounding the nipple), a breast mass, or an abscess. Fibrocystic breast changes may also produce nipple discharge (discussed above).

Further evaluation is necessary if you have a nipple discharge, particularly if it is bloody. Your doctor will examine your breasts for lumps and obtain a mammogram and ultrasound. Microscopic analysis of the fluid (cytology) may be performed. Some doctors use galactography, which demonstrates ducts by instilling contrast. An intraductal papilloma may be detected by exerting pressure circumferentially around the margin of the areola. When pressure is applied to the affected duct, discharge is expressed. There may be tenderness overlying the involved duct. A papilloma may be palpable, although this is less common.

The treatment of nipple discharge varies with the cause. Infectious mastitis is treated with antibiotics. Ductal ectasia is treated with antibiotics, ice packs, and anti-inflammatory drugs. Surgical excision may be required if the condition persists or a mass develops. Papillomas are excised through minor outpatient surgery. Findings suspicious for cancer are biopsied (discussed below).

Is there anything I can do to prevent breast cancer?

There are many risk factors for breast cancer. Most of these are beyond your control. There is an increased risk in women with a strong family history of breast cancer, but we don't get to choose our genes. The risk is also greater in women with an early menarche (age you started getting periods) or late menopause (cessation of periods). This is also beyond your control. There is an increased risk in women who delay childbearing since the breasts are not fully developed until after the first pregnancy. The earlier you have your first child, the lower your risk will be for breast cancer. Breast-feeding has also been associated with a decreased risk of developing breast cancer.

Nutritional risk factors are within your control. Your risk of breast cancer increases as the amount of total fat in your diet increases. It also increases with alcohol consumption (greater than three drinks per week). Several studies have shown an association between vitamin D deficiency and breast cancer. Supplementing your diet with 1000 IU of vitamin D may be of some benefit. There is a relationship between weight and breast cancer, especially in postmenopausal women. Maintaining a healthy diet that is low in fat and alcohol and high in fruits and vegetables may keep your weight down and reduce your risk of breast cancer. Vegetables containing indole-3-carbinol (broccoli, Brussels sprouts, cabbage, collard greens, cauliflower, kale, mustard greens, turnips, and rutabagas), a natural compound that appears to be anti-carcinogenic, may be of particular benefit. Indole-3-carbinol (400 mg daily) can also be taken as a supplement. Laboratory research suggests that this compound may help prevent certain cancers. However, keep in mind that there are no well-designed studies in humans to confirm this assessment. Regular exercise may also reduce your risk.

There is always controversy as to the role of estrogen and pro-gesterone in the development of breast cancer. There may be a small increase in the detection of localized breast cancer (confined to the breast) in current users of the birth control pill. However, this may be primarily explained by the fact that women using birth control pills are examined annually. If there is an increase, it disappears within ten years after stopping the pills. On the other hand, birth control pills clearly and substantially reduce your risk for both endometrial cancer and ovarian cancer. The role of menopausal hormone replacement therapy in the etiology of breast cancer remains more controversial. The best current evidence indicates a small excess risk of breast cancer with hormone replacement therapy, especially if a synthetic proges-terone is included in the regimen (see chapter 13).

Women who are at high risk for breast cancer can use hormonal chemoprevention to reduce their risk of breast cancer by approximately 50 percent. Tamoxifen, raloxifene (Evista), and exemestane (Aromasin) are all used for this purpose. A gynecologist, breast surgeon, medical oncologist, or genetic counselor can calculate your lifetime risk for breast cancer. If your lifetime risk for breast cancer is greater than 20 percent, chemoprevention should be at least considered. Your doctor can review the side effects for each of these medications.

Is my risk of breast cancer increased if my mother had breast cancer? When should I get genetic testing?

Family history is definitely important in assessing your risk of breast cancer. If you have a first degree relative (mother or sister) who develops breast cancer, your risk may be doubled. This is particularly true if the cancer presented before menopause. Inherited breast cancer generally presents at a younger age than nonfamilial cancer. If there are multiple female members of your family with either breast or ovarian cancer, your risk may be 50 percent or higher. The inherited tendency can be transmitted through the maternal or paternal side of your family through various gene mutations, the most common being BRCA1 and BRCA2 mutations. Genetic testing is available to screen men and women for these abnormalities. Genetic testing is generally recommended in each of the following situations:

- A woman who develops breast cancer under the age of forty or under the age of fifty if there are other family members who have had breast or ovarian cancer
- A personal history of ovarian cancer (especially if presenting at a young age) or family history of ovarian cancer in multiple relatives
- A family history that includes two first degree relatives with breast cancer or three or more first and second degree relatives
- A family history of male breast cancer
- A personal history of bilateral breast cancer
- A person of Ashkenazi Jewish background (Eastern European) with a family history of anyone developing breast or ovarian cancer
- A person who has a relative test positive for a BRCA1 or BRCA2 mutation
- A family history of malignant melanoma and pancreatic cancer
- A patient who has a "triple negative" breast cancer (see below)

What can you do if it is determined that you have a BRCA1 or BRCA2 mutation? Self breast exams should be done monthly and breast exams by a qualified healthcare provider should be performed every six months. Annual mammography, breast MRI, or both should begin at an early age (determined by the age at which breast cancer developed in your relatives, but no later than age twenty-five to thirty). Risk reduction mastectomy (removal of both breasts) should be considered, especially in women with a BRCA1 or BRAC2 mutation which convey a 45–70 percent lifetime risk for breast cancer. This reduces the risk of breast cancer, but does not eliminate it because surgery may leave behind breast tissue along the chest wall. Studies indicate that risk reduction mastectomy does decrease your risk by more than 90 percent. Nipple-sparing mastectomy, new breast reconstruction techniques, and improvements in implants have made this a more acceptable option. Use of anti-estrogen therapies like tamoxifen, raloxifene, and exemestane can also be considered to reduce the risk. Unfortunately, women with BRCA1 and BRCA2 genetic mutations have a higher incidence of developing "triple negative" breast cancers. These cancers do not test positive for estrogen receptors and are not prevented with anti-estrogen therapy. Prophylactic removal of your ovaries and tubes should be undertaken after childbearing is complete, usually between ages thirty-five and forty, because BRCA1 and BRCA2 mutations dramatically increase your risk for ovarian cancer (up to a 30–50 percent lifetime risk). Your hormones can be temporarily replaced until you are closer to the natural age of menopause. Birth control pills are also used in premenopausal patients to reduce their risk of ovarian cancer.

BRCA Positive
Three Different Responses

Lexi is a thirty-five-year-old dynamo. She is a "can-do" woman who aggressively and assertively tackles any hurdle life places before her. Her mother developed breast cancer at age fifty-four. Lexi has not been overly concerned about her mother's breast cancer. After all, it was discovered early and her mother has now been a survivor for twenty years. However, when her older sister Judy develops breast cancer at age forty-one, she tests positive for a BRCA1 mutation. Lexi immediately goes for testing herself and is found to have the same BRCA1 mutation. Her uncompromising nature kicks into high gear. This mutation will not get the best of her. Lexi decides to undergo a bilateral mastectomy with reconstruction. She has her tubes and ovaries removed laparoscopically and starts hormone replacement therapy to prevent premature menopause.

Darci is a fifty-two-year-old postmenopausal woman. Her mother died of breast cancer in her sixties. She has never had much contact with her mother's relatives because they live in Germany. However, more recently her brother Ted developed an interest in genealogy. He discovers that their mother had a sister who developed breast cancer and that Darci's maternal grandmother died from cancer that spread throughout the abdomen. The information on this is limited, but there is a suggestion that the cancer started "in the female pelvic organs." Darci is not overly inclined to pursue this further, but she also doesn't want to be left in the dark, so she decides to see a genetic counselor. The counselor recommends genetic testing and Darci tests positive for a BRCA2 mutation. She consults a breast surgeon, but is not willing to accept the removal of her breasts.

Darci decides to undergo laparoscopic removal of her tubes and ovaries. After all, they're not functioning at this point. However, losing her breasts is a different story. After discussing her options with the breast surgeon and a medical oncologist, she decides to go on tamoxifen to lower her risk of breast cancer. She agrees to get mammograms and breast MRI imaging on an annual basis staggering the two at six month intervals. She will be more diligent at self breast examination and will have the breast surgeon perform a breast exam every six months. She also commits to a lifestyle that maximizes risk reduction.

Lilly is a forty-year-old artist who spins beautiful pottery creations. Lilly does not interact with the traditional healthcare community and has always felt more comfortable embracing a holistic, natural approach to her health. She knows that there is a strong family history of breast cancer, but does not think that it will affect her. After all, she's not like her other relatives who abuse their bodies. Lilly exercises regularly, doesn't smoke, avoids alcohol, and only eats organic, vegetarian food. One day, her teenage daughter Pella comprises a family tree for her social studies class. Pella discovers that many of her great aunts died at an early age from breast cancer, as did her grandmother. She searches the Internet and discovers material on hereditary breast and ovarian cancer syndrome. Quite upset, she confronts her mother, but Lilly is not concerned. After all, she seems to take after her father, not her mother, and her mother never really took care of herself the way Lilly does. Lilly does not want to get genetic testing. Five years go by before Pella gets the best of her mother. Pella insists that she has the right to know if her mother has a mutation because it may also affect her. Finally Lilly's maternal instinct, or maybe just guilt, gets the better of her and she gets genetic testing. She is found to have a BRCA1 mutation. She is not, however, willing to use any artificial means to prevent the development of cancer. She will continue to exercise, keep her weight down, avoid alcohol, and eat vegetarian, all of which decrease the risk of breast cancer. She sees a holistic practitioner who places her on indole-3-carbinol supplements. She will perform self breast exams and assures Pella that if she finds a lump, she will get it evaluated. Pella is also tested and fortunately tests negative for the BRCA mutation.

How can I tell if I have breast cancer?

There are no symptoms associated with early breast cancer. Early detection is only possible with self breast exams, exams performed by qualified healthcare providers, and screening mammograms (with or without other imaging techniques). The most common physical finding is a painless, hard lump. If you or your physician detects a lump, it must be investigated (see below), even if your mammogram is normal. Other signs include the following:

- *Discharge from your nipple, particularly if it is bloody*: However, remember that most bloody discharges are from intraductal papillomas, which are not cancerous. Don't panic!
- *Nipple inversion*: If your nipples normally point outward, nipple inversion (a nipple pulled inward) is considered ominous. This does not apply to women with chronically inverted nipples.
- *Particular skin changes*: Sometimes the skin overlying a breast cancer develops the texture of an orange peel (called *peau d'orange*). Dimpling of the skin may be caused by an underlying cancer. Finally, inflammatory cancers may cause the breast to appear red and swollen, although there are non-cancerous conditions that also present with inflammation.
- *A lump in your axilla (armpit)*: This may reflect an enlarged lymph node from breast cancer.

You should perform self breast examinations monthly. Premenopausal women should do the exam early in their cycle to avoid the increased lumpiness and tenderness experienced premenstrually. Lie on your back and place one arm over your head. With your other arm, reach over and examine your breast. You should use a pattern such as concentric circles to ensure that no area of the breast is missed. Include the armpits in your examination. Keep your fingers flat and the pressure light to maximize your ability to sense changes in the breast tissue. Perform the same procedure on the opposite breast. Some women find the examination easier in the shower or bath when your skin is wet and slippery. Ideally, you should perform the exam in upright and recumbent positions.

The next part of the exam is visual inspection. Stand in front of a mirror with your arms behind your head. Look for any changes in the size or shape of your breasts. Identify any change in the skin texture or color as well as any dimpling of the skin. Make sure there is no inversion of the nipples. If there is any discharge, note its color.

Remember that the primary responsibility for your health rests with you. Any abnormalities should be brought to the doctor's attention. The survival rate with early breast cancer is excellent. Self breast exams, coupled with physician exams and mammography, provide you with an excellent chance for early detection.

When is a breast biopsy necessary?

Most solid lumps should be biopsied or removed. If it has a non-cancerous appearance on mammography, your physician may choose to follow it with frequent examinations and mammography. However, most doctors will recommend biopsy. Scattered calcifications (calcium deposits) in breast tissue are common and usually do not warrant biopsy. However, suspicious clusters of microcalcifications (very tiny calcifications) are biopsied. If a lump is cystic, a biopsy is not usually necessary. Biopsies can be performed in several different ways.

Fine needle aspiration is a procedure done in the office with a syringe and needle. It is only done if the doctor can feel a discrete lump. The doctor passes a needle through the lump several times while aspirating. This collects cells that are then analyzed for cancer. The reliability of this varies tremendously, depending on the doctor's level of experience. Fine needle aspiration collects cells, but not an actual piece of tissue (in distinction to those techniques described below).

Core needle biopsy is a procedure that collects breast tissue in the core of a large needle. If the mass is not palpable (cannot be felt during your exam), stereotactic core biopsy can be performed under radiologic guidance. You lie prone on a table with the breast extended through an opening in the table. The suspicious area is identified through imaging. A radiologist or breast specialist advances the biopsy needle to the abnormal spot and the needle collects tissue for analysis. Core needle biopsy may also be performed under ultrasound (using sound waves to image your breast) or MRI guidance.

Open biopsy is performed in the operating room as an outpatient. If a lump is palpable, an incision is made and the lump removed entirely (excisional biopsy) or partially (incisional biopsy). If the lump is not palpable, a needle is first placed into the mass under radiologic guidance. The surgeon can then follow the needle down to the mass or other suspicious areas seen on mammography.

Your doctor may choose any of the above methods to evaluate a breast abnormality. The current consensus among breast cancer specialists is for using minimally invasive core needle biopsies for initial diagnosis. If excisional biopsy is recommended, it is reasonable for you to ask why a minimally invasive biopsy is not possible.

Do I need to have my entire breast removed if there is cancer?

Surgery has undergone quite an evolution over the past century. Dr. William S. Halsted devised the radical mastectomy and reported his success with this procedure in 1894. A radical mastectomy removes all the breast tissue, along with the overlying skin and underlying muscles. The axillary lymph nodes are also removed. Radical mastectomy remained the treatment of choice until the 1970s. Earlier diagnosis of breast cancer emerged with the use of self breast exams, physician exams, and mammography. It became evident that less radical surgery could be successful. This led to a shift toward the modified radical mastectomy that preserves the pectoralis muscle (the large muscle in the front of the chest, under the breast). More recently, studies indicated that often the breast can be conserved. If the breast cancer is early and does not appear to be multicentric (arising from multiple areas within the breast), it can be removed while preserving the rest of the breast. This is referred to as a lumpectomy. A lumpectomy is usually followed by radiation (see below) of the remaining breast tissue. Breast-conserving surgery is not indicated in all cases. You must discuss this with your doctor to see if it is a reasonable choice.

Mastectomy vs. Lumpectomy

Lumpectomy followed by radiation is likely to be equally effective as mastectomy for women with only one site of cancer in the breast and a tumor under 4 cm, presuming the margins are clear (no cancer cells in the tissue surrounding the tumor). Presuming you meet the above criteria, the following factors may enter into the decision that you and your surgeon make regarding the surgical approach for your cancer:

Do you want to conserve your natural breast? Lumpectomy offers the advantage of preserving much of the appearance and sensation of your breast. However, in cases where there will be great distortion of the breast with lumpectomy, mastectomy with reconstruction may be a better choice.

Do you want your breasts to match as much as possible in size? Your surgeon can assess how much distortion will occur from a lumpectomy and can discuss with you the reconstructive options available for lumpectomy, when there will be significant distortion, and mastectomy.

How anxious you are about cancer returning in the same breast. The risk of local recurrence of your cancer is slightly higher after lumpectomy. This does not tend to decrease your likelihood of survival since a mastectomy can be performed if there is local recurrence in the same breast.

Your feelings about radiation. You are likely to need anywhere from five days to seven weeks of radiation therapy (five days per week) after lumpectomy. Radiation may create its own cosmetic distortions, such as changing the texture of the breast and the color and texture of skin overlying the breast. Radiation therapy may also affect the timing of reconstructive procedures and may limit your reconstructive options. There are shorter, more localized radiation treatments that have less likelihood of causing breast distortion (see below), but these are not universally available at this time and are still investigational.

Your feelings about surgery. A mastectomy takes longer and is more extensive than a lumpectomy. Mastectomy requires a longer recuperation and has a greater potential for post-surgery side effects. More surgery will be required if reconstruction is chosen after mastectomy.

Where you live; where you go for treatment; when and where your surgeon was trained. Mastectomies are more common in the Midwestern and southern parts of the United States compared with other regions in the country. Lumpectomies are more commonly performed in university-based hospitals than community hospitals.

In the past, dissection and removal of the lymph nodes under your axilla (armpit) accompanied either a mastectomy or lumpectomy. This axillary dissection of lymph nodes was crucial in determining the risk of metastasis (spread of the cancer). The status of the lymph nodes is also important when choosing additional therapy after the surgery. Sentinel node biopsy is a newer approach used for assessing lymph nodes. A radioisotope or dye is injected into the breast. It is followed to the first lymph node(s), referred to as the sentinel node(s). A small incision is made to excise this node, or grouping of nodes, and if there is no cancer, further lymph node dissection is avoided. This has proven to be reliable and is a great asset since lymph node dissection can create axillary scarring, pain, and swelling in the arm.

I hear they can reconstruct your breast. Is that true?

Breast reconstruction is a major advance in the rehabilitation of patients undergoing mastectomy. Breast conservation surgery (lumpectomy) is not always possible. Loss of your breast can be psychologically devastating. A woman may feel deformed, resulting in low self-esteem. Thirty to forty percent of women report a loss of sexual desire or reduction in arousal following mastectomy. This is not because of marital estrangement. Most relationships remain intact and, on occasion, even strengthen. The disruption in sexual functioning is more a product of your body image and the perception of disfigurement that accompanies mastectomy. Breast reconstruction re-creates the breast and restores a woman's sense of femininity and sexuality.

Traditionally, breast reconstruction was delayed until it was determined that there was little risk of recurrence. There was also concern that reconstruction would interfere with the detection of local recurrences. This has not been found to be true. Breast reconstruction can often be performed immediately following the mastectomy, thereby limiting you to one hospitalization. Reconstruction may involve the placement of an implant, or reconstruction of a breast from muscles and skin rotated onto the chest from your back or abdomen. Not all physicians agree that immediate reconstruction is best. They feel your risk of surgical infection is increased and your recuperation delayed. Not every woman is a candidate for immediate reconstruction, but you should certainly discuss it with your physician before your mastectomy.

Not all women perceive mastectomy as disfiguring. You may feel comfortable wearing an external prosthesis. This is certainly reasonable and has the advantage of decreasing the amount of surgery. You can always change your mind and undergo breast reconstruction later.

Why do I need radiation therapy after a lumpectomy?

Cancer cells can be present in the breast tissue surrounding the lumpectomy site. These cells can create a local recurrence or enter your lymphatic system or bloodstream and create recurrence of the cancer elsewhere in the body. Radiation is given to eradicate cancer cells remaining in the breast after lumpectomy. Over the past three decades, the most common method of administering radiation has been through an external beam directed at the entire breast. The radiation is administered daily over a period of five to seven weeks and is usually well tolerated. You may experience some degree of fatigue over the course of treatment. Local effects include skin changes (dryness, redness, or tanning), swelling, and muscle stiffness. Most effects from the radiation resolve within a few weeks after the completion of treatment, although swelling, hardness, and skin discoloration may persist longer. Severe complications from radiation can occur, but are rare. Some facilities may use accelerated whole breast irradiation, which delivers a higher dose of radiation over a shorter period of time, ranging anywhere from one to three weeks. More recently, some facilities have started to use accelerated partial breast irradiation

(APBI), which only delivers radiation to the lumpectomy site and a small amount of surrounding normal tissue. The radiation can be delivered through a balloon catheter (ex. MammoSite) that your surgeon places into the cavity remaining after your lumpectomy, or it can be delivered through a series of catheters that are placed in rows or bundles into the lumpectomy site. Radiation is delivered over five to seven days and then the catheter(s) is removed. Partial breast irradiation avoids damage to the skin, pectoralis muscle (under your breast), and chest. There is also less potential for a change in the shape or texture of your breast when compared with whole breast radiation. Not everyone is a candidate for APBI. You will have to check with your breast surgeon or oncologist to see if you are a candidate. Another recent advance in breast irradiation is intraoperative breast irradiation. Radiation is delivered in the operating room at the time of your lumpectomy. This is certainly the most convenient way of receiving your radiation, but long-term studies will be needed to see if this achieves the same results as more traditional approaches.

Radiation therapy may also be recommended after mastectomy to destroy any breast cancer cells that remain at the mastectomy site. During breast removal, it's difficult to take out every cell of breast tissue, especially the tissue behind the skin in the front of the breast or back along the muscle behind the breast. The following high-risk factors may lead your doctor to recommend radiation treatment after mastectomy:

- The cancer is 5 cm or larger (the cancer can be one lump, a series of lumps, or even microscopic clumps that together are 5 cm or larger)
- The cancer has invaded the lymph channels and blood vessels in the breast
- The removed tissue has a positive margin of resection
- More than three lymph nodes are involved or there is extracapsular extension, which indicates that cancer cells are moving beyond the lymph nodes

- The cancer invades the skin (with locally advanced or inflammatory breast cancer)

Based on these risks, about 20–30 percent of people are considered at high risk for recurrence after mastectomy and radiation would be recommended.

When is chemotherapy necessary?

Some women with very early breast cancer can be treated with surgery alone or lumpectomy with radiation (see above). However, many women will receive chemotherapy after their surgery for breast cancer. Microscopic cancer cells can travel to other areas of the body, even when it appears that the cancer is confined to the breast. These cells cause recurrence of the cancer if they are not treated. Doctors try to look at the "biological behavior" of individual cancers to determine the need for chemotherapy. Breast cancer in premenopausal women can spread quickly if not treated aggressively. Most premenopausal women will receive chemotherapy as part of their treatment regimen. Postmenopausal women who have estrogen receptor negative tumors (ER–, see below) may also receive chemotherapy. Even estrogen receptor positive (ER+) cancers may be treated with chemotherapy if they are advanced at the time of diagnosis. Your surgeon will consult a medical oncologist for help in deciding whether chemotherapy or hormonal therapy is necessary. Tests like Oncotype DX and MammaPrint can help your oncologist decide whether an early stage cancer warrants additional treatment with chemotherapy.

Occasionally, "neoadjuvant" chemotherapy is started before surgery. This is usually done when the cancerous lump is large and it is suspected that cancer cells have already spread beyond the breast. The preoperative chemotherapy may shrink the size of the lump, therefore allowing more conservative surgery.

Chemotherapy is usually given for four to six months, but may be given longer when treating advanced disease. Side effects from chemotherapy vary, depending on what agent is used. The most common side effects are nausea, vomiting, and hair loss. Medications are given to control the nausea. Most chemotherapeutic agents suppress your bone marrow, which makes your blood cells, so these drugs can lead to anemia and poor blood clotting and can make you more susceptible to infections. During chemotherapy, your blood counts are monitored closely, and sometimes special drugs are administered to boost the bone marrow.

Targeted therapy, using a drug called Herceptin (trastuzumab), may also be a part of your treatment regimen. HER2 receptors tell cells to grow and divide. In some breast cancers, HER2 is overexpressed (the cancer cells have many more HER2 receptors than usual). Herceptin is then given to selectively bind to these receptors, thereby stopping cell growth.

What is hormonal therapy?

"So what's this estrogen receptor stuff all about?" Your cancer will be tested to see if there are estrogen and progesterone receptors on the surface of the cancer cells. If your cancer is ER+, an anti-estrogen called tamoxifen (Nolvadex) may be given to decrease your risk of recurrence. Tamoxifen has typically been given for five years, but recent research demonstrates additional benefits when its use is extended to ten years. Side effects are usually mild and do not require discontinuation of therapy. The most common adverse reactions include hot flashes, nausea and vomiting, menstrual irregularities (in premenopausal women), vaginal discharge, and skin rash.

Tamoxifen does have risks associated with its use. There is a small increased risk of thrombophlebitis (blood clots in your veins). You are also more likely to develop endometrial polyps and endometrial cancer when treated with tamoxifen. Tamoxifen acts as an anti-estrogen with breast tissue, but similar to estrogen with endometrial tissue. This may seem quite disturbing. "What are they trying to do, trade one cancer for another?" Fortunately, most endometrial cancers bleed while still early and are curable with hysterectomy. If you are on tamoxifen and experience abnormal bleeding or any bleeding after menopause, tell your gynecologist, who will then investigate in order to rule out an endometrial polyp or cancer. The small possibility of endometrial cancer should not deter you from using tamoxifen. The benefit in reducing your risk of breast cancer recurrence clearly outweighs the small risk for endometrial cancer. Since tamoxifen binds to estrogen receptors elsewhere, investigators have also looked at its potential impact on the heart and bones. It appears to protect against osteoporosis and have no adverse cardiovascular impact.

More recently, oncologists have used a newer class of medications called aromatase inhibitors (Femara, Arimidex, Aromasin) in the treatment of estrogen receptor positive breast cancer in postmenopausal women. In postmenopausal women, estrogen is no longer made by the ovaries but is still made in fatty tissues elsewhere in the body. Studies have shown that obese women have a higher risk of recurrence of ER+ tumors. This may be caused by excess estrogen production from their fat stores. Aromatase inhibitors block this estrogen production effectively. There is evidence that aromatase inhibitors are more effective than tamoxifen. Often they are given to the postmenopausal patient in place of tamoxifen. Some oncologists may still give tamoxifen for five years and then add an aromatase inhibitor for another five years. Because aromatase inhibitors do not inhibit estrogen production from the ovaries and can stimulate ovarian cyst formation, they are not used in premenopausal women unless their ovaries are removed or chemically suppressed. Adverse effects of aromatase inhibitors include joint pain or inflammation, osteoporosis (bone loss), hypercholesterolemia (high blood cholesterol), and vaginal atrophy (thinning and dryness of the walls of the vagina). Cholesterol and bone density levels can be monitored during therapy and abnormal findings treated if necessary.

A Typical Breast Cancer Patient??

We begin this with a double question mark because in reality there is no such thing as a "typical" patient. Every woman presents with a unique set of factors and circumstances that will influence the course of her cancer treatment. Having said that, Jean's cancer care illustrates many of the elements described in this chapter.

Jean is a woman who turned sixty a few months ago. She has generally taken good care of herself. She eats a more healthy diet than most, doesn't smoke or abuse alcohol, and exercises a fair amount. She has always had normal breast exams and normal mammograms, until now. This time her mammogram suggests a breast density. She returns for additional views of the breast and a breast ultrasound, which confirms that there is a suspicious area. Her gynecologist sends her to Dr. Capshaw, a surgeon who specializes in breast cancer. After reviewing the films, Dr. Capshaw agrees with the radiologist and recommends a core needle biopsy under ultrasound guidance. The biopsy returns showing an invasive ductal breast cancer. The pathology specimen is tested and found to be positive for estrogen receptors and progesterone receptors and negative for HER2 receptors.

Dr. Capshaw discusses the results with Jean. The cancer appears to be relatively small at 1 cm and the pathology report does not indicate any aggressive characteristics, so Jean and Dr. Capshaw decide to perform a lumpectomy with a sentinel node biopsy. At the same time, Dr. Capshaw refers Jean to a nurse navigator who will help Jean coordinate additional appointments with a radiation oncologist and medical oncologist. The nurse navigator will also provide Jean with educational materials, access to support groups, and access to other organizations such as the American Cancer Society, which may be helpful in providing additional services.

Jean undergoes her lumpectomy without any complications and two sentinel nodes are negative. She then sees Dr. Punjab, the radiation oncologist. He explains to her that she will undergo five weeks of external radiation to the breast in order to eliminate any remaining cancer cells, and she agrees.

She also sees Dr. Marsalis, the medical oncologist. He recommends that she begin anti-estrogen hormonal treatment with Femara, an aromatase inhibitor. He explains that Femara may have side effects including joint pain, vaginal irritation, and bone loss. However, if tolerated, it will significantly reduce her risk of the cancer returning. Dr. Marsalis also has the pathology department send her breast tissue out for a relatively new test, Oncotype DX, which will help them decide if her cancer is likely to be aggressive. If the score is high, Dr. Marsalis would recommend that Jean consider chemotherapy. Fortunately, Jean's score indicates that she is at a low risk for recurrence.

Jean will continue to follow up with her various doctors on a regular basis. They will perform regular breast exams and she is also instructed to perform self breast exams. She will continue with mammograms on a regular basis and breast MRI exams may also be recommended. Because her cancer was early, no other imaging procedures will be performed at this time. However, additional imaging will be performed if she develops any symptoms that may be associated with metastatic breast cancer (ex. chest or abdominal or bone pain, shortness of breath, a new lump).

Jean is still upset that she developed breast cancer. However, she is thankful that her care progressed relatively smoothly and is thankful that her cancer was diagnosed early and does not have aggressive characteristics. She feels assured that her chances of survival are very good.

I was told I have CIS. Is that the same as breast cancer?

There are two types of CIS. Lobular carcinoma in situ (LCIS) means that abnormal cells are growing in the lobules, or milk-producing glands, at the end of breast ducts. "In situ" means that the abnormal growth remains inside the lobule and does not spread to surrounding tissues. Despite the fact that its name includes the word *carcinoma*, LCIS is not a breast cancer and it does not directly progress into cancer. However, it is an indicator that a person is at a higher-than-average risk for developing invasive breast cancer in the future. Patients with this condition should be followed more closely and breast MRI should be included in their surveillance. They should consider chemoprevention with tamoxifen, raloxifene, or exemestane which will decrease their risk for developing breast cancer.

Ductal carcinoma in situ (DCIS) is a noninvasive ductal breast cancer, meaning breast cancer that remains in the duct and hasn't spread to surrounding tissues. However, unlike LCIS, DCIS is an obligate precursor to invasive breast cancer and therefore requires treatment. The most common treatment for DCIS is lumpectomy and radiation. If the tissue tests positive for estrogen receptors, then anti-estrogen hormonal therapy may also be given. If the DCIS is large or multifocal (found in more than one spot), mastectomy may be recommended. Chemotherapy is not given with DCIS because it has not invaded other tissues. DCIS spans a spectrum from indolent grade 1 DCIS (the cells are closer in appearance to normal breast cells and grow slower) to high grade III DCIS (the cells look more atypical or bizarre and grow faster) and treatment is tailored appropriately.

How do you treat breast cancer that has spread to other parts of the body?

Perhaps the worst fear that women harbor is the fear that their cancer has spread beyond the breast to other places in the body. In the not-too-distant past, only 10 percent of women were still alive five years after the progression of metastatic cancer into places like the bones, lungs, or liver. However, with the development of new, targeted drugs, as many as 40 percent of women with recurrent or metastatic breast cancer survive at least five years.

The approach to metastatic breast cancer will vary depending on one's receptor status. If the metastatic cancer is ER+, then hormonal treatment like tamoxifen or one of the aromatase inhibitors (see above) will be given. Herceptin will be used to specifically target cells that overexpress the HER2 protein, something that happens in about one of every four breast cancers. Chemotherapy will be used for the ER– and HER– cancers.

Chemotherapy for metastatic disease is different from the aggressive regimens used for early stage breast cancer. Early stage breast cancer is often treated with relatively high doses of multiple chemotherapeutic drugs. For metastatic cancer, oncologists usually prefer to use sequential single-agent chemotherapy. Their goal is obtaining enough of a response rate to control the tumor while having minimal impact on the quality of a woman's life. Newer treatment approaches have reduced the often painful symptoms of the disease. Supportive care has gotten a lot better so that the symptoms that people have from treatments and progression of the disease are much more controlled. In addition to chemotherapy, adjunctive drugs may be given. The most common examples of this are bisphosphonates (Aredia, Zometa, Reclast). These drugs are normally used to prevent and treat osteoporosis. In metastatic cancer patients, they slow down damaging metastatic bone disease that leads to fractures. Occasionally, radiation or surgery may be used to treat metastatic disease located in a specific localized area.

Coping with the uncertainty of life with metastatic breast cancer affects different women in different ways. Some women want to continue working full-time for as long as possible, which often helps keep their focus away from the illness. Other women say, "Okay, since I may have a limited amount of time, I don't want to spend it in my office. I'd rather travel, enjoy my hobbies, and spend time with my family." Everyone has different priorities, and there is no one right answer for coping with metastatic breast cancer. Many women will obtain support from counselors, therapists, or group therapy sessions, which can usually be found through cancer centers. Women can also find support online at web-based support groups such as BCMets (www.bcmets.org), one of the oldest and largest. One of the most important things for women with metastatic breast cancer to remember is that there is always exciting progress being made through research in this field. Approaches being worked on now may be something available to you in the near future. While there are no guarantees, this is certainly possible.

If you have breast cancer and would like additional information or support, contact the following resources:

BreastCancer.org: www.breastcancer.org

Reach to Recovery, American Cancer Society: www.cancer.org/Treatment/SupportProgramsServices/ reach-to-recovery

Y-Me National Organization for Breast Cancer Information and Support: www.Y-me.org

National Cancer Institute: www.cancer.gov/cancertopics/types/ breast

Bright Pink: www.brightpink.org

American Society of Clinical Oncology: www.cancer.net/patient/ Cancer+Type/Breast+Cancer

American Society of Breast Surgeons: www.breastsurgeons.org

13

MENOPAUSE AND HORMONE REPLACEMENT: THE GREAT DEBATE

When will I reach menopause?

As forty rolls by, thoughts turn to menopause. There is an assumption that menopause is just around the corner. Half of the women asking this question are looking forward to menopause and getting rid of "that damn period." The other half are dreading its arrival. The average age of menopause is fifty-one. The majority of women will completely cease menstruation between ages forty-eight and fifty-five. However, it is not rare for a woman to stop menstruating as early as forty or to persist into her late fifties. There does appear to be a correlation with the age of your mother's menopause. If you begin to skip periods and start to develop hot flashes or night sweats, menopause is approaching. At this point you are considered perimenopausal. Menopause is the complete cessation of periods for one year.

Why do I have trouble sleeping?

Jenny looks at her clock again. You've got to be kidding me, *she says to herself.* It's only four o'clock. The last time I looked it was three o'clock. Before that, one o'clock. How is it possible to feel exhausted and never sleep? Sometimes it makes sense, like when I get night sweats. But other times I seem to wake up for no good reason. This must be because of menopause.

Up to 75 percent of menopausal women have sleep problems. Perimenopausal and postmenopausal women report difficulty in falling asleep, problems staying asleep with frequent awakenings, and early-morning awakenings. Hormonal changes, hot flashes and night sweats, mood disorders (especially depression or anxiety), sleep-disordered breathing, and normal changes that develop with aging all contribute to the problem. Abnormal sleep can affect your mood and ability to function the following day. Sleep disturbances can also affect your ability to concentrate.

The three most common sleep disorders, obstructive sleep apnea (OSA), restless leg syndrome, and insomnia, are all increased in menopause. The most common manifestations of OSA are loud and persistent snoring, pauses in breathing observed by a bed partner, and excessive daytime sleepiness. If you have these symptoms, your doctor should refer you to a sleep laboratory for confirmation. Mild OSA may be helped by weight loss and sleeping on your side instead of your back. Mild to moderate cases can sometimes be treated with an oral appliance that opens your airway. The most common treatment for significant OSA is a CPAP machine that delivers pressurized air through the nose or through the mouth in order to keep the airway open as you sleep.

Restless legs syndrome is noticed as an irresistible urge to move your legs, often accompanied by unpleasant "twitching" sensations in the legs. There is usually an urge to move and the unpleasant sensations are temporarily relieved by movement or rubbing the legs. The condition is found more commonly in patients with iron deficiency, certain neurologic conditions, and a positive family history. It is aggravated by stimulants (including caffeine), certain medications (especially SSRI antidepressants), and sleep deprivation. Medications used to treat this condition include dopaminergics (drugs that increase dopamine, a neurotransmitter), opioids (narcotics), anticonvulsants (anti-seizure medication), and benzodiazepines (antianxiety medication).

Insomnia is the recurrent and persistent inability to obtain sleep of sufficient length or quality to produce refreshment for the following day. It can be characterized by difficulty falling asleep or difficulty staying asleep. During perimenopause, 40–50 percent of women develop insomnia primarily because of hot flashes and other symptoms. Hormone replacement with estrogen often improves sleep. Women who need to take progesterone with their hormone replacement (women who still have a uterus) will do better with natural progesterone (Prometrium) than synthetic progesterone, such as Provera. Medications can help with insomnia, but the first step to correcting insomnia is to develop proper sleep habits. If you are having trouble falling asleep or staying asleep at night, try the following suggestions:

- Maintain a regular sleep schedule. Try to go to bed and wake up at the same time every day, including weekends. Sleep only as much as you need to feel refreshed during the following day.
- Avoid caffeine, remembering that caffeine is found in coffee, tea, chocolate, and cola drinks. Caffeine can stay in your bloodstream for up to six hours so it should be limited to the morning and early afternoon.
- Avoid nicotine (smoking or nicotine-containing smoking cessation products) before bedtime. Nicotine is a stimulant that affects sleep.
- Avoid alcohol. This seems counterintuitive since alcohol often relaxes us and makes us sleepy. Unfortunately, alcohol affects normal sleep patterns and therefore may cause you to wake up during the night.
- Eat regular meals and avoid late meals and snacks.
- Exercise regularly, but not in the two to three hours before bedtime.
- Incorporate regular stress-reducing activities into your life such as prayer, meditation, and yoga. These can be done before bedtime to help initiate a restful sleep.
- Use your bed for sleep and sex only. It is not a good idea to use your bed to watch television, listen to the radio, or read.
- Make sure that your sleeping environment is relaxing. Your bed should be comfortable and the room should not be too hot, too cold, or too bright.

- Avoid emotionally upsetting conversations and activities before bedtime.
- If you find yourself waking up and looking at the clock, hide it.
- If you are unable to sleep, turn on the light, leave the bedroom, and do something different, like reading a boring book. Return to bed when you get sleepy.
- Get up at your regular time every morning, no matter how little you slept.
- Consider seeing a sleep specialist. A doctor who specializes in this area can help you decide whether additional studies (such as evaluation in a sleep lab), lifestyle changes, or medications would be helpful.

What is a hot flash?

Joe thinks his wife Irene is losing her mind.

"What is wrong with you?" Joe asks. "It's thirty-five degrees outside and you're running around the house opening windows. Last night you got up to turn the fan on and then two hours later got up to turn the fan off. All night long it was covers on and then covers off. You're driving me nuts."

"I can't help it," Irene complains. "These hot flashes are driving me crazy. I couldn't wait until I stopped getting periods, but now that I have, it's terrible. I suddenly get hot and then next thing you know I'm soaking through my clothes. If this is menopause, I hope it ends soon."

"You seem miserable," responds Joe. "Neither one of us is getting any sleep. Why don't you go see Dr. Sussman? Maybe she can give you something for this."

Irene is experiencing hot flashes. Hot flashes, also referred to as hot flushes, are sudden, warm, flush feelings throughout the head, neck, and chest area. They may be quite dramatic. Often they appear with sweating, particularly at night. They may also be accompanied by insomnia, dizziness, or palpitations. A generalized sense of warmth or intolerance to heat is not considered a hot flash. Hot flashes are directly related to a reduction in estrogen production. They are usually most prominent after menstruation has ceased completely, but may begin while you are still intermittently getting periods.

Why is sex painful since I stopped getting periods?

Rob and Liz are attempting intercourse when Liz scrunches up her face with an agonizing expression.

"What's wrong?" asks Rob. "You look miserable."

"Nothing, just keep going," Liz responds, trying to sound reassuring.

"No, I can't continue with you looking like you're in pain. Something's wrong."

"I'm just really dry. I don't seem to get wet anymore and my vagina hurts a little when we have sex," Liz admits.

"Well, to be honest, it hasn't been much fun for me either," Rob responds. "Your vagina feels like sandpaper."

"Why haven't you said anything before this?" asks Liz, a little surprised at her husband. Rob has never been one to keep quiet about his needs before.

"I don't know. I guess I thought that this is the way it's supposed to be after menopause," says Rob, looking a bit perplexed.

"Well, I'll go buy a lubricant. Maybe that will do the trick," suggests Liz.

"If it doesn't, promise me you will go see Dr. Paxton. We can't be the only couple with this problem. Maybe he will have some ideas."

You've stopped getting periods. Terrific! Now you don't have to worry about getting pregnant. This should be a shot of adrenaline into the ol' sex life. But wait, something isn't right. Intercourse is painful. You have vaginal dryness and burning. What's happening? You probably have vaginal atrophy.

Estrogen sustains the lining of the vagina, referred to as the vaginal mucosa. Without estrogen, the mucosa thins and loses its normal elasticity. The normal moisture of the vagina is reduced, causing dryness and irritation. Over time (months to years), the caliper of the vagina diminishes. All of these factors lead to painful intercourse. The vagina may even burn or itch without sexual activity. This is called atrophic vaginitis. The lining of the bladder also atrophies in menopause. This may cause symptoms of urinary burning or urgency.

Atrophic vaginitis is corrected with estrogen replacement. Within several months of beginning estrogen replacement, the vagina will regain its normal elasticity and lubrication. Even very small amounts of estrogen cream administered vaginally once or twice weekly can reverse atrophic changes. Nonhormonal moisturizing products (Gyne-Moistren, Replens, Luvena, RepHresh) are also available to help those with vaginal dryness. They are particularly useful for women who have absolute contraindications to estrogen replacement (see below). Products are also available that enhance lubrication during intercourse such as Lubrin, Vagisil Intimate Moisturizer, Astroglide, and what seems like a thousand different K-Y products. Experiment to see which one you prefer. All of these nonhormonal preparations are available over the counter in the feminine hygiene section of your pharmacy or supermarket. We recommend staying away from lubricants that add additional ingredients (such as chemicals designed to spice up your sex life) since these may cause an allergic or irritant reaction.

I don't seem to have any sex drive. Is that because of menopause?

Lucy feels bad for her husband Al. She knows Al would like to have sex more often. It's just that she doesn't care about sex anymore. She used to have a great sex drive. Now she'd just as soon see him go out with his buddies. Lucy doesn't think there's anything wrong with their relationship. She loves her husband, and if he makes advances, she accommodates him. She doesn't know what's wrong and wonders how she can get her sex drive back.

Decreased libido, or sex drive, is frequently seen in menopause. You may also experience diminished sensitivity to sexual stimulation of the nipples and clitoris. Decreased arousability can then reduce your capacity for orgasm. This may be secondary to a decrease in ovarian hormone production. Estrogen replacement may help this problem, although sex drive in women correlates more with testosterone production. Women commonly think that androgens, such as testosterone, are male hormones. However, the ovaries and adrenal glands of women make small amounts of testosterone and other androgens. If decreased sex drive is a significant problem for you in menopause, your doctor can begin estrogen replacement. Estrogen, given orally or vaginally, may indirectly improve sex drive by improving vaginal lubrication and comfort, thereby making sex more enjoyable. If this does not correct the problem, a small amount of testosterone can be added to the hormone replacement. Although substantial evidence suggests that testosterone therapy improves sexual well-being in postmenopausal women with loss of sex drive, there is currently no FDA-approved testosterone replacement product for women in the United States (although this is likely to change, so ask your doctor). There is one product, Estratest, that combines estrogen and testosterone for hormone replacement. However, oral testosterone products are not generally recommended for women since they may adversely affect lipid levels (like cholesterol) or induce insulin resistance (like diabetes). Until there is an approved transdermal product, pharmacists can compound a testosterone cream or ointment under the direction of your gynecologist.

The potential risks of testosterone replacement include a small chance of masculinizing side effects such as increased facial hair, male pattern baldness, acne, deepening of voice, and clitoral enlargement. Don't let us give you the wrong impression. It is very uncommon to see any of these effects from the doses of testosterone used to increase libido. There is no evidence from current studies that transdermal testosterone therapy in formulations designed for women adversely affect lipid levels, carbohydrate metabolism, blood pressure, or blood coagulation. Testosterone treatment may increase bone density and lean body mass (muscle) while reducing body fat in postmenopausal women. Whether testosterone therapy raises breast cancer risk is a concern that is unanswered. Although there is no evidence to date that transdermal testosterone therapy increases the risk of breast cancer in postmenopausal women, well-designed studies have not been of sufficient size or duration to permit a clear conclusion.

Decreased libido often arises from factors unrelated to hormone production (see chapter 4). Medical conditions such as depression, iron deficiency, and hypothyroidism should be excluded. Medications, particularly antidepressants and antipsychotics, should be reviewed for their possible impact on sex drive.

Menopause is a time of transition. You may have children leaving the house, a change in the location of your work (from the house to the workplace or vice versa), a new career, or a partner undergoing his own changes. All of these can lead to stress and changes in your relationship, which can impact your sex drive. Make sure that you make time for each other, both in the house as well as getting away together. Try to embrace some new, fresh adventures or hobbies that can help build, or rebuild, intimacy. Ultimately, sex is more about intimacy than lust. If you sense that intimacy between you has waned, work on it. If you don't know how, seek the help of a therapist.

I feel depressed. Does menopause cause that?

Menopause is not associated with depression in the majority of women. However, decline in the production of ovarian hormones may induce mood disturbances in some women. In menopause, women may present with depressed mood, fatigue, irritability, anxiety, and sleep disturbances. It is not known whether these are directly attributable to the decrease in estrogen. Some of them may be secondary to the physical symptoms of menopause (hot flashes, night sweats, insomnia). There is no doubt that there are hormone receptors in the brain. Animal studies indicate that changes in hormone levels alter the activity of neurotransmitters (chemicals in the brain). This alteration could induce depression or other mood disturbances in susceptible women. Women at high risk for depression during menopause include those with a past history of depression (or severe premenstrual mood disorder) and those with a family history of depression.

Menopause occurs during midlife, a time of transition. Women who have previously invested time and energy into raising children must redefine their role and explore other avenues for fulfillment. Midlife is often accompanied by other stresses. You may have to care for infirm parents. Health problems may develop for you or your spouse. Friends may be lost through illness or relocation. Coping with these and other midlife challenges may be difficult and lead to mood disturbances.

Your personal perspective on menopause and the views of our society influence your ability to confront menopause. For some women, the thought of losing their reproductive capacity is upsetting. It diminishes their sense of femininity and impacts their self-esteem. It certainly doesn't help that North American society is youth oriented. Negative stereotyping of aging women promotes an "over-the-hill" mentality. It is interesting that women usually have an easier transition through menopause in cultures that place value on advancing age (increased privileges and stature).

You don't have to know whether your mood changes are directly attributable to declining ovarian function. Presuming you don't have any contraindications (ask your doctor) and you are aware of the risks and benefits of hormones, your doctor can begin hormone replacement. It certainly appears that the administration of estrogen enhances mood in many women during menopause. Lack of general energy and a diminished sense of well-being may result from testosterone deficiency. When this is the case, adding testosterone to the hormone replacement regimen may benefit mood more than estrogen alone. If you magically turn into a new person, the mood changes were probably related to the decrease in your hormones.

Another approach, particularly if mood changes are severe, is evaluation by a psychologist or psychiatrist. Given the fact that there are other risks associated with hormone replacement therapy, it is not unreasonable to consider the use of an antidepressant preferentially over hormone replacement.

As you approach menopause, consider all the positives. The departure of your children creates more time for you to explore new activities and hobbies. It may give you the opportunity to reenter the workforce or devote more time to your current job. Perhaps you can finally travel to those places that were inaccessible while the children were at home. You and your husband may have the chance to spend more time alone, thereby strengthening your relationship. Your sex life may flourish now that you are freed from concerns about unplanned pregnancy. There is no substitute for experience. You have acquired wisdom and insight throughout your life that enable you to tackle challenges that weren't approachable in your youth.

What is the latest update on hormone replacement therapy?

Irene is thrilled. She saw Dr. Sussman, who started her on hormone replacement therapy. Finally she is sleeping through the night. Joe has noticed a dramatic improvement in her mood and she can work through the day without fanning herself and worrying whether she will soak through her clothes. She meets her childhood friend Peggy at the Red Lobster for lunch. She and Peggy have known each other since they were children and share everything.

"*I feel so good,*" *begins Irene.* "*I saw Dr. Sussman two months ago and he started me on hormones. I finally feel normal again.*"

"*Aren't hormones dangerous?*" *asks Irene.* "*My doctor said he won't prescribe hormones in menopause because there were studies that showed too many risks.*"

"*Well, according to Dr. Sussman, the risks are fairly small. In my case, I don't think I had any choice. I was turning into a basket case with those horrible hot flashes and sweats. Don't you get them?*"

"*I guess I get some, but nothing that I can't handle. Can't you get something else?*" *persists her friend.* "*I saw them advertising something called Remifemin on TV. You don't need a prescription and it's all natural, so it must be safer than hormones.*"

"*I asked Dr. Sussman about that. He said that none of the over-the-counter products would be strong enough to treat severe hot flashes and sweats. According to him, none of the herbal products are approved by the FDA and none of them have been studied for safety over a long period of time. For now, I'm just going to stay on the hormones. They've turned me into a new person and I like that person much better than the one who had hot flashes,*" *Irene states defiantly.*

"*Just don't stay on them forever,*" *responds Peggy, who is unconvinced.*

"Dr. Sussman says we'll take it one year at a time. Just because I need them now doesn't mean that I have to stay on them forever. If I'm doing well, he will decrease the dose next year."

Prior to the year 2000, it was standard for gynecologists to recommend hormone replacement therapy for all postmenopausal women. "Observational" studies, those observing women over many years, found that hormone replacement therapy (HRT) helped protect against heart disease. Since heart disease kills more women than all other diseases combined, it was natural to think that HRT was beneficial. However, several randomized clinical trials, studies that are felt to be more scientific in their design, were published and seemed to indicate that there was no cardioprotective benefit to hormone replacement therapy. The most noteworthy of these studies, the Women's Health Initiative (WHI), was published in 2002.

The WHI study found that there was an excess risk for heart attacks, strokes, breast cancers, and blood clots in the leg or lung. They did find that there were fewer hip fractures and fewer cases of colon cancer, but the overall risk of hormone replacement therapy outweighed those benefits. It is important to realize that the excess risks found were fairly low:

- Seven additional cardiac events per ten thousand women per year of use
- Eight additional strokes per ten thousand women per year of use
- Eight additional cases of breast cancer per ten thousand women per year of use
- Eighteen additional cases of blood clots per ten thousand women per year of use

The WHI only looked at a particular hormone replacement therapy that combined Premarin (conjugated estrogens) and Provera (a synthetic progesterone). A second arm of the study looked at women who were using Premarin alone (women who have had a hysterectomy do not require progesterone). The women taking Premarin alone did not have a higher risk of breast cancer or heart disease. However, they still had an excess risk for strokes and blood clots. Following the WHI, physicians began to recommend hormone use only for short periods of time in women with severe menopausal symptoms. Women already taking HRT were encouraged to stop their hormone replacement.

More recently, scientists have asked, "How could there be so many discrepancies between the findings of prior observational studies and the newer randomized clinical trials?" The answer may be in the timing of hormone replacement therapy. Observational studies tended to follow women who started hormones close to their menopause and continued them for long periods of time. The randomized clinical trials tended to enroll women further from their menopause and followed them for a shorter number of years. Analysts have looked more closely at the WHI and have found that the risks are very different for women in their fifties than women in their sixties and seventies. Women in their fifties enrolled in the WHI study were not found to have an excess risk of cardiac events, and in fact appear to have a cardioprotective benefit (leading to an overall lower mortality rate). Likewise, the excess risk for stroke is not seen until the sixth decade of life. Looking at breast cancer risk, there is still a small excess risk for breast cancer in women using combination HRT (both estrogen and progesterone), but not in the women taking estrogen alone for a relatively short number of years. While there was still a small excess risk for blood clots for women in their fifties, more recent studies suggest that this risk may be eliminated, or significantly reduced, by using non-oral preparations of estrogen, such as an estrogen patch or gel.

The other major benefits of estrogen relate to quality of life issues. Hot flashes, night sweats, and vaginal dryness are most effectively eradicated through estrogen replacement. The increase in facial hair often seen with menopause is decreased with estrogen replacement. Genital prolapse (see chapter 15) is also less likely with hormone replacement. Additional symptoms that may improve with hormone replacement include insomnia, palpitations, mood disturbances (see above), decreased sex drive, achy joints, and urinary frequency. These symptoms are not always related to menopause. However, when they are caused by menopause, estrogen replacement is beneficial. Quality of life issues are not addressed as medical benefits when studies evaluate hormone replacement, but your doctor should certainly take them into consideration when helping you decide whether hormone replacement therapy is right for you.

So what reasonable conclusions can be derived about the risks and benefits of using hormones in menopause? The latest analysis would suggest that while there is still a small risk for increasing breast cancer and blood clots with combination HRT, there may be a cardioprotective benefit in women in their fifties that outweighs those risks. While it would still not be recommended to use HRT in women without menopausal symptoms, many gynecologists now feel more comfortable using HRT in women in their fifties who are symptomatic. Reanalysis of the WHI data would still suggest that we should not begin HRT in women in their sixties or seventies. There will be some women in that age group who have sufficiently severe menopausal symptoms to recommend continuing HRT, but that should be the exception, not the rule.

What type of hormones should I take? How are they given?

The premenopausal ovary produces estrogen, progesterone, and a small amount of androgens such as testosterone. Almost all the benefits of hormonal replacement derive from estrogen. Therefore, estrogen is the foundation of any hormone replacement regimen. However, unopposed estrogen (without progesterone) increases the risk of endometrial cancer (cancer of the inside lining of the uterus). Women who have not undergone hysterectomy must also take progesterone to balance the effects of estrogen on the endometrium. Women with decreased sex drive, fatigue, or a diminished sense of well-being may benefit from the addition of testosterone, although each of these symptoms is often unrelated to sex hormones. Most physicians do not routinely add testosterone to their hormone replacement regimen.

Hormones are given in many formats. Pills, patches, implants (under the skin), injections, creams, suppositories, vaginal rings, and intrauterine devices have all been used. Oral administration (tablets or capsules) and transdermal products like skin patches and gels are the most common modalities for estrogen replacement in the United States. Estrogen tablets and gels are generally used daily. The patch is changed once or twice weekly. Patients with gastrointestinal distress from estrogen tablets may do better with the transdermal approach. There are potential advantages in using transdermal estrogen in women with gallbladder disease, headaches, high blood pressure, hypertriglyceridemia (high triglycerides), and diabetes. There is also evidence to suggest that women using transdermal estrogen have less risk for venous blood clots, stroke, and heart attacks. Women who get skin reactions from the transdermal products may do better with tablets. Women using estrogen primarily for vaginal symptoms should use an estrogen product that is designed for intravaginal placement.

Not all estrogens are the same. Traditionally, the most common estrogen used in replacement regimens in the United States has been Premarin, which is actually a composite of many estrogens derived from the urine of pregnant horses. Decades of experience with Premarin provided physicians with confidence in its use. Most of the studies in the United States that have evaluated the effects of estrogen on women have looked at Premarin. More recently, physicians are trending toward the use of estrogens that are similar to those found naturally in women. These are either synthesized or obtained from plant sources. Each physician tends to have his or her preference, and there is not sufficient evidence to support the superiority of one brand over another. Most hormone replacement regimens provide you with estrogen continuously.

There is more variation in how physicians give progesterone. If you had a hysterectomy, there is usually no need for progesterone. Remember, progesterone is only given to decrease the risk of endometrial cancer. In certain situations, such as hormone replacement after hysterectomy for endometriosis, progesterone may also be given. There are two basic regimens for giving progesterone. The cyclic regimen provides you with progesterone for ten to fourteen days periodically (every one to three months depending on the dose of estrogen). You will typically get a menstrual period after the progesterone is stopped each month, but cannot get pregnant. However, many women aren't thrilled with the prospect of resuming periods. For that reason, many physicians have switched to a continuous regimen. In the continuous regimen, you receive a smaller amount of progesterone every day. Up to 40 percent of women will have erratic bleeding initially on this regimen. However, by the end of one year, 80 percent of women will no longer have any bleeding. The most common progesterone prescribed is medroxyprogesterone acetate (Provera, Cycrin). Natural progesterone (Prometrium) may also be given, particularly when women experience side effects from the synthetic progestins. Natural progesterone appears to have some health advantages over synthetic progesterone (see below).

What about bioidentical hormones?

Dr. Thornton has just finished his seminar on menopause. Ashley and June, participants in the seminar, strike up a conversation while finishing their coffee.

"So I came here to learn more about hormone replacement," Ashley says. "Are you taking any hormones?"

"Yes, I believe in bioidentical hormone replacement," responds June. "I see a doctor who specializes in bioidentical hormones."

Ashley looks perplexed. "I don't understand the whole bioidentical hormone craze. According to Dr. Thornton, the estradiol and progesterone he prescribes are identical to the hormones my ovaries used to make. Doesn't that make them bioidentical?"

"Not really. Bioidentical hormones include estriol, which is safer than prescription estrogen. My specialist, Dr. Schaeffer, also measures my salivary gland hormone levels, which gives him a better appreciation for the hormone levels found in actual tissues rather than the bloodstream. It's all very sophisticated. He checks my levels every three months and adjusts my prescription so that it is just right. I'm sure that my body will age better if I continue these hormones."

"Have there been good studies showing that this is a better way to give hormone replacement?" asks Ashley. "Dr. Thornton mentioned that these products compounded by a pharmacist aren't reviewed by the FDA. How do we know that they are safer than normal hormone replacement?"

"Well, they must be because Dr. Schaeffer is a specialist in this area and he tells me that they are safer," June says, rather defensively.

"How much are you paying for these bioidentical hormones?" asks Ashley.

"I pay forty dollars a month for the hormones and one hundred every time Dr. Schaeffer gets the salivary gland hormone levels."

"Well, I'm glad you're happy with your hormone replacement," Ashley comments, "but I think I'll stick to a prescription product covered by my health plan."

Periodically, you will see promotion of a concept referred to as *bioidentical hormones*. The name is actually a bit of a misnomer. The hormones that are identical to those produced by your ovary before menopause are estradiol and progesterone. Both of these are available in FDA-approved formulations. When people refer to bioidentical hormones, they are usually referring to an estrogen product that is a combination of two or three estrogens, dominated by estriol, a weaker estrogen that is produced in large quantities during pregnancy. Proponents of estriol suggest that it does not increase breast cancer risk, in contrast to the more potent estradiol, and even go as far as suggesting that it may protect against breast cancer. While there is some intriguing science behind this theory, we do not have randomized, prospective clinical studies to support this contention. At this time, there is no FDA-approved estriol product. Hormone replacement regimens that include estriol must be compounded by a pharmacist. While this may be reasonable, there is at least the potential for more variability in the product you are receiving and you will pay out-of-pocket for your hormone replacement. Insurance companies do not generally cover products that are not approved by the FDA. At this point, the American College of Obstetrics and Gynecology and the North American Menopause Society do not support the use of compounded estrogen preparations.

Bioidentical, natural progesterone is available as Prometrium, which is FDA approved. There is some evidence that natural progesterone may be a better progesterone for use in hormone replacement therapy. Some of the beneficial things we see estrogen do for the heart, such as improving cholesterol and dilating coronary vessels, is offset when one adds a synthetic progesterone like Provera. This does not happen when natural progesterone is added. In the laboratory, breast cell proliferation seems to be induced by synthetic progestins, but not natural progesterone. However, once again, we do not have randomized, prospective studies to demonstrate the superiority of natural progesterone over synthetic progestins in hormone replacement therapy regimens. Prometrium is compounded in peanut oil, so it is contraindicated in patients with a peanut allergy.

You will also see natural progesterone cream promoted as an alternative to standard hormone replacement therapy. The best-designed scientific studies have shown little or no benefit of progesterone cream over placebo in the resolution of menopausal symptoms. The transdermal absorption of progesterone and the amount of actual progesterone in creams varies tremendously. If you would like to use a progesterone cream alone, there is little or no risk in doing so, but it is not recommended to use progesterone cream for the purpose of protecting the endometrium in women who are taking estrogen replacement.

You will often see proponents of bioidentical hormone replacement promoting salivary gland hormone levels. Salivary gland hormone levels vary tremendously and should not be used to adjust hormone replacement. Hormone levels obtained through blood work is also not necessary. Hormone replacement is adjusted based upon the control of symptoms. The dose of hormones you receive will be determined by the lowest amount of estrogen required to control your symptoms. If reasonably large doses of estrogen do not appear to relieve your symptoms, blood work will help your doctor determine if you are absorbing the estrogen properly. Otherwise, blood work for hormone levels is not necessary.

Do I have to wait until I stop getting periods to begin hormone replacement therapy?

You are still getting fairly regular periods, but you have noticed progressively worsening hot flashes and night sweats. Perhaps your mood swings are off the charts. You're wondering if this could be menopause, but your doctor says, "No, you are still getting periods." To be fair, you both are correct. By definition, you are still producing premenopausal levels of estrogen. You will no longer menstruate when the estrogen levels fall into the menopausal range. However, if you are producing estrogen with greater variability, you can still experience menopausal symptoms. If the symptoms are severe, there is no reason why you can't begin hormone supplementation as long as it's balanced with both estrogen and progesterone. Some physicians will provide you with hormone supplementation in similar fashion to postmenopausal hormone replacement regimens. Others will recommend low-dose oral contraceptives if you do not have any contraindications to their use. Low-dose oral contraceptives are a particularly good choice if you also have heavy or irregular periods.

Is there an age at which it is too late to start hormone replacement therapy?

The ideal time to start hormone replacement is immediately after menopause. The most recent evidence would suggest that hormones begun shortly after menopause pose little or no additional adverse risk for strokes and heart attacks. This does not seem to be the case in later decades. Data from the Women's Health Initiative study suggests an excess cardiovascular risk in older women (beginning in the sixth decade for stroke and the seventh decade for heart attacks). Current recommendations promote the use of hormone replacement therapy only for the indication of menopausal symptoms, and only for the shortest amount of time necessary. The emergence of new menopausal symptoms in the sixth and seventh decades of life (symptoms that were not there at the time of menopause) is extremely rare and unlikely to be related to sex hormone deficiency. Hot flashes or night sweats that develop for the first time late in life are more likely related to other medical conditions (ex. thyroid disease), medications, or instability of the autonomic nervous system.

Should I avoid hormones because they cause cancer?

Sally and Tony have been happily married for thirty-three years—well, at least until now.

"I'm not going on those damn hormones! They give you cancer!" Sally exclaims, glaring at her husband.

"Well you have to go on something," Tony counters, just as determined. "You're bitching about hot flashes all day long and not getting any sleep. You're screeching at the kids and I can't take it anymore. You need to do something. Go see Dr. Johnson."

"I'll go and talk to him," concedes Sally, "but don't expect me to change my mind."

The Women's Health Initiative study found a small excess risk for breast cancer in women using Prempro, a combination of con-jugated estrogens (Premarin) and a synthetic progesterone (Provera). In one hundred women, this would result in one to two additional breast cancers developing over a period of twenty years of hormone use. Obviously this risk is much less if hormones are used for a lim-ited time, and has very little impact if hormones are only used for two to three years during the menopausal transition. Interestingly, the Women's Health Initiative did not find an excess breast cancer risk in women using estrogen alone and in fact found a lower risk for breast cancer in that group. This would suggest that the synthetic progestin Provera, in contrast to natural progesterone, was the primary culprit in causing breast cancer, not the estrogen. Other observational studies would suggest that long-term use of estrogen alone (ten to fifteen years or more) may increase the risk of breast cancer, although not nearly as much as combination hormone replacement therapy (estrogen and progesterone together). There is a suggestion that natural progesterone may not have the same adverse impact on breast cancer risk as synthetic progestins, but this is yet to be proven in well-designed studies. Women who still have their uterus must add progesterone to their hormone replacement regimen. Otherwise there is an excess risk for endometrial cancer, cancer of the inside lining of the uterus. Adding progesterone eliminates the excess endometrial cancer risk when given appropriately.

Use of hormone replacement in menopause is always a balance between the severity of symptoms versus potential excess risks. Because the excess cancer risk is relatively small, you may be a good candidate for hormone replacement therapy if your symptoms are severe enough to adversely impact your ability to function at work or in the home or your relationships with other people. Because the risk slowly increases with time, it makes sense to periodically reduce your dose of hormone replacement therapy, and eliminate its use when symptoms abate, or at least become more tolerable.

What side effects will I get from hormone replacement?

The two most common complaints we receive from women beginning hormone replacement are bleeding and breast tenderness. If you are given continuous hormone replacement therapy (designed to avoid periods), intermittent bleeding is not unusual when hormone replacement therapy is first begun and tends to disappear over time. If it persists beyond the first year, further investigation would be appropriate to rule out other pathology. Breast tenderness is another common complaint. It is most likely to be a problem if you had severe, premenstrual breast tenderness before menopause. The tenderness usually disappears after menopause, only to return when hormone replacement is started. Breast enlargement may

> **Myths about Hormone Replacement**
>
> *Hormones make you gain weight:* *No! Eating poorly and lack of exercise make you gain weight. If anything, hormone replacement may reduce that midriff bulge.*
>
> *Hormones put hair on your face:* *Menopause puts hair on your face. Hormone replacement lessens the likelihood of this happening.*
>
> *Hormones have too many side effects:* *Actually you are far more likely to have beneficial effects than adverse effects.*
>
> *Hormones are dangerous:* *The risk from taking hormone replacement for a limited time in your fifties is fairly low, certainly no riskier than driving a car.*
>
> *Hormones will keep me young:* *Sorry, you're still going to age, but women on hormone replacement often feel much better than those who are not.*

also occur. Breast tenderness from hormone replacement sometimes improves over time. Lowering the dose of hormones will sometimes decrease the tenderness. Decreasing caffeine consumption (coffee, tea, colas, and chocolate), supplemental Diindolylmethane (DIM, 100–300 mg per day), vitamin E (400–800 international units, or IU, per day), evening primrose oil (3–4 gm per day), and Ginkgo Biloba (60–240 mg) have all been tried in women with premenstrual breast tenderness and appear to help some women. They can be tried in the postmenopausal woman with breast tenderness associated with hormone replacement. Nonprescription pain relievers containing acetaminophen (Tylenol) or ibuprofen (Advil, Motrin) should also be considered. If severe, adding a small amount of testosterone to the hormone regimen may reduce the breast tenderness.

Gastrointestinal distress including nausea, cramping, and bloating may be experienced as a side effect of hormone replacement. These tend to dissipate over time and may also be reduced by changing to a different brand of estrogen or a different method of administration (transdermal versus the oral route) and also by reducing the dose.

Less common side effects include headaches, mood disturbance, skin changes (particularly a spotty darkening of the skin when exposed to the sun), and fluid retention. You are also more likely to develop gallbladder disease on oral hormone replacement therapy, an adverse effect that does not appear with transdermal estrogen (patches, creams, gels).

Before starting hormones, advise your doctor if you have:

- *A history of breast cancer or breast biopsies reflecting an increased risk for developing breast cancer*
- *A history of endometrial cancer*
- *A history of endometriosis*
- *Gallbladder disease*
- *Hypertension (high blood pressure)*
- *Diabetes*
- *Ongoing liver disease (hepatitis)*
- *A history of blood clots in your veins*

"What about weight gain? Aren't those hormones going to make me gain weight?" You may gain weight, but it probably won't be caused by the hormone replacement. Many women will gain weight at this time in their life whether or not they use hormone replacement. Some of this may be related to menopause itself, some related to decreasing activity levels as we age, and some related to increased consumption. (Are you going out to eat more now that the kids are out of the house?) You must either eat less or exercise more to keep your weight stable. Refer to chapter 1 for additional suggestions.

Most women tolerate hormone replacement with little or no side effects. You are far more likely to experience beneficial effects (decreased hot flashes and night sweats, prevention of vaginal dryness, improved sleep, better mood) than detrimental effects. The possibility of getting a side effect should not prevent you from considering hormone replacement. If you develop a side effect that cannot be managed, you can always discontinue the therapy.

Are there women who can't take hormones?

Some women are not candidates for hormone replacement therapy. Traditionally, women with a history of breast or endometrial cancer cannot use hormone replacement. The risk of recurrence may be increased if estrogen is given under these circumstances. Some physicians will consider hormone replacement if the cancer was very early (your risk of recurrence is low) or you have been free of disease for a long time (usually considered to be at least five to ten years). This is very controversial, and the vast majority of physicians will avoid hormone replacement if you have had either of these cancers. Historically, deep vein thrombosis (DVT) has been a contraindication to hormone replacement. DVT is the formation of blood clots in the large veins of your legs. We're talking about the deep veins in your legs, not the superficial veins that are readily visible. Blood clots in the deep veins can travel to your lungs (pulmonary embolism), which is potentially life-threatening. Estrogen has effects on various factors responsible for regulating blood clotting. There are large observational and case cohort studies showing that transdermal estrogen does not increase the risk of DVT in the same way that oral estrogens do. However, most physicians will not prescribe any type of hormone replacement therapy for a woman who has had a DVT or is predisposed to developing blood clots. If there is any reason to suspect that you may be at an increased risk for DVT (usually based upon family history), further testing can be performed.

Women have an increased risk of gallbladder disease with oral hormone replacement therapy. If you currently have gallbladder disease or asymptomatic gallstones, hormone replacement may not be in your best interest. This disadvantage must be weighed against the benefits of the hormones to your quality of life. Keep in mind that you can live perfectly fine without your gallbladder. If you are miserable from your menopausal symptoms, hormone replacement should still be considered. In this situation, we recommend a transdermal estrogen preparation, which is much less likely to alter gallbladder function.

Diabetes (high blood sugar) and hypertension (high blood pressure) are two diseases that were previously considered "relative contraindications" to hormone replacement. Neither of these is currently considered to be a contraindication. Transdermal estrogen (patches, creams, and gels) may be a better choice than oral preparations if you have either of these conditions.

Active liver disease (hepatitis) may also contraindicate the use of hormones. Estrogen is metabolized (eliminated from your system) by your liver, so it must be used with caution when there is liver dysfunction.

What else can I take for my symptoms other than hormones?

Donna and Ginger are swimming buddies. They meet at the local YMCA every Wednesday morning to swim laps. Donna notices a clear patch on Ginger's abdomen, something she hadn't noticed before.

"What's that on your belly?" Donna asks. "Are you sick?"

"No, I'm fine," responds Ginger. "The patch is for hormone replacement. Do you remember how miserable I was a few weeks ago with hot flashes? Dr. Hernandez gave me this estrogen patch. It's been wonderful. I'm a new woman."

"I would never take hormones," replied Donna. "I think that they're dangerous. I've been taking Estroven. You know, the one that's advertised on TV? I think it's been helping me and it has to be safer than hormones since you don't need a prescription."

"Dr. Hernandez isn't a big fan of herbal products," responds Ginger. "He doesn't think they are very effective for women with severe symptoms. He also doesn't like the fact that herbal products aren't approved by the FDA and don't have long-term safety studies. I don't think the risks of hormone replacement are too bad, and I only plan on taking them for a few years."

"You could be right," acknowledges Donna, "but I always feel more comfortable using natural products."

What can you do if you or your physician decides that hormone replacement is not an option but you have menopausal symptoms? Changing your diet by lowering fat intake and increasing fruits and vegetables may help reduce hot flashes and night sweats. Weight loss will also reduce vasomotor symptoms. Vaginal moisture can be somewhat restored with the use of nonhormonal over-the-counter products (Replens, Gyne-Moistren, RepHresh, Luvena, lubricants).

There are several types of nonhormonal prescription medicines that have been used to reduce vasomotor symptoms (hot flashes and night sweats). The most commonly prescribed alternatives to hormone replacement therapy are products that would normally be used for depression, SSRIs and SNRIs. One of the better studied of these medicines, and the one that we tend to prefer, is venlafaxine (Effexor). Other SSRIs that have been studied for this purpose include fluoxetine (Prozac), paroxetine (Paxil), citalopram (Celexa) and sertraline (Zoloft). Women who are taking tamoxifen for the treatment or prevention of breast cancer must be careful in choosing their SSRI medication. Prozac, Paxil, and Zoloft significantly inhibit the enzyme that converts tamoxifen to its active metabolite, thereby decreasing its effectiveness. Effexor, Celexa, Lexapro, and Luvox only weakly inhibit the enzyme and are better choices for women on tamoxifen.

Clonidine (Catapres) is usually used for treating high blood pressure. However, it has also been used as a treatment for hot flashes and night sweats. It is administered either orally or as a patch changed weekly. Gabapentin (Neurontin), a drug more typically used for seizures or nerve pain syndromes, is a more recent addition to the list of medications used for menopausal symptoms. It is important to understand that none of these medications are without risk or potential side effects, so their use must be discussed with a physician prior to their consideration.

We're often asked about the use of "natural" products for the treatment of hot flashes. All of the products listed below have advocates within the complementary and alternative medical (CAM) community. As you will see, many of these have had mixed results when subjected to scientific scrutiny.

- *Phytoestrogens*: Numerous plants have estrogen-like substances called phytoestrogens, the most common being isoflavones. Advocates of phytoestrogens propose that these are safer because they are far less potent than prescribed estrogens. Foods high in phytoestrogens include soybeans and soybean products such as soy milk and tofu. Phytoestrogens are also derived from some vegetables and berries as well as grains, seeds, and sprouts. Well-designed scientific studies in humans are rare, and those that do exist are conflicting in their conclusions. Women who want to consume phytoestrogens should do so through food products rather than supplements, and should aim for 100 mg of isoflavones or 25 g of soy protein per day. For more information, visit www.hss.edu/files/Soy_Phytoestrogens.pdf.
- *Red Clover*: Red clover is a member of the legume family and contains at least four estrogenic isoflavones. These have been extracted into a product called Promensil. Most studies have

not found Promensil to be significantly better than placebo in relieving hot flashes.

- *Black cohosh*: Black cohosh is perhaps the most commonly found ingredient in over-the-counter products promoted for menopause (Estroven, Remifemin). There have been many studies looking at black cohosh. Many of these studies have design weaknesses and more research is needed. Although definitive evidence of significant benefit is lacking, black cohosh does appear to be safe and may have efficacy in the treatment of menopausal symptoms in some women. It should be administered initially at 20–40 mg twice daily. It may take four to eight weeks to feel an effect. Adverse effects are rare and include GI upset, headache, and dizziness. In laboratory studies, black cohosh appears to suppress rather than stimulate breast cells and appears to have an inhibitory effect on the estrogen receptors of breast cancer cells. However, there is no long-term study looking at the safety of black cohosh beyond twelve months in patients with or without breast cancer.

- *Ginseng*: There is no evidence to support the use of ginseng for the treatment of hot flashes and night sweats. However, one well-designed study looking at panax ginseng showed significant improvement in symptoms of depression and sense of well-being. Panax ginseng should not be taken with stimulants because it may cause headache, breast pain, diarrhea, or bleeding. The recommended dosage is 100 mg of a standardized extract twice daily for three out of four weeks.

- *Dong quai*: Dong quai has a long history of traditional use in menopause and menstrual disorders in Asia. However, there is no evidence to support the use of dong quai as a single agent in the treatment of menopausal symptoms. Its use in combination with other herbs, as it has been traditionally used in Asia, has not been well studied.

- *Kava kava*: Evidence has shown that 100–200 mg three times per day (standardized to 30 percent of kavalactones) decreases anxiety, irritability, and insomnia associated with menopause.

Kava kava is often combined with other components such as black cohosh and valerian for the management of menopausal symptoms. Kava kava has the potential for significant, albeit rare, side effects. Cases of hepatotoxicity (liver toxicity) so severe as to require liver transplant have been reported. Other adverse effects include dermatitis and a movement disorder similar to Parkinson's disease. Because of these adverse effects, it has been removed from many European markets. We don't recommend using it, but if you do, be aware of the risks and avoid taking it in conjunction with other anxiety-reducing agents, alcohol, and acetaminophen, and have liver function tests performed periodically.

- *St. John's wort*: St. John's wort has been used primarily as an antidepressant. It is used in Germany for menopausal mood swings. St. John's wort appears to be beneficial in mild to moderate depression with 60 percent improvement in mood, energy, and sleep with a dose of 300 mg three times per day. It is not effective in reducing hot flashes and night sweats. St. John's wort should only be started after consulting with a physician since it has multiple drug interactions.

- *Chasteberry*: Chasteberry has a long history of use in the treatment of menopausal symptoms, although its efficacy in menopause has not yet been demonstrated through well-designed studies.

- *Ginkgo*: Ginkgo Biloba is often promoted for the improvement of libido in menopausal patients. In studies, Muira Puama plus ginkgo had a significant effect in 65 percent of patients studied, but further trials are needed. Adverse effects include GI upset and headache. Ginkgo has drug interactions and anticoagulant effects, so it should only be taken after consulting your physician.

- *Vitamin E*: Vitamin E has been recommended for the treatment of hot flashes dating back to the 1940s. However, more recent studies investigating vitamin E at 200–600 IUs have failed to show an effect. Higher doses (1,200 IU) may be effective, but vitamin E is an anticoagulant and doses this high cannot be recommended. Vitamin E is still commonly recommended in the CAM community. If you would like to try it, do not exceed 800 IU and do not use it in conjunction with anticoagulant medications.

- *Hesperidin*: Hesperidin is extracted from citrus fruit and is purported to improve vascular integrity. One study that combined 900 mg of hesperidin, 300 mg of hesperidin methyl chalcone, and 1,200 mg of vitamin C was found to be effective in reducing or eliminating hot flashes. The most common side effects are GI upset and headache. The long-term safety of hesperidin has not been evaluated.

- *Evening primrose oil*: One study found a reduction in night sweats but no reduction in daytime hot flashes. More studies are needed.

- *Pure pollen extract*: Femal (two tablets daily; also known as Serelys), a pollen extract has shown a modest reduction in hot flushes in two small studies and appears to be safe.

Progesterone creams are also available over the counter today, some with micronized progesterone (which is natural progesterone, derived from plant precursors) and others with only wild yam extracts. Manufacturers may claim that these wild yam precursors have progesterone-like effects, which is misleading. There is no pathway by which the human body can convert wild yam precursors to progesterone (although this can be done in the laboratory). Micronized progesterone is absorbed across the skin, but you need a lot of cream to achieve progesterone levels comparable to those found during a normal menstrual cycle. Using progesterone cream alone poses no significant risks. However, using progesterone cream as a substitute for prescribed progesterone in a hormone replacement regimen can be dangerous. These products may not adequately balance the effects of estrogen on the endometrium.

Various changes in your lifestyle may help you cope with hot flashes. Women definitely notice worsening of their menopausal symptoms under stressful circumstances. Exercise, yoga, and meditation are several activities that you can try when you are under stress to help decrease the frequency of your symptoms. These also increase your general sense of well-being. You can also be taught progressive relaxation techniques. Relaxation techniques for hot flashes can be found at the National Center for Complementary and Alternative Medicine through the National Institute of Health website: www.nccam.nih.gov/health/stress/relaxation.htm. Studies on acupuncture and menopausal symptoms are mixed. Generally, acupuncture is safe. If menopausal patients are interested in exploring this as part of their management plan, it is reasonable to do so. Alcohol, caffeine, and hot or spicy foods will increase hot flashes and night sweats, so it makes sense for you to avoid these. Wear breathable clothing like cotton and dress in layers so you can add or remove layers as needed. Do the same with bedding. In place of a comforter, use several lighter blankets, which will give you more flexibility.

What are those new drugs that are supposed to replace estrogen, and are they safer?

Imagine a drug that has all the benefits of estrogen but none of the risks. It protects your bones, reduces your risk of heart disease, and extinguishes those hot flashes without any effects on your breasts or uterus. Okay, the dream is over; no such drug exists. However, scientists are evaluating phytoestrogens (see above) and other compounds that aspire to meet those lofty goals. Some of these compounds, called SERMs (selective estrogen receptor modulators), mimic estrogen in some areas of the body while blocking it in others.

Raloxifene (Evista) was the first SERM to gain approval from the FDA for menopausal women. It prevents osteoporosis and bone fractures, has no adverse impact on your uterus, and reduces your risk of breast cancer. Overall it does not appear to cause excess risk for your heart, although there appears to be a small excess risk for stroke. Like oral estrogen, it causes an excess risk for DVT. More importantly, it does not treat vasomotor (hot flashes and night sweats) menopausal symptoms. In fact, it increases the frequency, although not the severity, of hot flashes. It is therefore not indicated for the treatment of menopausal symptoms. It is a reasonable drug to be considered in women for the prevention of osteoporosis, particularly those who are at excess risk (see the question on osteoporosis).

Osphena (ospemifene) is a recently approved SERM indicated for the treatment of painful intercourse in menopausal women. However, it may increase your risk of blood clots, stroke, and endometrial cancer (cancer of the inside lining of the uterus). Additional side effects include vaginal discharge, muscle cramps, hot flashes, and sweating. It has not been adequately studied in women with a history of breast cancer. Considering all of this, it does not seem to be an improvement over using small amounts of vaginal estrogen, which provides the same benefit. Fortunately, there are many SERMs in development and there is certainly a possibility for one to contain most of the benefits of estrogen without most of the risks.

Tibolone is a drug that is commonly used in menopausal women outside of the United States. It is approved in ninety countries for the treatment of menopausal symptoms and forty-five countries for the prevention of osteoporosis. It has not been approved by the FDA in the United States, although it may be in the future. Metabolites of tibolone have estrogenic, progestational, and androgenic properties. Tibolone decreases hot flashes and night sweats, treats vaginal dryness, and increases libido. It also prevents osteoporosis and bone fractures. The data on breast cancer is mixed. Observational studies have tended to show an increase in breast cancer. On the other hand, a well-designed study looking at older women (sixty to eighty-five) showed a substantial decrease in breast cancer. The cardiovascular data on tibolone is a bit murkier. It decreases total cholesterol and triglycerides, which should potentially be a benefit, but it also reduces good cholesterol (HDL cholesterol). Overall, it does not appear to significantly increase the risk for deep vein thrombosis (blood clots) or myocardial infarction (heart attacks). However, tibolone increases the risk for stroke. If it eventually gets approved in the United States, tibolone would seem to be a reasonable choice for treating menopausal symptoms in relatively young women (those in their fifties) who do not have additional risk factors for stroke such as high blood pressure, smoking, and diabetes.

How can I tell if I have osteoporosis and what can be done to prevent it?

The diagnosis of osteoporosis can be made through a variety of tests that measure bone density. The most common test used is a DEXA scan. If your doctor sends you for a bone density study, he or she is most likely sending you for a DEXA scan. Current guidelines from the National Osteoporosis Foundation recommend that women get their first bone density study at age sixty-five unless they have the following risk factors:

- Thin body build (small bones)—Less than 127 pounds or a BMI less than twenty-one
- Current smokers—Another reason to quit. Smoking is particularly hard on your bones.
- History of a parent with a fracture—Did Mom start to lose height and develop a curvature in her upper back? Did she fracture her hip? If so, she had osteoporosis, which may increase your risk.
- A personal history of bone fracture
- A postmenopausal woman with a medical cause for bone loss, such as the ongoing use of anti-inflammatory steroids (ex. Prednisone) and hyperparathyroidism (the parathyroid gland regulates calcium metabolism)
- Rheumatoid arthritis
- Consumption of three or more units of alcohol per day (one unit is twelve ounces of beer, four ounces of wine, or one ounce of liquor). Moderate alcohol intake does not have an adverse impact on bone density and actually may slow down bone loss.

Additional risk factors that your doctor may take into consideration include:

- White or Asian race—Osteoporosis is found less frequently among African-American women.
- Inadequate calcium intake—Women rarely consume adequate quantities of calcium. Your peak bone mass is reached by age thirty-five. If your diet was deficient in calcium before thirty-five, your risk of osteoporosis is increased substantially.
- Insufficient exercise—Your bone density is maintained through regular exercise, particularly weight-bearing exercise such as walking, cycling, and dancing.
- Late menarche (age of onset of periods) or early menopause (cessation of periods)
- Anorexia—Women with a history of anorexia are more likely to have low bone density from inadequate diet and decreased estrogen production.
- The use of additional medications other than steroids that may be associated with bone loss including anticonvulsants (anti-seizure medications), furosemide diuretics ("water pills" used for fluid retention and high blood pressure), thyroid replacement (used for an underactive thyroid), proton pump inhibitors (used to treat GI reflux and ulcers), and aromatase inhibitors (used in the prevention and treatment of breast cancer). If you require these medications, you should consider special measures to decrease bone loss.

A proper diet is important in the prevention of osteoporosis. Teenagers should increase their dietary intake of calcium. The teen years are critical bone-building years. Unfortunately, most teenage girls do not drink large quantities of milk. In fact, many drink soda, which is actually harmful to bones. Women ages twenty-five to fifty should have a daily calcium intake of 750 mg. After menopause, the requirement increases to 1000–1200 mg. Consuming foods rich in calcium is preferable to calcium supplements. There is currently great debate over whether calcium supplements should be used to supplement dietary calcium in order for women to achieve their recommended daily dose. The National Osteoporosis Foundation recommends augmenting dietary calcium intake with supplements as needed to reach 1200 mg per day. However, recent studies suggest that there may be a small increase in strokes and heart attacks in older women taking calcium supplements. Extrapolating from the data of those studies, there would be six additional cardiovascular events (stroke or heart attack) for each thousand women taking calcium supplements. There may also be a small increase in the risk of renal calculi (kidney stones). For these reasons, many practitioners have stopped routinely recommending calcium supplements or lowered the amount they recommend, and are placing a stronger emphasis on obtaining calcium through food. If you have trouble getting calcium through food, we would suggest Citracal with vitamin D and magnesium. In order to avoid large amounts of calcium entering your body all at once, we would recommend that you split tablets, taking them at different times of the day.

Foods Containing Calcium

	Amount	Calcium (milligrams)	Fat (grams)
Cheese	1 ounce	150–220	6–9
Cottage cheese	1 cup	210	9.5
Hard ice cream	1 cup	175	14
Milk	1 cup	300	whole, 8; low-fat, 5; skim, 1
Low-fat yogurt	1 cup	350–400	2.5–3.5
Almonds	1 ounce	66	16
Scallops, steamed	3 1/2 ounce	115	1.4
Shrimp, raw	3 1/2 ounce	63	0.8
Broccoli, cooked	2/3 cup	88	0.3
Spinach, cooked	1/2 cup	83	0.3
Kale, cooked	3/4 cup	187	0.7
Turnip greens, cooked	2/3 cup	184	0.2
Beans, canned	1/2 cup	68	3.2
Green beans, cooked	1 cup	62	0.2
Chickpeas (garbanzos)	3 1/2 oz	75	2.4
Sweet potato, baked	1 small	40	0.5
Figs, dried	5 medium	126	1.3
Raisins	5/8 cup	62	0.2
Orange	1 medium	56	0.1

Vitamin D is also critical for calcium absorption and bone mineralization. Some women get sufficient vitamin D from exposure to the sun or diet (fatty fish, butter, egg yolks, liver, and fortified milk), but vitamin D deficiency is fairly common. We recommend that all postmenopausal women get a 25-OH Vitamin D blood test to ensure that they are not deficient in vitamin D. Postmenopausal women should get 800–1000 IU of vitamin D daily. Vitamin D supplements are available separately if you are not getting enough with your food or calcium supplement.

Exercise is effective at slowing the loss of bone in menopause. Some studies indicate that it may even be able to increase bone density. The best exercises are those that are weight-bearing in nature such as walking, bicycling, dancing, and step climbing. Also, exercises against resistance and weightlifting are good. Exercise also helps develop your muscles, which can help you burn calories more efficiently and often improves balance, thereby reducing falls and preventing fractures. Obviously the

Why Talk about Osteoporosis?

Consider these facts from the National Osteoporosis Foundation:

- Ten million people in the United States have osteoporosis. Eight million are women.
- Women can lose 20 percent of their bone mass in the first five to seven years after menopause.
- There are approximately 300,000 hip fractures and 550,000 vertebral fractures in the United States annually.
- A woman's risk of hip fracture is greater than her combined risk of breast, uterine, and ovarian cancer.
- Twenty-four percent of hip fracture patients over the age of fifty die in the year following their fracture.
- At six months after a hip fracture, only 15 percent of patients can walk across a room unassisted.

aerobic components of your exercise program (those that increase your heart rate) have the added benefit of maintaining a healthy heart.

What medications are used to treat osteoporosis?

Ellen fills her mother's medication organizer at the beginning of every week. Her mother, Lydia, is in her mid-eighties and starting to get forgetful. Ellen notices a new medication.

"What's this pill for, Mom?" asks Ellen. "I don't remember seeing it before. When did you get it?"

"Dr. Simpson gave it to me yesterday," her mother replies.

"It couldn't have been yesterday. We didn't go to Dr. Simpson yesterday," says Ellen, convinced her mother is confused.

"Yes, I did. You were busy, so Abigail took me. The pill is for my bones. Dr. Simpson is afraid I'm going to fall and hurt myself, so she is putting me on this to keep my bones strong. I'm supposed to take it once a week."

"You're not going to take that medicine," Ellen declares. "I've heard bad things about those drugs. They rot away your jaw and cause fractures in your legs. I saw an ad on TV from a law firm saying these drugs are harmful."

"I don't know about your generation," Lydia says, beginning to get angry, "but my generation doesn't let lawyers tell doctors what they should and shouldn't do. I'm sure Dr. Simpson wouldn't have given me this if it wasn't necessary."

"Well, that may be," says Ellen, "but I can't say that I trust doctors and drug companies as much as you do. Let me call Dr. Simpson and see why you need this."

As we saw above, osteoporosis is a common condition affecting a large proportion of the population, especially women. The estimated cost of osteoporosis-related fractures is 20 billion dollars per year. This begs the question, "What can we do to prevent and treat osteoporosis?" Estrogen is very effective at slowing down bone loss, but in view of its additional risks, it is not recommended solely for that indication. Fortunately, there are many other very effective agents for the prevention and treatment of osteoporosis.

Bisphosphonates are a group of drugs that inhibit bone breakdown. Alendronate (Fosamax, Binosto) was one of the first and is still probably the most widely used nonhormonal medication for the prevention and treatment of osteoporosis. Risedronate (Actonel) and ibandronate (Boniva) are two other commonly used oral bisphosphonates with the advantage that they can be taken monthly instead of weekly. A more recent entry is zoledronic acid (Reclast), administered as an annual intravenous infusion. Most of the oral bisphosphonates are taken with a full glass of water upon waking up in the morning before you consume anything else. After taking them, you must remain upright (No, you can't go back to bed!) and cannot eat or drink anything for at least thirty to sixty minutes (longer is better) for optimal absorption. Atelvia is a newer form of risedronate that can be taken after breakfast. The most common side effects of oral bisphosphonates are GI upset (especially reflux) and bone, joint, and muscle pain. Reflux with these medications can lead to the development of esophagitis. In most cases, patients will develop heartburn symptoms before this happens and they can be switched to an intravenous bisphosphonate such as Reclast or one of the other agents listed below. The most common side effects of Reclast are flulike symptoms, fever, muscle and joint pain, headache, and GI upset. Side effects with Reclast are somewhat less disconcerting since you will only receive the infusion annually and each successive infusion tends to have fewer side effects than the first.

Osteonecrosis of the jaw (dead bone in the jaw becoming exposed through the gum with inflammation and pain) and atypical femoral fractures (fractures in the thigh bone) are two complications of bisphosphonates that have been widely publicized even though they are rare. Both of these can be seen after prolonged use of bisphosphonates (generally regarded as greater than five years). Ninety-five percent of bisphosphonate-related osteonecrosis of the jaw has occurred in cancer patients receiving high doses of intravenous bisphosphonates, especially after undergoing dental procedures that will involve the bone (tooth extraction, implant). The incidence of osteonecrosis of the jaw occurring in patients taking oral bisphosphonates without these conditions is probably no more than two to five per ten thousand women per year. If your doctor or dentist wants to be ultra-careful, he or she can ask you to hold your bisphosphonate for three to six months before and after dental procedures that will enter the bone. You should also maintain good oral hygiene and regularly visit your dentist for preventive care.

Atypical femoral fractures that occur in the mid part of your femur are also rare. There were no occurrences of this type of fracture in the sixty thousand women enrolled in the initial studies of Fosamax, Actonel, and Boniva. The risk of this type of fracture occurring is probably no more than one per ten thousand women per year. If you have significant osteoporosis with a high risk of hip fracture or spinal compression fractures, your benefit from continuing bisphosphonates well exceeds the risk associated with their use. Having said that, there are many doctors who will give patients one to two years off bisphosphonate therapy after five years (or more) of use. If bone density is poor or declining further after the medication is stopped, it can always be restarted or your doctor can switch you to a different class of osteoporosis medicine such as Forteo (see below).

Raloxifene (Evista) was the first SERM to gain approval from the FDA for menopausal women. SERMs bind to estrogen receptors in the body and in some areas act like estrogen, while in other areas act like an anti-estrogen. They prevent osteoporosis and bone fractures, have no adverse impact on your uterus, and reduce your risk of breast cancer. Evista does not cause an excess risk for heart attacks, but there is a small increase in the risk for stroke. Evista also causes an excess risk for deep vein thrombosis (blood clots in your veins) and its most common side effects are hot flashes and muscle cramps. Evista is generally well tolerated and is a reasonable drug to be considered in women for the prevention of osteoporosis.

Prolia (denosumab) is an example of a different class of medication that also helps you retain bone mass. It is administered as a subcutaneous injection every six months. Prolia is convenient and very effective, but does have potential risks, such as lowering your blood calcium level. You should have blood work to check your calcium level before starting Prolia and should take calcium and vitamin D supplements while undergoing treatment. Prolia may weaken your immune system, increasing your risk for serious infections. Skin problems such as rash, dermatitis (inflammation of your skin), and eczema have been reported. The most common side effects seen with Prolia are back pain, pain in your arms or legs, hypercholesterolemia (high cholesterol), muscle pain, and bladder infections. Since it is rather new, it is unknown whether Prolia will increase the risk of osteonecrosis of the jaw or atypical femoral fractures with prolonged use.

Forteo (teriparatide) is different than Prolia and the bisphosphonates. While they work primarily by helping to reduce bone turnover, thereby maintaining the bone mass you already have made, Forteo actually builds new bone. It is administered as a daily subcutaneous injection. While this sounds intolerable, it is really not that bad. The injection uses a tiny needle, so at most you feel a little pinch. Forteo is usually reserved for people with particularly severe osteoporosis. It can only be administered for two years. Sometimes patients develop a drop in their blood pressure when changing position after starting Forteo. This may be associated with a fast heartbeat, dizziness, or feeling faint. It usually disappears after the first few doses. Forteo can increase your blood calcium level, so your doctor will check your blood calcium level before you start using it and may not use it if you have a history of kidney stones. Your doctor may choose not to use Forteo if you are also on digoxin (used for a variety of heart conditions) since it increases the risk of digoxin toxicity. Common side effects include nausea and pain in the joints, bones, or muscles.

Calcitonin (Miacalcin, Fortical) is a drug that is generally administered by nasal spray that decreases the breakdown of bone. It also appears to have an analgesic (pain relieving) effect in women with spinal compression fractures. The FDA has recently determined that the risks of Calcitonin outweigh its benefits. There appears to be slightly higher rates of cancer and a relatively poor track record for decreasing fractures.

Another advance in the management of bone loss is the use of the FRAX calculator in women with osteopenia (bone loss that is less severe than osteoporosis). The patient's age, weight, height, gender, bone density score, and certain specific additional risk factors are entered into a calculator, which then gives the doctor your ten-year risk of developing any fracture and your ten-year risk for hip fracture. You and your doctor can then make a more reasonable decision as to whether you should start medication.

Some doctors measure various biochemical markers of bone formation and bone breakdown to help with the diagnosis and management of osteoporosis. He or she may also order lateral spine X-rays to detect spinal compression fractures in the spine.

For additional information, visit:

National Osteoporosis Foundation: www.nof.org

14

WHERE'S THE NEAREST BATHROOM?

Why do I always have to run to the bathroom?

Scene: Turnpike

> *Gladys: "When's the next rest stop?"*
> *Harry: "Why?"*
> *Gladys: "I have to go to the bathroom."*
> *Harry: "Didn't you just go?"*
> *Gladys: "Yeah, but I have to go again."*
> *Harry: "Can't you wait until you get home?"*

Harry is convinced that his wife Gladys could write a book entitled Bathrooms Across America. *He's not kidding. Gladys knows where every bathroom is within a hundred-mile radius. At the supermarket, it's between the butcher section and the produce section; make a left and it's the first door on the right. At Macy's, it's on the third floor between home furnishings and women's petite. It only has one stall, so don't wait too long. She has every rest stop on the New Jersey Turnpike timed to the nearest minute and the nearest tenth of a mile.*

Does this sound familiar? It seems as if you're always running to the bathroom. You know where all the bathrooms are located. Your children have started to kid you about it. You may have an unstable bladder, commonly referred to as overactive bladder (OAB). An overactive bladder wants to contract before you are ready to void. It causes an increase in the frequency of voiding as well as a sense of urgency. When severe, it is associated with urgency incontinence. You start to lose urine before you can make it to the bathroom. The unwanted bladder contractions may occur spontaneously or be triggered by a specific event, such as the sound of running water. The uninhibited contractions may be secondary to conditions that cause inflammation or irritation to the bladder (infection, stones, estrogen deficiency). They can also result from diseases that affect the nervous system (stroke, dementia, Parkinson's disease, multiple sclerosis, spinal cord injury). Most often there is no identifiable source for the unstable bladder.

If you have urgency incontinence, you should see a gynecologist, urologist, or gynecologic urologist. (How fancy can you get?) Some conditions that cause incontinence can only be diagnosed with specific testing. The doctor will probably perform a cystoscopy and cystometrogram (CMG). These are described below. He will also obtain urine for analysis. These studies can help rule out underlying conditions that may be inducing the unwanted bladder contractions.

Okay, you've been evaluated and there is no obvious cause for the overactive bladder. Now what do you do? Start by eliminating caffeine (coffee, tea, chocolate, colas), alcohol, hot spices, acidic foods (tomato and citrus products, or use them with Prelief, an over-the-counter product designed to neutralize acid in foods), and artificial sweeteners from your diet. Alternatively, keep a food diary and see which items increase your bladder urgency. Your doctor may also have a more extensive list of possible culprits. If you take a prescribed diuretic, ask your doctor if it can be stopped and replaced by a different type of medication or reduced. If you must take a diuretic, time it so that you will be home. The first approach to treating an unstable bladder is bladder retraining. We have to get you back to the point where you are controlling your bladder, not vice versa. Pick a time interval that you can successfully wait between voiding. This may be as low as half an hour. For purposes of discussion, let's say you choose one hour. For one week, you must go to the bathroom every hour on the hour and empty your bladder. If you are successful without any accidents, add fifteen minutes to the next week. Every week that you are successful, add fifteen more minutes until you get to a reasonable interval (at least three to four hours). This method of training using timed voiding really does work, but (and this is a big *but*) you have to be very motivated to follow through with the schedule. You do not have to wake yourself at night to comply with the schedule. (Let's not get too crazy!)

Another goal is for you to learn how to control the sense of urgency until it subsides. What's happening now is that you run to the nearest bathroom as soon as you feel the urge. That seems like the right thing to do. After all, you don't want to have an accident. Wrong! You've just let your bladder win. Your running to the bathroom only heightens the sensation of a full bladder. Running to the bathroom also stimulates the bladder muscles, thereby inducing contractions. Burgio, Pearce, and Lucco recommend the following six steps in their book *Staying Dry: A Practical Guide to Bladder Control* (highly recommended):

- Stop what you are doing and stay put. Sit down when possible, or stand quietly. Remain very still. When you are still, it is easier to control your urge.
- Squeeze your pelvic floor muscles quickly several times (described below). Do not relax fully in between.
- Relax the rest of your body. Take a few deep breaths to help you relax and let go of your tension.
- Concentrate on suppressing the urge feeling.
- Wait until the urge subsides.
- Walk to the bathroom at a normal pace. Do not rush. Continue squeezing your pelvic floor muscles quickly while you walk.

If you are menopausal, estrogen replacement may reduce your urgency and frequency. Estrogen sustains the inside lining of the bladder and urethra, referred to as the mucosa. Without estrogen, the mucosa atrophies (similar to the vaginal mucosa). This can produce increased frequency, urgency, and burning with urination. Small amounts of estrogen applied vaginally, which doesn't have the same risks as systemic estrogen, can help correct the mucosal atrophy.

When all else fails, there are medications that help reduce bladder irritability. These medications increase bladder storage capacity and reduce the number of unwanted contractions. You're thinking, *Hey, this sounds great. Just give me those magic pills and my problem will be solved.*

Unfortunately, there's a catch. (Isn't there always?) Most of these have annoying side effects. The most common side effect is dry mouth. Hard candy or chewing gum may help with the dryness. Other side effects include palpitations, constipation, blurry vision, and decreased sweating. They cannot be used in women with some types of glaucoma, unstable heart disease, or conditions associated with blockage of the bowel or bladder. There are many choices when it comes to overactive bladder medications. Some of the more recent products may be slightly more effective with fewer side effects, but not dramatically so. Your bladder did not become unstable overnight, and it may not regain its stability with medications immediately. We recommend that you try one of these medications for at least two to three months before you decide whether it is helping you or not. If you have intolerable side effects from one of the medications, let your doctor know. He or she can try another. One of these medications, oxybutynin, is now available over the counter under the name Oxytrol. Myrbetriq (mirabegron) is a newer drug for overactive bladder, approved by the FDA in June of 2012. It works on a different type of bladder receptor than most of the other drugs. It may increase blood pressure and is not recommended for patients with uncontrolled hypertension (high blood pressure). The FDA has also approved Botox for OAB. The Botox is injected into the bladder muscle through a cystoscope (a telescopic instrument used to look into your bladder) and can be repeated every three months. Sacral nerve stimulation, described below when we address interstitial cystitis, can also be used in OAB that seems to be refractory to all other treatments.

Is it normal to get up at night to go to the bathroom?

Getting up once during the night is not unusual. More than once isn't typical and is referred to as nocturia. There are many reasons for nocturia, some of which are obvious. Of course we'll mention them anyway.

Many people consume beverages in the late evening. It may be the first time all day they have had the opportunity to sit down and relax. Reading a good book with a cup of tea sounds just perfect. Others don't drink adequate amounts of liquids throughout the day. They make up the difference in the evening hours. Unfortunately, those liquids will come back to haunt you in the middle of the night, requiring several trips to the bathroom. Try to drink more throughout the day and restrict the amount of fluids consumed in the late evening. This is particularly true of caffeinated and alcoholic beverages, which have diuretic properties (help your kidneys get rid of fluid). Do not take a prescribed diuretic ("water pill") within two to three hours of bedtime.

Some women retain fluid throughout the day when they are on their feet. You can recognize this as swelling in your legs, particularly ankles and feet, and tight shoes. When recumbent at night, the fluid finally makes its way out of the legs and up to the kidneys where it is eliminated. This results in extra trips to the bathroom. In this situation, a prescribed diuretic taken in the late afternoon or early evening may be able to help the kidneys excrete the retained fluid prior to bedtime. You should consult your doctor to exclude more serious conditions that cause fluid retention. Your doctor can also rule out other diseases, such as diabetes, that cause frequent urination.

Women with overactive bladders will also note increased nighttime frequency and urgency. Refer to our discussion above on the unstable bladder.

Why do I lose urine when I cough or sneeze?

Barbara and Connie play tennis together at Kingston Racquet Club. They are walking onto the court when Bonnie blurts out, "Wait a minute, I have to go back."

"What's the problem?" asks Connie.

"I have to put on a pad," responds Barbara. "If not, I'll be totally wet by the time we're done."

"I used to have that problem," Connie responds. "It was terrible. You know how often I get bronchitis. Every time I coughed, I would wet myself."

"What did you do to fix it?" asks Bonnie. "My gynecologist says that I need surgery. I'm not sure that I'm ready for surgery. I only have the problem in certain situations."

"I started doing Kegel exercises," Connie replies.

"I heard those don't work very well." Bonnie is skeptical.

"They didn't work very well until I really committed to them, but now that I do them every day, things have gotten much better. I hardly have any leakage when I cough."

Have you ever heard a woman exclaim, "Don't make me laugh or I'll have an accident!" How about, "I laughed so hard that I wet myself"? They probably weren't kidding. Losing urine with a cough, sneeze, or laugh is common and referred to as urinary stress incontinence (USI). It is usually caused by inadequate support under the bladder neck, where the urethra enters the bladder. Childbirth, age, postmenopausal loss of estrogen, and a lifetime of lifting and pushing have conspired to destroy the support in this region. Even your genes may have betrayed you. Fair-skinned women (northern European) and Asian women have a particularly high likelihood of developing stress incontinence, as well as prolapse disorders (see below). Activities that may produce incontinence include coughing, sneezing, laughing, running, jumping, and dancing. All of these cause the bladder neck to descend, and urine can escape.

Urinary stress incontinence is cured by restoring the support at the bladder neck. Some of this support is provided by the muscles of your pelvic floor. One of these muscles, the pubococcygeus (throw that one at your gynecologist if you really want to show off), can be strengthened to help with bladder neck support. You can strengthen it through Kegel exercises. First you must identify the proper muscle. Place one or two fingers in the vagina. Now squeeze the pelvic muscles until you feel them tighten around your finger. Those are the muscles used in Kegel exercises. It is the same muscle group that enables you to voluntarily shut off your stream of urine or prevent the passing of gas. Try to contract these muscles without contracting your abdominal muscles. Place your other hand on your abdomen to make sure that it remains soft while you contract the pelvic muscles. Squeeze the pelvic muscles for a count of three, and then relax for a count of three. Repeat this fifteen times during one session and try to do three sessions daily. Every week, increase the length of time that you hold your squeeze until you reach a count of ten. However many counts you are contracting the muscle is the same amount of time that you will wait between squeezes. When you can reliably identify the correct muscles, you don't have to do these exercises with your fingers in the vagina. You can do them while waiting in line for the train or while sitting at a traffic light. You can do them almost anytime. As long as you're not grimacing, who's going to know? Pilates and yoga also help to correct the alignment and strength of your pelvic floor muscles.

There are also fancy gadgets to help train the muscles involved in pelvic support. A manometer (a device that measures pressure) can be used to provide feedback. It registers the amount of pressure generated when you squeeze the pelvic support muscles. Pelvic floor exercises are more effective if you have this feedback. Many of these devices will also deliver an electrical impulse to help stimulate the muscles (InTone, SenseRx, FemiScan). In addition to strengthening the pelvic floor muscles, electrical impulses can inhibit involuntary bladder contractions. Therefore, these devices are also of benefit in the treatment of an overactive bladder (see above). Your doctor may utilize the services of a gynecologic physical therapist or nurse practitioner for instituting these therapeutic devices. Weighted vaginal cones (tampon-like devices) are also useful. You are provided with a set of cones that are of the same shape and size but gradually increasing in weight. You place a cone in the vagina and retain it for fifteen minutes twice daily. The cone can only be held in place if you correctly tighten the pelvic support muscles. The weight of the cone is increased until you can successfully retain the heaviest cone.

Unfortunately, most of the support at the bladder neck is provided by fibrous tissue. You can't exercise fibrous tissue back into shape. Once it is torn or stretched, it cannot be restored without surgery. There is not a lot you can do to make this tissue stronger. A healthy diet helps. Estrogen replacement after menopause also strengthens the tissue. Even small amounts of vaginal estrogen will be effective. However, most of its strength is predetermined by genetics. In other words, you're born with either strong or weak fibrous tissue.

Mechanical devices may be used to elevate the bladder neck. In one form or another, these are designed to either increase support at the bladder neck (specially designed pessaries) or block leakage (FemSoft insert). They have only had a fair amount of success and tend to come on and off the market fairly quickly. For mild situational incontinence, use of a tampon may also be of some help by elevating the bladder neck. With the advent of less invasive surgical approaches, most mechanical devices have fallen by the wayside.

If conservative measures don't correct the incontinence, surgery is recommended. Traditionally, urinary stress incontinence surgery required reasonably major surgery with significant sized incisions. However, there has been a gradual evolution away from these larger procedures to those which are now classified as minimally invasive. The most common procedures use a small strip of mesh that is threaded through very tiny incisions (transobturator, or TOT, sling or transvaginal, or TVT, sling procedures). This type of surgery is 80–90 percent successful and can be performed either as an outpatient or at most with an overnight stay.

The single most important factor in determining the success of surgery is proper patient selection. Although it is not universally recommended, we strongly encourage urologic evaluation prior to surgery. If you have genuine stress incontinence, your chances of success with surgery are great. If your incontinence is related to other causes, such as an unstable bladder, the surgery will probably not be successful. In fact, you may worsen after surgery.

Stress incontinence may also be related to an intrinsic defect in the urethral sphincter mechanism. The urethral sphincter is comprised of the muscles in the wall of the urethra as it passes into the bladder. If these don't keep the urethra closed, you will lose urine with any activity that increases the pressure in your abdomen (laugh, cough, and sneeze). This type of defect can be more resistant to standard treatment. Some medications can strengthen urethral tone. They usually contain either phenylpropanolamine (Ornade) or pseudoephedrine (Sudafed). Many over-the-counter decongestants and appetite suppressants contain one of these two medications. They must be used cautiously in individuals with high blood pressure, cardiac disease, or hyperthyroidism. Side effects include palpitations, nervousness, headaches, and insomnia. Doctors also inject collagen (the stuff that makes up fibrous tissue) or synthetic beads directly into the wall of the urethra to correct intrinsic urethral defects. These injections help the urethra close more effectively. They can be performed as an outpatient under the guidance of a cystoscope. Often repeat injections are necessary for optimal benefit. Finally, your doctor may recommend a TOT or TVT sling procedure as described above, although sling procedures in patients with intrinsic sphincter deficiency have a somewhat lower success rate compared with patients who have genuine urinary stress incontinence.

Why do I keep getting bladder infections?

Bladder infection, or cystitis, is a fairly common infection. The urethral meatus (opening) is located just above the opening of the vagina. Since the vagina has many bacteria, it is not surprising that these organisms gain access to the bladder. This is particularly true with intercourse. It is not uncommon for women to get a bladder infection during their honeymoon ("honeymoon cystitis") from the increased sexual activity. Isn't that a heck of a way to celebrate your new marriage!

The occasional cystitis can be treated with antibiotics and forcing fluids. Over-the-counter bladder analgesics like Uristat or AZO can be added to reduce pain. Ideally, you should have a urine culture performed if you present with symptoms of infection (frequency, urgency, and burning). Not all infections respond to the same antibiotic. Your doctor can choose the correct antibiotic if a culture is done. Recurrent bladder infections should prompt your doctor to order additional studies. First, you should get urine cultures every time there is an infection. A repeat culture should be obtained two weeks after finishing the antibiotics. If the same bacteria are still present on culture after treatment, then it probably did not respond to the original antibiotic. This may be resolved by taking a different antibiotic. If the infection appears to clear each time (negative posttreatment cultures), then you are dealing with reinfection.

Frequent reinfection (three to four times per year) may be a sign of a more serious underlying condition. You should see a urologist for additional studies. You may have a congenital defect in your urinary tract (born with a faulty design in your plumbing). You might have bladder or kidney stones or a bladder or urethral diverticulum (sac or pouch opening out from the bladder wall). The doctor will probably perform cystoscopy and might order an IVP (see below) or CT scan of your kidneys. He may also want to perform a cystometrogram (see below) to evaluate your bladder function. Often no source for the recurrent infections is found. In this situation, you may be given methenamine (Urex, Hiprex), which has nonspecific antibacterial activity, or a daily prophylactic antibiotic to prevent future infections. When used for prevention, broad-spectrum antibiotics (antibiotics that seem to kill everything) should be avoided. Long-term use of broad-spectrum antibiotics increases the risk of your body developing bacteria that are resistant to antibiotics.

"What else can I do to avoid recurrent infections?" If the infections are induced by sexual activity, it is recommended that you empty your bladder after intercourse. You may also be instructed to take an antibiotic after intercourse. Prevent urethral injury by using a lubricant (such as K-Y Jelly) if there is inadequate natural lubrication. With recurrent infections, make sure you drink plenty of liquids throughout the day and empty your bladder on a regular basis. After voiding, wipe only from front to back. Good hygiene is essential in preventing recurrent infections. You and your partner need to keep the genital and anal areas clean. Showers are better than baths. Avoid tight clothing and wear cotton rather than synthetics. Synthetics trap heat and moisture (a lovely environment for bacteria), whereas cotton breathes. In postmenopausal women, estrogen replacement (even just vaginal estrogen) may help prevent recurrent infections.

Everyone has heard of cranberry juice, but does it really work? Scientists have found compounds in cranberry and blueberry juice that inhibit bladder infections, so it's probably worth a try. Cranberry tablets (300–400 mg twice daily) are available over the counter. Many natural compounds are promoted for the prevention of urinary tract infections in the complementary and alternative community. Those that have at least some scientific studies supporting their use include uva ursi (short-term only), berberine (0.5 gm–1 gm daily), green tea extract (250–500 mg daily), mannose, and probiotics (see chapter 5). Acidification of the urine with vitamin C (1–3 gm orally three to four times daily) may also be of some benefit.

What are those tests the doctor wants me to do?

Your doctor has forewarned you that additional tests will be required to diagnose the cause of your bladder problem. Now what exactly does he or she have in mind? Some of those words the doctor was throwing around sounded rather ominous. Let's spend some time examining these tests. What is involved? What can they accomplish?

- *Cystoscopy* (also cystourethroscopy): Cystoscopy is a procedure in which a doctor inserts a thin telescope through the urethra into the bladder. This enables him or her to look directly into the bladder for evidence of tumors, stones, diverticuli (see above), or inflammatory conditions. He or she can also visualize how well the urethral sphincter closes. Insertion of the cystoscope may cause discomfort. The doctor may use a numbing ointment or sedation to lessen the pain. Occasionally, the procedure is done under anesthesia as outpatient surgery. You may have some burning and frequency with urination after the procedure. A small amount of blood in the urine afterwards is not unusual. If these persist more than twenty-four hours, notify your doctor; you may have an infection. Sometimes doctors give an antibiotic after the procedure to prevent infection.
- *Cystometrogram*: A cystometrogram measures the pressure in your bladder as it is filled. It also evaluates your bladder capacity and looks for unwanted bladder contractions (bladder spasms). A catheter is placed in the bladder through

the urethra. Sometimes more than one catheter is placed, and the doctor may also insert a catheter into the rectum to measure abdominal pressure (gee, this just keeps getting better and better). Your bladder is then filled with water or carbon dioxide. The doctor asks you to indicate your first sense of bladder filling (first sensation). You then tell him or her when it feels as if you must void (bladder capacity). As the bladder is filling, the doctor looks for involuntary contractions. Women with urgency incontinence (overactive bladder) will demonstrate first sensation at lower bladder volumes and exhibit involuntary contractions. This test can also detect neurologic problems that cause abnormal bladder function (inadequate sensation or poor contraction of the bladder muscles).

- *IVP* (intravenous pyelogram): An IVP is a radiologic test that lets your doctor visualize the collecting system from the kidneys down to (and including) the bladder. He or she can evaluate the position and integrity of the ureters (the tubes connecting your kidneys to the bladder—not to be confused with the urethra). Certain disorders (kidney stones, congenital defects) are visualized well with an IVP. The test is performed in the radiology department. A radiologic dye is injected intravenously and X-rays are taken as your kidneys excrete the dye. Most people tolerate this test well, but you can have a severe reaction if you are allergic to iodine or shellfish. If you know of such an allergy, inform your physician.

- *Voiding cystourethrogram*: A radiologic test to evaluate the structure and function of your urethra and bladder. The bladder is filled with dye through a catheter. X-rays are taken of you standing, bearing down, and voiding. A voiding cystourethrogram may help diagnose structural support problems or intrinsic urethral defects (see above section on stress incontinence).

- *Urethral pressure profile*: This test compares the pressure in your bladder to that in the urethra. A pressure catheter is placed into the bladder. A small amount of water is placed into the bladder and the pressure is measured. The catheter is then withdrawn into the urethra and the pressure measured at several points along the urethra. The pressure in the urethra must be greater than that in the bladder if you are to remain continent. Low urethral pressures may be associated with stress incontinence.

- *Q-tip test*: A Q-tip is placed into the urethra. You are then asked to strain (bear down). If there is inadequate support of the bladder neck and urethra, the angle of the Q-tip will change. This is seen in women with stress incontinence.
- *Marshall test*: You are asked to bear down or cough with a full bladder. Your doctor looks through the vagina for descent of the bladder neck and loss of urine. He or she then elevates the bladder neck and has you cough or strain again. If there is no more leakage, you probably have genuine stress incontinence. Surgery that elevates the bladder neck (see above) should solve your problem.
- *CT (or CAT) scan*: A CT scan of the abdomen or pelvis may be ordered, particularly if your doctor needs to rule out a kidney or bladder tumor.
- *Ultrasound scan*: Ultrasound may be used to image the kidneys, ureters, and bladder and can also be used to see if you are completely emptying your bladder after voiding.

"You've got to be kidding! You don't really expect me to go through all of these. I'd rather live with my incontinence." Let's not panic. It isn't very likely that you will have to undergo most of these tests. Your doctor will only submit you to those that are necessary for your particular situation. Most of these tests sound worse than they are in reality. Of course, that's easy for us to say.

If you would like more information on incontinence, consider the following resources:

National Association for Continence: www.nafc.org

Continence Restored, Inc: 203-348-0601

My doctor says I have interstitial cystitis. What's that?

Jenny meets her mother, Gloria, at Tiffany's Diner every Sunday morning before they go to church. Both women usually enjoy this time together, but this morning Jenny looks unusually downcast.

"What's wrong?" her mother asks.

"Nothing, Mom; I'm fine."

"You're not fine. I'm your mother. You might be able to fool other people, but I know that something is going on with you, so let's have it."

"I'm just so tired of being in pain all the time. My pelvis feels like it's on fire. It hurts when I go to the bathroom and it feels like I have to go all the time. It even hurts when I have sex," responds Jenny, looking quite miserable.

"How come this is the first time I'm hearing about this?" asks Gloria, clearly upset.

"I don't tell you everything, Mom. You have your own medical issues to worry about. You don't need to be worrying about me."

"I'm your mother," Gloria replies. "Worrying about your children comes with the territory. You shouldn't hide things from me. You need to see a doctor about this. Did you see your gynecologist? What did he have to say?"

"I saw Dr. Schaeffer. He did an exam, got cultures, ordered blood work, looked at my urine, and got a pelvic ultrasound. He told me everything is normal and that I don't have a gynecologic problem. He sent me to a urologist."

"What did he say?" asks her mother, obviously concerned.

"The urologist was a woman, Dr. Washington. She looked at my urine and put an instrument into my bladder to take a look. She said everything looked normal. When I asked her why I go to the bathroom so often and why it hurts, she told me that I must have an irritable bladder. She put me on a medicine to relax the bladder, but all it did was make my mouth dry so I stopped it."

"It sounds like you're really hurting," responds her mother. "Is there anything else that can be done?"

"I went to see another gynecologist, Dr. Lewis, for a second opinion," begins Jenny. *"She looked at the records of the other doctors and told me that the only thing left to do was a laparoscopy, so that's what we did."*

"What's a laparoscopy? That sounds scary."

"It's a procedure in the operating room where they knock you out and put a telescope in your belly to look at your pelvic organs."

"You had surgery and didn't tell me?!" Gloria exclaims, obviously hurt by this revelation.

"I didn't tell you because I knew you would freak out. Ed went with me. It's not a big deal. In any case, it wasn't very helpful. Dr. Lewis said that all my pelvic organs look fine."

"You poor thing. I don't know what to tell you. I guess it's good that all your tests were normal. Maybe it's something that will just go away on its own," says her mother, trying to sound reassuring.

"Maybe, but it's been going on for almost a year now. That's the worst part. I have no idea why this is happening and if it'll ever get better."

Welcome to the frustrating world of interstitial cystitis (IC), also referred to as painful bladder syndrome (PBS). Interstitial cystitis is an inflammatory bladder disorder that can cause urinary frequency and urgency, decreased bladder capacity, dyspareunia (painful intercourse), and suprapubic (just above your pubic bone) or pelvic pain. If you have these symptoms and no obvious cause has been identified (infection, stones, tumor, unstable bladder, gynecologic diseases), IC/PBS must be considered. Nobody knows for sure what causes interstitial cystitis, and women often have symptoms for years before an accurate diagnosis is made. Most research into the cause of IC has focused on decreased levels of protective substances that line the bladder wall or increased leakiness through the lining that protects your bladder wall.

There are other medical conditions that seem to be associated with IC/PBS, including inflammatory bowel disease, systemic lupus, irritable bowel syndrome, vulvodynia (see chapter 11), allergies, endometriosis (see chapter 8), and fibromyalgia. Each of these has been described in at least some studies to be more common in people with IC/PBS, but there is no evidence that any of these conditions is the cause of IC/PBS. Women with this condition are also more likely to have had frequent urinary tract infections or prior gynecologic surgery.

The diagnosis of interstitial cystitis is usually made by cystoscopy. Under anesthesia, a telescope is introduced into the bladder through the urethra. The bladder may initially look normal, or there may be ulcerations of the inside lining (mucosa). The urologist will then stretch the walls of the bladder by filling it with water, a process called hydrodistention. Small hemorrhagic areas called glomerulations may then be seen. A bladder biopsy may be taken and sent for analysis. The biopsy may show inflammation or fibrosis (scarring) if you have interstitial cystitis. Another test performed for diagnosis of this condition is called the potassium sensitivity test (PST). In this test, your doctor places two solutions—water and potassium chloride—into your bladder, one at a time. You're asked to rate on a scale of zero to five the pain and urgency you feel after each solution is instilled. If you feel noticeably more pain or urgency with the potassium solution than with the water, your doctor may diagnose interstitial cystitis. People with normal bladders can't tell the difference between the two solutions. Because both of these diagnostic techniques are either invasive or painful, some doctors are now willing to proceed with treatment on the basis of severe bladder symptoms, presuming no other cause for the symptoms can be discovered.

No one specific treatment for interstitial cystitis has been found to work for everybody. Hydrodistention (mentioned above) provides temporary relief of symptoms in 30 percent of women. Some foods and beverages appear to aggravate the symptoms of interstitial cystitis. Alcohol, caffeine-containing beverages, chocolate, citrus fruits, tomatoes, and spicy foods seem to be the prime offenders. Avoid these and any other foods that consistently worsen your symptoms. Bladder training (as outlined above in our discussion of the unstable bladder) will also help some women. Other conservative support measures include stress management, hypnotherapy, biofeedback, and electrical stimulation therapy. Medical regimens are used with varying degrees of success. Elmiron (pentosan polysulfate sodium, for those of you with a chemistry degree) is approved by the FDA for the treatment of interstitial cystitis. Elmiron is generally well tolerated, although side effects may include nausea, diarrhea, headaches, and reversible hair loss. Even after therapy has begun with Elmiron, symptoms may persist for a long time because the sensory nerves in the bladder have been hyperactive and take a long time to return to their normal state of activation. Therefore, doctors recommend giving up to one year of Elmiron treatment in mild IC/PBS and two years in severe IC/PBS before deciding if the drug is effective or not. Having said that, between one-third and two-thirds of patients will improve after three months of treatment. Anti-inflammatory medications, antidepressants, antihistamines, and antispasmodic drugs are all used by physicians with varying degrees of success. An example of this is Urelle (also Uribel) that combines analgesic, antiseptic, and antispasmodic drugs. Some forms of treatment include the installation of medication or chemicals directly into the bladder. Approximately 90 percent of women will respond to medical treatment, although several different agents may be necessary before success is achieved.

Transcutaneous electrical nerve stimulation (TENS) uses mild electrical pulses to relieve pelvic pain and, in some cases, reduce urinary frequency. Electrical wires are placed on your lower back or just above your pubic area and pulses are administered for minutes or hours two or more times a day, depending on the length and frequency of therapy that works best for you. In some cases a device that delivers electrical impulses will be inserted into the vagina.

Another possible nerve stimulation treatment is sacral nerve stimulation. Modulation of your sacral nerve roots, which regulate bladder sensation and function, may reduce feelings of urinary urgency that accompany interstitial cystitis. With sacral nerve stimulation, a thin wire placed near the sacral nerves delivers electrical impulses to your bladder, similar to what a pacemaker does for the heart. If the procedure successfully lessens your symptoms, a permanent device may be surgically implanted.

When all else fails, surgery may be recommended. Cystoscopy with either fulguration (burning) or excision of the ulcerations which are sometimes present in interstitial cystitis can be done as outpatient surgery. Enlarging the bladder (augmentation cystoplasty) may help reduce urinary frequency and urgency in those individuals that have a small bladder capacity. Although this may increase bladder capacity, patients may have difficulty emptying it (usually requiring intermittent catheterization) and still have bladder pain. When symptoms are severe and intractable, urinary diversion can be performed. In this procedure, the bladder is no longer functional. Instead, the urine is diverted to a pouch constructed from intestinal tissue. Strong consideration should be given to removing the bladder (cystectomy) if diversion is elected. Urinary diversion without cystectomy increases the chance of persistent pelvic pain after surgery. Urinary diversion with cystectomy is only considered when there is end-stage bladder disease that is refractory to medical management.

Interstitial cystitis is a frustrating condition for you and your doctor. You may have symptoms for years before an accurate diagnosis is rendered. Various treatment regimens may be tried without significant or lasting improvement. You have to be persistent in exploring a variety of treatment modalities. Using the available treatments, most women will ultimately find relief.

For further information on interstitial cystitis, visit:

Interstitial Cystitis Association: www.ichelp.org

Interstitial Cystitis Network: www.IC-network.org

European Society for Study of Interstitial Cystitis: www.essic.eu

15

PELVIC PROLAPSE: THE "DROPPED BLADDER"

What is that bulge down there?

It's been a long time, but Joe is feeling vigorous. He finally discovered the wonders of the magic blue pill. He eagerly climbs into bed with Angie. They start to snuggle and just when he's getting excited, something horrible appears.

"There's something coming out of your vagina!" Joe exclaims.

"What are you talking about?" asks Angie, totally baffled.

Joe continues, "There's something bulging out of your vagina. It looks like you're giving birth to an alien or something. I'm not getting near you till that thing gets checked out."

"Well, I don't feel anything abnormal," says Angie, "but I'll get it checked out. Now you've got me worried."

No, Angie's not giving birth to an alien, but she does have a "dropped bladder" or what doctors call a cystocele. Many women later in life develop pelvic prolapse with descent of the uterus, bladder, or rectum down the vagina. Most women don't have much in the way of symptoms from this until something starts protruding from the opening of the vagina. You feel a mass bulging when you wipe yourself and you're scared out of your wits! Your first thought is that you must have a tumor, but it is much more likely that you have pelvic prolapse. Pelvic prolapse (also called pelvic descensus or pelvic relaxation) is descent of the pelvic organs from inadequate support. Failure of the support between the vagina and the bladder leads to a cystocele. A rectocele occurs if support is insufficient between the vagina and the rectum. The uterus drops if its supporting ligaments deteriorate (uterine descensus). Inadequate support at the top of the vagina produces vaginal vault prolapse (the vagina turns inside out and protrudes). Finally (Is there no end to this madness?), you can develop an enterocele. An enterocele is a herniation between the walls of the vagina and rectum. We could describe these defects all day and you still wouldn't be able to visualize them. This is one situation where a picture really is worth a thousand words. Your gynecologist can show you a picture of these defects to give you a better idea of what we're talking about.

How did this happen?

Your uterus, bladder, and rectum are supported by fibrous tissue (also called connective tissue) and ligaments (not as firm as ligaments that are in joints). They are also supported by the levator ani muscles that comprise the floor of the pelvis, referred to as the pelvic diaphragm. Stretching and tearing of these tissues during childbirth results in permanent damage to your pelvic support. A lifetime of straining and bearing down (pushing and lifting heavy objects) also causes stress on these structures. Connective tissue deteriorates with age and menopause (secondary to decreased estrogen). Over time, the cumulative stress of these factors produces pelvic prolapse.

Inherent constitutional factors (size and shape of the pelvis and the quality of the connective tissue) play a large role in the predisposition for prolapse. Northern Europeans, Egyptians, and women from India are particularly prone to developing prolapse. It appears less frequently in African-American women. The predisposition for prolapse also appears to be familial. If your mom has pelvic support problems, your risk is increased.

What symptoms will I have from prolapse?

Symptoms vary according to the size and type of defect. Mild to moderate relaxation of pelvic support is common and usually not associated with any symptoms. As the prolapse progresses, you will begin to feel a bulging sensation or pressure in the lower vagina. Some women liken this sensation to sitting on an egg. You also may experience a "pulling" sensation or cramping in the lower abdomen, groin, pelvis, and lower back. Symptoms are usually accentuated by standing and lifting. You may have difficulty emptying your bladder with a cystocele. This can cause frequent bladder infections. Incomplete evacuation of bowel movements may be secondary to a rectocele. A rectocele does not produce constipation. Constipation commonly coexists with a rectocele, but is not caused by it. Women often find that manual elevation of their cystocele or rectocele facilitates the emptying of these organs.

I lose my urine. Is that because of my dropped bladder?

Patients and doctors often incorrectly attribute incontinence to a cystocele. A cystocele, by itself, does not usually cause incontinence. If the cystocele is massive and totally prolapses beyond the opening of the vagina, you may experience overflow type incontinence. The capacity of the bladder has been exceeded and it cannot empty. The pressure in your bladder builds up until the urine begins to overflow out of the urethra. If there is very poor support of the tissues under the bladder neck, you may have stress incontinence.

If you have incontinence, don't assume that it is related to your cystocele. The incontinence must be evaluated as a separate entity as outlined in our section on bladder disorders.

Is pelvic prolapse dangerous?

There is nothing particularly dangerous about pelvic prolapse. Aggressive treatment is not required for minor degrees of relaxation. Begin preventive measures to keep the prolapse from worsening (see below).

A cystocele associated with recurrent bladder infections should be corrected. Bladder infections can ascend to the kidneys or into the bloodstream, which causes more serious problems.

If there is protrusion beyond the opening of the vagina, ulceration of the tissue will eventually occur. The tissue will deteriorate, ulcerate, bleed, and possibly become infected. This does not happen overnight, so don't panic. However, you should proceed with definitive correction of your prolapse if it extends beyond the outer lips of the vagina.

What can I do to keep my prolapse from getting worse?

Mild degrees of pelvic relaxation do not require aggressive intervention. However, you can help prevent it from worsening. A group of muscles, collectively called the levator ani, provides support for the rectum, vagina, and bladder. This is also referred to as the pelvic diaphragm or pelvic floor. These muscles are strengthened through Kegel exercises. These exercises, as well as other techniques used to strengthen the levator ani, are outlined in our section on bladder disorders (see page 314).

Postmenopausal women should consider hormone replacement therapy if they have pelvic relaxation. Estrogen prevents atrophy of the vaginal and bladder mucosa (the inside lining of the vagina and bladder). Estrogen also appears to maintain the integrity of pelvic connective tissue (fibrous tissue that provides the majority of the support to pelvic structures). Small amounts of vaginal estrogen will provide these benefits with little or no risk to other areas of the body.

If you have pelvic relaxation, you should restrict heavy lifting, pushing, and pulling. Any activity that increases your abdominal pressure is likely to worsen your condition. When lifting, use your legs (squat close to the object and straighten your legs to lift), not your abdominal muscles. Fill your grocery bags and laundry baskets half full. Avoid carrying the grandchildren. Place them on a couch next to you if you want to snuggle. If you go on a walk with them, use a stroller. Stop moving furniture when you clean. Get your children or husband to do it (they must be good for something). While you're at it, have them lug that heavy vacuum cleaner upstairs. Better yet, buy another vacuum for upstairs. These are just some examples of activities that you may need to modify.

Medical conditions that induce chronic coughing or constipation may worsen pelvic prolapse. Your doctor and you should try to correct these if possible. Weight reduction may also be of benefit in those who are very heavy. If you have not already done so, stop smoking. Girdles should not be worn in women with pelvic prolapse. The girdle increases abdominal pressure, which places downward pressure on the pelvic organs.

How is prolapse corrected?

When your prolapse has progressed beyond the opening of the vagina, it is unlikely that Kegel exercises or other therapeutic techniques will be of much benefit. You must proceed with surgical correction or a pessary. A pessary is a silicone device designed to provide support that is inserted into the vagina. Ring-shaped pessaries are the most common, but other shapes are also available. Some pessaries are inserted and removed by a health professional. Others are designed to permit self-insertion and removal. The primary advantage of a pessary is that it is not surgery. There is no significant risk in using a pessary. The pessary is fit in the doctor's office. It should not be uncomfortable and should relieve most of the pressure you were experiencing from the prolapse. However, the pessary is a foreign object. Because of that, you gradually develop an increased discharge, often with a foul odor. Trimo-San is a cleansing deodorant gel that may be used with a pessary to decrease the discharge. Your doctor will ask you to return to the office on a regular basis (approximately every three months). At that time, the doctor or one of his or her assistants will remove the pessary and clean it. He or she will also clean the vagina and inspect it for any sign of ulceration. Sometimes the pessary will cause an ulceration of the vaginal mucosa (lining). This is particularly true if the mucosa is thin from estrogen deficiency. Postmenopausal women can decrease the likelihood of vaginal ulceration with estrogen replacement. Even small amounts of vaginal estrogen cream can help sustain the vaginal walls, thereby decreasing the risk of ulceration. Pessaries that are self-inserted are less likely to cause abnormal discharge or vaginal ulceration. Usually, you insert the pessary in the morning and remove it at night. It can also be removed for intercourse.

Surgery is the most definitive approach to correcting prolapse. Let's face it. Pessaries can be a pain in the neck. Surgery provides you with the opportunity to get the problem solved conclusively. The type of surgery varies according to the type of prolapse. We'll briefly review the most commonly used operations. You will have to consult your doctor to assess which of these might be appropriate for you.

- Vaginal Hysterectomy—If the uterus descends significantly, it is removed through the vagina by vaginal hysterectomy. The supporting ligaments of the uterus are then reattached to the top of the vagina for support. If these ligaments appear inadequate, a vaginal vault suspension may also be performed (see below).
- Anterior Colporrhaphy (anterior vaginal repair)—This is an operation for the correction of a cystocele (dropped bladder). An incision is made through the mucosa (lining) of the vagina to gain access to the supporting tissue of the bladder. This supporting tissue is then brought under the bladder to lift it higher. Other operative procedures performed at the same time might include a separate procedure for bladder neck suspension (to correct stress incontinence) and reattachment of support tissue to the sidewalls of the pelvis (paravaginal repair).
- Posterior Colporrhaphy (posterior vaginal repair)—This corrects a rectocele. An incision is made through the vaginal mucosa overlying the rectum. Supporting tissue is then brought over the rectum to reduce the rectal bulge.
- Perineorrhaphy—This procedure corrects a defective perineum (the area between the opening of the vagina and the anus). Your perineum is composed of muscles and connective tissue that provide support for the lower portions of the vagina and rectum. Connective tissue and muscles that help support the vagina, rectum, and bladder connect to this area. Often it has been damaged through childbirth and must be rebuilt at the time of surgery.

- Vaginal Vault Suspension—If there is inadequate support at the apex of the vagina after hysterectomy, the vagina inverts and descends outward (like turning your pocket inside-out). This must be corrected by resuspending the top of the vagina. Some doctors open the top of the vagina and attempt to re-create support from ligaments that previously supported the uterus. Other physicians suspend the vagina to the sacrospinous ligament, a firm ligament found inside the pelvis. These two operations are done by a vaginal approach (no abdominal incisions). A different approach using an abdominal incision or laparoscope involves suspending your vagina to your sacrum (tailbone) using mesh.
- Enterocele Repair—An incision is made through the vaginal mucosa to expose the enterocele. The hernia sac is excised and the space between the rectum and the vagina closed.

More recent innovations in pelvic support surgery have brought us laparoscopic approaches to correct some of these defects. Graft insertion using natural tissue from an animal (ex. pig dermis) and mesh procedures have also been developed with the hope of increasing the long-term success of surgery. Surgical approaches will vary from physician to physician and may be performed by your gynecologist, urologist, or a new specialist, the urogynecologist. Every approach has its own set of advantages and disadvantages, which you should discuss in detail with your physician.

It is important that your doctor perform a thorough examination prior to surgery. All support defects should be corrected at the time of surgery. Let's look at an example to illustrate this important point. You may have a profound cystocele that bothers you greatly. In your mind, only the cystocele needs to be repaired. However, other defects (rectocele, uterine descensus, or enterocele) may coexist. If they are less pronounced, you will not be aware of them. However, if not repaired, they will worsen and require repair later.

It is also important for your doctor to identify any coexisting bladder problems. If there is poor support at the bladder neck, you may have either overt (obvious) or occult (hidden) stress incontinence. With occult stress incontinence, you have inadequate support of the bladder neck (refer to our section on bladder disorders). However, there are no symptoms of incontinence because your cystocele has "kinked" the urethra in a way that prevents leakage. If the cystocele is repaired without adequately elevating the bladder neck, you will have stress incontinence after the surgery. (That's just great! You've solved one problem and created another.) If your doctor is aware of this situation, he or she can make certain adjustments or additions to the surgery that will prevent postoperative stress incontinence. A simple test can be performed in the office to diagnose occult stress incontinence. Come to the office with a full bladder. The doctor can introduce his fingers or a pessary vaginally to elevate the bladder (thereby simulating a surgical repair). The doctor then looks for incontinence while you cough or bear down.

Another bladder condition that may be affected by surgery is the overactive bladder. The bladder is likely to be more "spastic" after surgery with increased urgency and frequency. This is usually temporary and controllable with medication. As the inflammation and swelling from surgery abates, the bladder function should improve. Many gynecologists recommend urologic evaluation before surgery. It should be mandatory if you have any symptoms of bladder dysfunction (urgency, frequency, incontinence).

So how do you choose between a pessary and surgery? If your general health is good (no obvious contraindications to surgery) and you are looking for a definitive answer, you should probably proceed with surgery. If you want to avoid the risk of undergoing surgery, you're better off trying a pessary. If you don't like it, you can always change your mind and proceed with surgery. Women with severe medical problems should try to use a pessary. Your family doctor or internist can tell you if there is any increased risk of undergoing surgery with your particular set of medical conditions.

I hear that surgery doesn't always work. Why?

First, you need a doctor with extensive experience in vaginal reconstructive surgery. If your gynecologist is not experienced in vaginal surgery, he or she should refer you to someone else. However, there are factors beyond the control of your doctor. The doctor can only control the quality of your surgery. He or she cannot control the quality of your tissue. If your connective tissue is particularly weak, the surgery may fail (after all, you probably wouldn't have the problem to begin with if the tissue was strong). The doctor also cannot control the type of stresses that this tissue will endure after surgery. That's where you come into the picture. After surgery, you should modify activities that are likely to cause recurrence of the prolapse. These were discussed above in the section on prevention.

Most women who have reconstructive surgery do well. The majority of repairs hold up well over time. However, there are no guarantees with this type of surgery. Nobody can predict if your prolapse will recur after surgery. As mentioned above, doctors have begun inserting graft material or mesh in place of your weak fibrous tissue in order to increase the success rate. Ideally, insertion of mesh should provide a permanent repair. Because of this potential benefit, there has been a big push to use rather new mesh procedures, especially by urogynecologists (gynecologists with a subspecialty in urology). However, they are not without their own set of complications. There is a 5–10 percent risk of the mesh eroding through the vaginal mucosa. Often this exposed area of mesh needs to be removed, which may require additional surgery. Some women will also develop scar tissue around the mesh, which can cause pelvic pain, especially during intercourse. Graft material can be used in place of mesh and because it is natural, erosion is generally not an issue. In fact, over the period of one year, your body resorbs (absorbs by gradual breakdown) the graft, thereby limiting its potential complications. However, because graft materials are not permanent (like mesh), they may not increase the long-term success of surgery.

Ideally, you should postpone surgery until you have completed childbearing. Childbirth will damage the reconstructed pelvic support. Pelvic muscle exercises and pessaries may provide you with enough relief to get by in the meantime. If surgery really becomes necessary, there are procedures that resuspend the uterus (similar to those performed for vaginal vault prolapse). You should also postpone surgery if you are in circumstances that will require repetitive heavy lifting or straining, whether that is at home or work.

Three Women with Prolapse, Three Different Approaches

Ellie, June, and Alice all have severe pelvic prolapse. They all have relaxation of the uterus, bladder, and rectum that has progressed to the point where the pelvic organs appear at, or beyond, the opening of the vagina.

Ellie is eighty-one years old. Although she is in fairly good medical shape, she definitely does not want to undergo surgery unless it is critically necessary. She sees her gynecologist, Dr. Stone, and they agree on using a pessary. Ellie is no longer sexually active and does not want to have to insert and remove the pessary herself. Dr. Stone fits her with a ring pessary, begins vaginal estrogen to thicken the vaginal walls, and schedules a return visit for three months. At that time he will remove and clean the pessary, examine the vaginal walls for any sign of ulceration, and replace the pessary for another three months.

June is seventy-two years old. She has high blood pressure that is easily controlled with medication and no other significant medical problems. She figures to be around for at least another twenty years. After all, her mom lived well into her nineties. She really doesn't want to mess with a pessary for the rest of her life. On the other hand, she has seen an article in the newspaper reviewing complications of mesh procedures and more recently saw a TV ad from a law firm soliciting women who have had mesh procedures that have gone badly. She discusses this with her gynecologist, Dr. Kaufman, and they decide to proceed with surgery using more traditional techniques that do not employ mesh.

Alice is sixty years old. She is very active and thoroughly annoyed by her prolapse. There is no way that she is going to fuss with a pessary for the next thirty years. She discusses her situation with her gynecologist, Dr. Thompson. He compares the pros and cons of traditional reconstructive surgery with those of the newer mesh procedures. Dr. Thompson tells Alice that his traditional reconstructive surgery holds up well approximately 75–80 percent of the time. Alice feels strongly that she does not want to have to have surgery more than once, so Dr. Thompson refers her to a urogynecologist who is facile with mesh procedures. Alice is willing to accept a 5–10 percent chance of a significant complication related to the mesh because it offers the opportunity of greater long-term success.

16

WHEN YOU NEED SURGERY

What are the complications of surgery?

Dorothy has just been told that she needs a hysterectomy. Nothing conservative has helped her horrendous bleeding problems. She should have seen this coming as one treatment after another failed, but she remained in denial, hoping that hysterectomy wouldn't be necessary. Now that she's consigned to surgery, one question after another pops up. So what's next? Do I need a complete hysterectomy? Is this going to put me into menopause? How long will I be in the hospital? What complications will I get? How long will I be out of work? *Dorothy remembers Aunt Tilly who went in for a hysterectomy and came out with a colostomy bag. What if that happens to her?*

Do you know the definition of *minor surgery*? It's surgery performed on somebody else. It doesn't matter what anyone says: If you are going under the knife, it's a big deal. It is important for you to understand the potential risks that are associated with surgery, but you shouldn't obsess over the possibility of a complication. The risk of a serious complication is very low (1–3 percent or less depending on your surgery). In most cases, the benefit to be gained from your surgery far outweighs the small likelihood of a significant complication. Don't let your concern prevent you from proceeding with necessary surgery.

We will begin with entering the abdomen. After all, every surgery requires some way of getting into your abdomen or pelvis. Traditionally, most surgery was performed through an open incision in the abdomen whether it be vertical (between your pubic bone and navel) or horizontal (side to side, at the top of your pubic hairline, a.k.a. the bikini cut). Today, most gynecologic surgery is performed laparoscopically, through tiny incisions in your abdomen. The most significant complication related to entering the abdomen is injury to the bowel or bladder if these are adherent to the abdominal wall. This is unlikely unless you have a history of prior abdominal surgery or intra-abdominal infection (ex. ruptured appendicitis, diverticulitis, pelvic inflammatory disease). Your doctor will take special precautions under these circumstances.

The most common complication when operating inside the abdomen or pelvis is bleeding. Every organ in the body is supplied with blood vessels, and there will be some bleeding associated with all surgery. Occasionally, there will be a greater blood loss than expected. If you lose enough blood to compromise your health, the doctor may choose to give you a blood transfusion, either during surgery or shortly after surgery. Donated blood is currently screened for infectious diseases such as hepatitis and HIV, so your risk of acquiring an infection through a blood transfusion is very low.

The pelvic organs lie adjacent to other important structures including the bowel (large and small intestines), bladder, and ureters. Injury to these organs may occur during your surgery. The risk of injury is increased if these structures are adherent to the uterus, tubes, or ovaries. Prior surgery and inflammatory conditions such as diverticulitis (an infection that develops from little outpouchings protruding from the wall in your large intestine), appendicitis, and pelvic inflammatory disease (see chapter 5) will cause adhesions. Endometriosis (see chapter 8) is notorious for causing dense adhesions. Malignant tumors may adhere to, or invade, other organs. Doctors proceed very cautiously when encountering adhesions to avoid injuring adjacent structures. The vast majority of the time they are able to avoid injury to the bowel, bladder, and ureters. When there is an injury, it is usually immediately apparent and can be repaired. They may have to call upon the services of another type of surgeon such as a general surgeon, colorectal surgeon, or urologist if a repair becomes necessary. Although your surgery and recovery may be prolonged from these complications, adverse long-term consequences are uncommon. Most complications during surgery are discovered immediately and can be treated at that time. However, sometimes the complication isn't apparent at the time of surgery. If a complication is discovered after your initial surgery, it is possible that a second operation will be required to resolve the problem. Fortunately, this is a rare occurrence.

Nerves also run through the pelvis and abdominal wall. Injury to major nerves is uncommon. Nerve damage can be direct (from cutting a nerve) or indirect (from retractors, instruments that provide increased visibility by pulling tissue away from the operative field). Nerve damage may produce pain, dysesthesia (abnormal sensation), or numbness in the affected area. Rarely, the sensory and motor nerves to the legs are compressed. This can affect the ability of your leg to move properly. The nerve usually heals over time, although it may take several months for recovery. Physical therapy may be required to help restore normal function. This rather dramatic complication is very uncommon.

Incisional complications can occur after your surgery. A hematoma (collection of blood) can develop within your incision after surgery. Most hematomas will resolve spontaneously, but occasionally your doctor will have to drain the collected blood or reopen the incision to secure a bleeding vessel. Your incision can get infected from skin bacteria, despite the fact that your doctor prepares the skin with an antiseptic solution prior to surgery. If infection is present, it will be treated with antibiotics and if an abscess develops, it will be drained.

In patients with particularly poor support tissue in their abdomen, the closure of the incision can fail and the incision can reopen. This rare complication is referred to as an evisceration. If this happens, you will immediately return to the operating room where your doctor will use special closure techniques to reinforce the incision. Sometimes the incision appears to heal well, only to have a bulge or opening appear later. A bulge may indicate the presence of a hernia. An opening in your incision with persistent drainage may be a fistula, a false passage that develops within your incision. Fistulas and hernias are usually repaired during a second surgical procedure, often with the help of a general surgeon.

A keloid is an excessively thick scar that forms along your incision line. Some women are more prone to keloid formation than others. African-American women are particularly likely to develop keloids. While a keloid is not dangerous, it is unsightly. Doctors commonly recommend silicone gel sheets (ScarAway, NewGel, NovaGel) for keloids. Another common approach is the injection of cortisone-like steroids directly into the scar. Cryotherapy (freezing), radiation, fluorouracil (used in chemotherapy), interferon (proteins produced by your body's immune system), and Imiquimod (Aldara, an immune system modulator) have also been used with varying degrees of success (as a general rule, when you see a whole bunch of things being tried, it means no one thing succeeds particularly well). More natural remedies include Mederma (a botanical extract), Thiosinaminum 5C (a homeopathic product derived from mustard seed oil), calendula gel, lavender oil, vitamin E cream, and scar massage. If all else fails, it pays to see a plastic surgeon who may be able to perform a scar revision with better results.

Nerve entrapment is a rare but painful complication. It occurs when a nerve in the abdominal wall that was incised during surgery heals encased in scar tissue. This produces a focal area in the abdominal wall that can be exquisitely painful. Injections of local anesthetics and steroids into the scar tissue may provide relief. If not, surgery can be performed to free the nerve from its entrapment.

Postoperative complications include deep vein thrombosis (DVT—blood clots in your veins), urinary retention, intestinal ileus (decreased bowel motility), and pneumonia. Increased age, obesity, cancer, prior DVT, diabetes, cardiovascular disease, and varicose veins all increase your risk of DVT. If you have any of these risk factors, preventive measures should be utilized. Blood clots can usually be prevented through special compression stockings, perioperative heparin (a blood thinner), and early mobilization.

Decreased bowel motility is common after intra-abdominal surgery. The bowel seems to say, "Hey, I'm just not going to work for awhile." The normal motion that carries food down the intestine stops. This normally resumes spontaneously within two to seven days. Occasionally this will take longer. If you develop nausea and vomiting, a nasogastric tube will be placed to drain your gastric, biliary, and pancreatic secretions. Eventually, the bowel regains its motility. Rarely, adhesions cause a bowel obstruction. In this situation, there is an actual mechanical blockage of the bowel and surgery may be required to restore bowel function.

Urinary retention (inability to empty the bladder) may occur postoperatively, especially after reconstructive bladder surgery (ex. cystocele repair—see chapter 15). When this occurs, a catheter will be kept in place to drain your bladder until it is able to empty itself.

Sometimes patients do not breathe deeply after surgery. This is particularly true if you have a large abdominal incision. Without deep breathing, tiny segments of your lungs collapse. You may develop shortness of breath and a low-grade fever. If not corrected, pneumonia may follow. You may be given a device that helps you breathe deeply (incentive spirometer) after surgery and your nurses will encourage deep breathing and coughing after surgery to prevent this problem.

Infections that may develop in the postoperative period include urinary tract infection, pneumonia, "wound infection" (in the incision), and infection in the pelvis or abdomen where the surgery was performed. Prophylactic antibiotics are usually given around the time of surgery to reduce the risk of infection. Antibiotics are given afterwards if you develop a postoperative fever that is thought to arise from an infection.

"Okay, that's it! I'm never undergoing surgery. Just put down that knife! You aren't operating on me, not after telling me about all those complications." Concern over potential surgical complications can be healthy. It leads you to ask your doctor important questions that will better prepare you for surgery. Your doctor's awareness of potential complications reminds him or her to take precautions. However, don't let your concern evolve into a disabling fear that prevents you from undergoing necessary surgery. Life-threatening complications and those that necessitate additional surgery are very uncommon in gynecologic surgery. If the benefit of your surgery far outweighs the surgical risks, you should proceed with the operation.

Healthy Fear

No fear (inappropriate): Dr. Drew obtains a pelvic ultrasound from Lisa, a forty-year-old woman who last week experienced discomfort in the left lower abdomen. The pelvic ultrasound reveals a small cyst in the left ovary.

Lisa immediately reacts to the news. "Okay Doc, take it out. Let's get rid of that ovary right away. This could be cancer and I don't want to take any chances."

"Let's not overreact to this, Lisa. It looks like this is a simple cyst and more than 90 percent of those will disappear within a month or two," says Dr. Drew in a reassuring tone.

"But what if it's cancer?" responds Lisa. "I could be dead in a month or two!"

"First of all, that's not true. Waiting a couple of months will not make a difference. We don't want to do surgery unless it's really necessary. Most of the time surgery proceeds without complications, but there is always a chance of a complication. In your case, it is very unlikely that surgery will be necessary. We'll repeat the scan in two months. If the cyst has not disappeared or decreased in size, then we can readdress possible surgery at that time."

Excessive fear (inappropriate): Agnes, a seventy-year-old postmenopausal woman, has noticed that her lower abdomen is enlarging. She sees Dr. Utley, who orders an ultrasound revealing a large complex (solid and cystic) mass.

"Agnes, we have your scan back and it confirms what I felt on your exam. You have a large mass in your pelvis that is now rising up into your lower abdomen. We are going to have to operate and remove it."

"No way," begins Agnes. "You're not operating on me. I've heard of people going into surgery and never waking up. My sister had a D&C when she was forty and ended up with a perforated bowel. No way am I letting anyone operate on me. I'm not in any pain and I feel fine," she concludes defiantly.

"Agnes, there is a reasonable possibility that this could be ovarian cancer. If it is and you don't undergo surgery, you will die. I'm not saying that this has to be ovarian cancer but there is a reasonable possibility of it. On the other hand, serious complications from surgery are uncommon. You really need to reconsider this."

"I'll think about it," says Agnes, backing off a little. "I'll call you if I decide to have surgery."

Dr. Utley concedes. "Okay, Agnes, but don't wait too long. If you're not sure, you can get a second opinion. That would be reasonable, but deciding to do nothing is not reasonable."

Healthy fear: Gerry's uterus has been progressively enlarging from fibroids. She was putting off surgery as long as she could, but now it looks like she's five months pregnant. She is still five years away from menopause and Dr. Lutz has told her that the uterus will probably continue to grow until she reaches menopause. Dr. Lutz is recommending a hysterectomy.

"You know I have been putting this off, Dr. Lutz. For the last ten years I have been getting bouts of diverticulitis. I'm somewhat scared of getting a hysterectomy because of the inflammation and scar tissue that might be in my pelvis from the diverticulitis," says Gerry, hoping that Dr. Lutz will change her mind about the surgery.

"I'm glad you reminded me of that," Dr. Lutz responds. "There are precautions that we can take to minimize your risk. I will have you do a modified bowel prep to clean out your lower colon before the surgery. After the uterus has been removed, we will closely inspect your bowel to make sure that there has been no injury. If there is, we should be able to fix it right then and there. As an extra precaution, I will make sure that Dr. Steinway, one of our general surgeons, is available in case we need him to repair your bowel. Of course, I don't want you to worry too much. It is very unlikely that bowel injury will occur."

"Okay, that sounds reassuring," responds Gerry. "Let's go ahead and pick a date for the surgery. It will be nice to get rid of this bulge in my belly."

How long will I be in the hospital?

Three people die: a doctor, a schoolteacher, and the head of a large HMO. When they are met at the pearly gates by St. Peter, he asks the doctor, "What did you do on earth?"

The doctor replied, "I healed the sick and if they could not pay, I would do it for free." St. Peter told the doctor, "You may go in."

St. Peter asked the teacher what she did, and she replied, "I taught educationally challenged children." St. Peter then told her, "You may go in."

St. Peter asked the third man, "What did you do?" The man hung his head and replied, "I ran a large HMO." To this St. Peter replied, "You may go in, but you can only stay three days."

Well, if it were up to your insurance company, you'd probably be dropped down a chute straight from the recovery room into your car. Hospital stays have dramatically decreased in duration over the past few years. Procedures such as D&Cs (dilation and curettage), hysteroscopy, and laparoscopy are usually performed as outpatient surgery. Hospitalization for reconstructive vaginal surgery (see chapter 15) and major abdominal surgery such as an abdominal hysterectomy can be as short as two days. It is extended only if there is a severe postoperative complication (as defined by your insurance carrier). You may still need help after you are discharged. Social services, visiting nurses, and care management personnel at the hospital can help you make these arrangements. Ask your doctor if home care services will be necessary. Family members may be able to provide the care. If not, consider contacting the care management (social services) department of the hospital before you are admitted. If there will be difficulty in arranging home care, it's easier to solve the problem in advance rather than on the day of discharge.

Will I be "knocked out" during surgery, or can I have a local anesthetic?

The type of surgery often dictates which anesthesia is chosen. Some minor procedures can be performed under local anesthesia, or local anesthesia with sedation. Most gynecologic surgery, however, is performed under general anesthesia, which is administered intravenously, or regional anesthesia, given in the form of spinal or epidural anesthetics.

Meet the Anesthesiologist

In today's world, your first opportunity to speak with an anesthesiologist is minutes before you are rolled back for surgery. If you have concerns or questions about anesthesia, consider making an outpatient appointment with a member of the anesthesia department prior to the day of surgery.

General anesthesia will render you completely unconscious. While you are "asleep," an anesthesiologist (or, more commonly, a nurse anesthetist) inserts an endotracheal tube down your windpipe to help you breathe and protect you from aspirating (accidentally breathing stomach secretions into your lungs). When surgery is finished, the anesthetic agents are discontinued and you will wake up. Sometimes medications are given to reverse the effects of the anesthesia. If an endotracheal tube was used, it will be withdrawn when you are alert enough to breathe on your own (it may cause you to have a sore throat for a few days). You may feel nauseous from the anesthesia. This problem clears up on its own, but medications can be given if the nausea is severe.

General anesthesia has a low incidence of complications in healthy women. If your surgery involves general anesthesia, you will be instructed to refrain from eating and drinking for at least six hours before surgery, which allows your stomach to empty. General anesthesia may be riskier if you have significant cardiac or pulmonary disease. In these situations, regional or local anesthesia may be preferred.

For regional anesthesia (spinals and epidurals), a needle is inserted near the spinal cord and numbing agents, similar to those used in local anesthesia, are injected to anesthetize the nerves that supply sensation to the lower abdomen and pelvis. Feeling is also lost in the legs. Normal sensation is regained within several hours after surgery. During surgery, the patient remains conscious. Some women like the idea of not having to "go to sleep" whereas others abhor it. If surgery will take a long time, it may become difficult to lie in the same position. Often the anesthesiologist will provide sedation to keep the patient from becoming antsy.

Regional anesthesia does not increase the risk of aspiration. That is its major benefit compared with general anesthesia. It is also safer than general anesthesia for women with significant pulmonary disease (such as asthma). However, some surgeons do not find regional anesthesia satisfactory. If the nerves emanating from the spinal cord are not numbered adequately, some areas may not become completely anesthetized. Anxious patients may find it difficult to remain still and cope with the strange sensations caused by the anesthetic. Individuals with certain spinal or neurologic conditions may not be good candidates for regional anesthesia.

Headaches used to be a concern following regional anesthesia. Patients had to lie flat for twenty-four hours after surgery and even then might have gotten severe headaches (called spinal headaches) lasting for days or weeks. Newer techniques, however, have minimized the incidence of spinal headaches, and patients no longer must lie flat after surgery. Injury to the spinal cord from the needle is uncommon. Direct contact of the needle with the spinal cord or the exiting nerves may cause abnormal sensations such as burning, pricking, or numbness in the legs, but these go away spontaneously. Serious adverse reactions to the anesthetics may occur, but are rare.

When possible, local anesthesia is usually the safest form of anesthesia, but it can be used only in minor surgery. The choice between regional and general anesthesia is often based on the preference of the anesthesiologist and surgeon. The patient's general health or type of operation may dictate one over the other. The patient's personal preference may also influence the decision.

If you have concerns regarding your anesthesia, make an appointment with the anesthesiologist before your scheduled date of surgery.

Why do I need a catheter in my bladder?

Immediately before major surgery after anesthesia has been administered, a catheter is inserted through the urethra into the bladder. A small balloon at one end is inflated with water to prevent the catheter from slipping out. The catheter prevents the bladder from becoming overdistended with urine during the surgery. The catheter is attached to a collecting bag that accurately measures urine output. A normal output indicates that blood volume is satisfactory. A low output suggests the need for more intravenous fluids. The catheter is usually removed the day after surgery. Reconstructive vaginal surgery (see chapter 15) may require longer catheterization, whereas minor surgical procedures usually do not require catheterization at all.

What can I get to relieve pain after surgery?

Thanks to modern medicine, you'll experience less pain than women of previous generations. Some operations that used to be performed through large incisions can now be accomplished through small ones with the aid of laparoscopy. Some uterine surgery can be performed through the hysteroscope without any incision. Postoperative pain is diminished with these approaches and can often be controlled with oral painkillers.

There are several approaches to providing pain relief after major surgery. Traditionally, injections of narcotics were given, usually at four-hour intervals. This is still a reasonable approach for some women. The problem is that pain relief is excellent during the first hour or two after the shot, but diminishes significantly thereafter. By the time your next injection arrives, you may be in considerable pain.

Patient-controlled analgesia (PCA) is a solution to this problem. A narcotic is placed into an intravenous solution and connected to a pump. The patient presses a button to release a small amount of narcotic for pain relief. Pressing the button on a regular basis provides a continuous level of comfort. Overdosing is not possible because settings on the pump limit the total amount of narcotic that can be released.

Patients undergoing regional anesthesia may have narcotics administered through a catheter left in place near the spinal canal. This treatment is called epidural analgesia. Close monitoring by the nursing staff is required for safe administration of epidural narcotics. When used properly, it provides excellent, sustained pain control after surgery.

Narcotics can produce respiratory and central nervous system depression. Nausea, low blood pressure, and inability to empty the bladder are also potential adverse effects. Intramuscular injections, PCA, and epidural analgesics are usually discontinued after twenty-four to forty-eight hours. Oral painkillers are then given as necessary.

Pain and Nausea: The Dilemma

A large part of how you feel after surgery will depend on how much pain and nausea you have postoperatively. Unfortunately, narcotics tend to cause nausea. Different narcotics can be used, but it is not unusual for a patient to get nauseous from every narcotic tried. Your doctor can try several different medications to relieve your nausea. If they are successful, then you might be able to increase the amount of narcotics you use for pain. As a general rule, if you have a lot of pain and not much nausea, use more narcotics. If you have a lot of nausea and not much pain, use less. There are non-narcotic pain relievers, but they tend to be less effective and in some cases may increase the risk of postoperative bleeding.

Will I feel nauseous after surgery?

Effects of anesthesia, postoperative narcotics, or surgery itself can cause postoperative nausea. Nausea associated with the anesthetic disappears within the first six to twelve hours after surgery. Some of the newer agents used in general anesthesia are less likely to induce nausea. The anesthesiologist may give you medication toward the end of your surgery (before you "wake up") that will reduce postoperative nausea. The anesthesiologist or your gynecologist can also order antinausea medication in the recovery room for you. Nausea associated with narcotics can sometimes be managed by reducing the dose or changing to a different drug.

Pelvic surgery may cause a temporary decrease in bowel activity. Your bowels are less likely to be affected by laparoscopy and vaginal surgery. After major abdominal surgery, bowel motility may decrease to the point where you develop nausea and vomiting. Doctors routinely prescribe antinausea medication after major surgery, but you may have to request it. Don't wait until you're retching. If you feel nauseous, ask the nurse for medication.

When can I return to work?

The answer depends on the type of operation you've had. After minor procedures such as a D&C or hysteroscopy, you can return to work within a day or two. No incisions need to heal, and you really can't create any problems by resuming your work routine. You may experience cramping and bleeding that put you out of commission for a few days, but you'll quickly get back to normal. After laparoscopic surgery, most activities can be resumed within two to three weeks, and you can usually go back to work in two weeks, though it is difficult to give a general answer covering all such cases, since so many operations are now performed

> ### Caution!
>
> *Don't abuse your disability*
>
> *You may have an urge to extend your disability beyond that which is really appropriate. Trying to do so, however, may place your doctor at risk. If your employer or their disability insurance provider decides to challenge the amount of time allotted for your recovery and it is deemed excessive, both you and your doctor can be found guilty of insurance fraud.*

WHEN YOU NEED SURGERY • 351

laparoscopically. Following a laparoscopic tubal sterilization, your doctor may allow you to return to work within several days. However, you could be out of work for several weeks after a laparoscopic hysterectomy. Most gynecologists will tell you not to work or do any heavy lifting or pushing for four to six weeks after major abdominal surgery so that incisions will have sufficient time to heal. Any activity that increases pressure in the abdomen during the initial healing may increase your risk of developing a hernia. Major reconstructive vaginal surgery also requires restricted activity to ensure adequate healing and to reduce the risk of recurrence.

The nature of your work also influences the decision. If your job is mainly sedentary, you can go back fairly quickly. On the other hand, jobs that require heavy lifting or other strenuous tasks mandate a longer leave of absence.

Your employer's disability policy may also factor into the equation. Ask your employer or the director of personnel about their disability or sick-leave policy. If your time from work is not compensated, you will probably want to return as soon as it is medically safe to do so. However, if the policy is liberal, you may want to extend your absence until you feel stronger.

Your doctor cannot extend your absence unless there is a legitimate medical indication, such as a postoperative complication.

> ## The Bottom Line
>
> *After the first week or two, it is very unlikely that routine daily activities (other than intercourse) will cause a problem inside the abdomen or pelvis where your doctor operated. Many women with relatively sedentary jobs can return to work fairly quickly if desired. Most of the risk at this point lies in disturbing abdominal incisions. Laparoscopic incisions are not at great risk because of their small size. However, if you have a larger abdominal incision, avoid heavy lifting and straining at home or work. Adhering to this limitation may reduce your risk of developing a hernia.*

What restrictions will I have after surgery?

We can give you an idea of our restrictions, recognizing that every gynecologist has their own philosophy regarding necessary restrictions. You should stay home the first week after major surgery (substantial surgery done through a large incision, not laparoscopy or hysteroscopy). Take short walks inside or outside the house and rest, but do not confine yourself to bed. Complete immobility increases your risk of getting blood clots in your veins. It also turns your muscles into mush. You should limit climbing stairs to once or twice daily if possible and take the steps one at a time while holding onto a handrail. Light cooking that doesn't involve heavy pots and pans is reasonable. Cleaning is out! This is your golden opportunity to get your family involved in those mundane chores you always did that they took for granted before the surgery. With a little luck (and some good acting), you may even get them to continue after you have recovered.

During the second week, it is best if someone else drives you when you leave the house, and your trips should not be too strenuous. Go to a movie or restaurant. You deserve it. Gradually increase the amount of walking during the second week, but continue to limit heavy lifting and pushing. Make your trips to the grocery store brief and let someone else carry the bags.

You can gradually resume normal activities over the next several weeks and can start driving your car during the third week. You should refrain from exercise other than walking until six weeks after surgery. After that, gradually reintroduce exercise and sports. If a particular activity causes pain, stop. Wait a couple weeks and try again. Activities that involve heavier lifting can slowly be resumed. However, heavy exertion, such as moving furniture or heavy boxes, should be postponed for another few weeks.

Now for the big question: "When can I have sex?" Sexual intercourse can be attempted six weeks following major surgery. After hysterectomy or reconstructive vaginal surgery, wait until your doctor gives the okay at the postoperative visit, usually six weeks after surgery. He or she will examine the vagina at that time to see if it has healed sufficiently. If you have pain during intercourse, stop and wait several weeks. Persistent pain or bleeding during intercourse should be brought to the attention of your doctor.

There are usually no major restrictions concerning sex after minor vaginal surgery, such as a D&C or hysteroscopy. However, your doctor may limit intercourse and use of tampons for one or two weeks.

Restrictions after laparoscopy vary according to the nature of the operation performed. Simpler procedures, such as laparoscopic tubal sterilization, entail few restrictions. Complicated operations, such as laparoscopic hysterectomies, may carry restrictions similar to those mentioned for major surgery, although you can often resume normal activity in two to three weeks rather than four to six. Advanced laparoscopic surgery is a relatively new phenomenon, so there is less consensus on how quickly normal activities should be resumed.

What is robotic surgery?

Robotic surgery, also referred to as computer assisted surgery, has developed in order to perform minimally invasive surgery, such as laparoscopy, with precision. Robotic arms are placed into the abdomen through small incisions, similar to traditional laparoscopy, but the ends of the arms that actually perform the surgery are manipulated at a distance, combining surgical talent with computer assistance. Newer generations of doctors will probably train using robotic surgery more than traditional laparoscopy. The advantage of robotic surgery over traditional laparoscopic surgery is the ability of the robotic arms to articulate in a greater variety of directions and the improved visualization obtained through 3-D computer enhancement. A potentially huge advancement may be the ability of doctors to perform complicated surgery through minimally invasive techniques from remote locations, theoretically from anywhere in the world.

Drawbacks include the greater expense of robotic surgery ($1.4 million for the da Vinci surgical system and fifteen hundred dollars in disposable supply costs per procedure) and the learning curve for acquiring the requisite skills needed to smoothly operate the system (twelve to eighteen cases are probably needed to achieve facility with the system). Most gynecologic surgery can be performed cheaper and in shorter time using traditional laparoscopic techniques, presuming you have an experienced gynecologist. Don't intentionally seek out robotic surgery just because it is new and sounds cool. Before you seek out a facility that employs robotic surgery, ask your gynecologist if there is any significant benefit in doing so. However, there are gynecologic surgeries that clearly benefit from robotic surgery, especially cancer cases that entail lymph node dissection.

What is the difference between a complete hysterectomy and a partial hysterectomy?

A complete hysterectomy removes the entire uterus. It has nothing to do with the ovaries! We can't emphasize this enough. Often women think that a complete hysterectomy includes removal of the ovaries. Removal of the ovaries is called oophorectomy.

A partial hysterectomy (also called supracervical hysterectomy) involves the removal of part of the uterus. The upper portion of the uterus is removed including the endometrium and myometrium, but the cervix is left in place. Proponents of supracervical hysterectomy point out the following benefits:

- Most problems caused by the uterus (with the exception of cancer) occur in the upper part of the uterus, so there is no strong indication for removing the cervix if it is otherwise normal.
- The combination of Pap smears and HPV testing can adequately predict which patients are likely to develop a cervical problem in the future. In patients who are at low risk for future cervical cancer (those with normal Pap smears and negative HPV tests), there is no great need to remove the cervix.
- Retaining the cervix may help with pelvic support.

- Retaining the cervix prevents scar formation at the top of the vagina and shortening of the vagina, both of which can sometimes lead to painful intercourse.
- Supracervical hysterectomy is much easier to perform laparoscopically than total hysterectomy.
- Because the most difficult part of a hysterectomy is removal of the cervix, supracervical hysterectomy may reduce your risk of a complication.

Proponents of cervical removal feel that it is best to remove the cervix with the rest of the uterus in order to eradicate any future cervical problems, the most serious being cervical cancer. Also, sometimes the entire endometrium is not removed during supracervical hysterectomy. If this happens, a premenopausal woman may continue to have cyclic bleeding (although lighter) and a postmenopausal woman may still have a risk for endometrial cancer.

There is not an absolute consensus among gynecologists regarding this issue. Your best bet is to discuss the pros and cons of total versus supracervical hysterectomy with your doctor given the specific nature of your problem and your past history regarding any cervical issues. Keep in mind that if your cervix is left in place, regular Pap smears and HPV testing will be necessary in future visits to detect any abnormal cervical changes while they are still precancerous and curable.

When I have a hysterectomy, should my ovaries also be removed?

If your ovaries appear normal at surgery, they do not have to be removed during a hysterectomy. Even after the childbearing years are over, ovaries play an important role. Estrogen made by the ovaries protects the bones against osteoporosis and the heart against coronary artery disease. Their premature removal places a woman at risk for early onset of these medical problems. Removal of the ovaries also induces menopausal symptoms such as hot flashes, night sweats, and vaginal dryness.

So why in the world would you want to have your ovaries removed? The answer is plain and simple: avoiding ovarian cancer. You have a one in eighty chance of developing this cancer during your lifetime, and although it is not as common as some, it is not rare. Ovarian cancer is difficult to detect early. Only 25 percent of ovarian cancers will still be confined to the ovary when diagnosed. In addition to ovarian cancer, you may also develop benign (noncancerous) ovarian tumors. Even though you are unlikely to die from such a tumor, you still need additional surgery for its removal.

In the past, it was common to remove your ovaries at the time of hysterectomy once you reached your mid-forties. The thinking on this has changed over the last five to ten years with studies emerging that demonstrate a higher mortality rate in women who have their ovaries removed at the time of hysterectomy than women who retain their ovaries. Currently most authorities recommend that normal ovaries should not be removed. After menopause, it is more reasonable to remove the ovaries. At this point they are no longer producing estrogen so the main benefit of keeping them no longer exists.

Other factors also can influence this decision. If you have a long-standing history of ovarian problems (ex. cysts, endometriosis), it may be reasonable to remove your ovaries at the time of hysterectomy. If there is a family history of breast and ovarian cancers, your risk of developing ovarian cancer may be higher than average. In this situation, it is sensible to remove the ovaries. If this is done prior to menopause, hormone replacement therapy will be given until you reach the natural age of menopause (fifty-one).

How will the doctor perform my hysterectomy?

We're assuming that the decision to perform a hysterectomy has been finalized. If the hysterectomy is performed because of uterine prolapse (see chapter 15), the uterus will be removed vaginally. If it is being extracted to fight cancer, it will probably be removed through an abdominal incision, allowing your doctor to thoroughly explore the pelvis and abdomen to detect any spread of the cancer. An abdominal hysterectomy also permits the removal of lymph nodes if this is deemed necessary. With advancing techniques in laparoscopy, including robotic surgery, many gynecologic oncologists will now perform a total laparoscopic hysterectomy, with or without lymph node dissection, in patients with early stage endometrial (inside lining of the uterus) or cervical cancer. Surgery for ovarian cancer (which includes a hysterectomy) is still performed through a large incision.

Is Robotic Surgery Always Preferable?

With the advent of robotic surgery, there is an assumption that any surgery that can be performed this way is preferable to every other approach. The reality is that most gynecologists are very facile in traditional laparoscopic surgery, and most gynecologic surgeries can be performed just as quickly and safely using traditional techniques. It is reasonable for you to ask your surgeon if there is any benefit to having your procedure done utilizing robotic equipment, but most of the time there is not a tremendous advantage.

Doctors vary in their approach to hysterectomy for benign disease such as bleeding, fibroids, or endometriosis. Many doctors prefer to remove a very large uterus through a larger abdominal incision. A smaller uterus can usually be removed vaginally or through laparoscopic surgery. The larger the uterus, the more skill and experience are required to perform a vaginal or laparoscopic hysterectomy. A prior history of vaginal deliveries (as opposed to C-section deliveries or no deliveries) increases the probability that your doctor can remove the uterus from a vaginal approach since vaginal childbirth relaxes the ligaments supporting the uterus and allows easier access to it.

Will a hysterectomy put me into menopause?

Removal of the uterus does not change the production of female hormones. Hormones are produced by the ovaries. If the ovaries are not removed, you will not experience symptoms related to reduced hormone levels. You will no longer menstruate, but the hormones are still being produced.

A hysterectomy can make it more difficult to detect the onset of menopause. If you have symptoms of menopause, such as hot flashes, night sweats, and vaginal dryness, it may be obvious that the change is occurring. However, 25 percent of women don't experience significant menopausal symptoms. Your doctor can check hormone levels to assess your ovarian function after age fifty. However, this is not necessary. Hormone replacement therapy will actually be dictated by the degree of your menopausal symptoms, not hormone levels.

Why do I have to be examined if I had a hysterectomy?

Mary is out getting her mail when she sees her neighbor Lucille getting ready to leave.

"Hey Lucille," begins Mary. "Where are you off to?"

"I'm going in to see my gynecologist," responds Lucille. "Not my favorite thing in the world, but I don't want to take any chances."

"I'm lucky," replies Mary. "I don't have to go anymore. I had a hysterectomy."

"Are you sure?" asks Lucille. "My sister had a hysterectomy, but her doctor still wants to see her every year."

"Well, I think I'm good to go, but I guess I'll ask Dr. Kelton if he still wants me to see him. I just assumed that I didn't need to go after my uterus was removed."

There are many women like Mary who develop the misimpression that they no longer need a gynecologist after hysterectomy. In their mind, the only reason they were going to a gynecologist was to get a Pap smear, so after their uterus is removed, they feel it is no longer necessary to go. If your ovaries were not removed during your hysterectomy, it is especially important that you continue with pelvic exams. Ovarian tumors are difficult to detect and usually do not present with early symptoms. Pelvic exams are one way to keep a check on the ovaries.

If the ovaries were removed, your chances of developing gynecologic problems are certainly decreased, but not eliminated. Although they are less common, women can still develop vaginal and vulvar problems (see chapter 11). Periodic inspection of these areas is important. If you have a history of cervical or endometrial cancer, your doctor will perform a vaginal Pap smear at the time of your visit. He or she will not do this if your hysterectomy was performed for benign (noncancerous) reasons. The doctor will also perform breast and rectal exams during your annual visit. He or she will order necessary screening tests, including mammography. Important topics such as hormone replacement therapy, osteoporosis prevention, and bladder issues will be discussed at your visits.

If I have an ovarian tumor, does the whole ovary need to be removed?

The short answer is "not always." If you have a benign (noncancerous) cyst or tumor of the ovary, your doctor may be able to perform an ovarian cystectomy. In this procedure, the cyst is removed from the ovary, preserving the remaining normal ovarian tissue. If you have not yet had children or wish to have more, this approach is recommended. If your family is complete, preserving the ovary is not critical, assuming that your other ovary is normal. You only need one ovary to produce your female hormones. Removing the abnormal ovary will not cause premature menopause.

Sometimes technical factors encountered at surgery will dictate whether the entire ovary is removed. If the growth or cyst is exceedingly large, there may not be much normal ovarian tissue to preserve. In that situation, your doctor may elect to remove the whole ovary. The ovary's appearance may reflect the possible presence of cancer. If so, it is safer to remove the entire ovary. Finally, a complication, such as bleeding from the ovary, may require its removal.

After menopause, your doctor may also recommend removal of the other ovary even if it appears normal.

Will I need to take hormones after the surgery?

If both of your ovaries are removed, you will abruptly enter menopause, assuming you are premenopausal at the time of surgery. If your hormones are not replaced, you are likely to experience severe hot flashes and night sweats as well as other menopausal symptoms. Most doctors will provide you with hormone replacement therapy to ease this transition. Whether you ultimately continue with hormone replacement depends on many factors (see chapter 13). If one ovary is preserved, hormone replacement is not necessary. If you are menopausal at the time of surgery, no changes will occur after ovarian removal because the ovaries were not functioning before surgery.

Why do I need a catheter for so long after bladder surgery?

Surgery involving the bladder creates inflammation and swelling that can prevent it from emptying itself. A catheter is necessary to drain the urine until the swelling subsides. This may be as short as one or two days or as long as two to three weeks in duration. The bladder may also be positioned differently after the surgery, which may inhibit it from emptying. With time, it will adjust to its new position.

Doctors vary in their approach to catheterization. Some will place a catheter through the urethra, whereas others will place it in the bladder through the abdominal wall. Doctors may also use intermittent catheterization, a procedure in which you are taught to catheterize yourself. You're probably thinking, "You've got to be kidding!" However, it is surprisingly easy for most women to learn this technique. You can catheterize yourself at periodic intervals (usually every four hours) until you are able to empty your bladder normally.

Why am I losing urine after my bladder surgery?

Perhaps your surgery repaired a dropped bladder. Or perhaps it corrected stress incontinence. Your catheter is finally removed and you are ready to rejoice. But what's this? All of a sudden you feel as though you have to run to the bathroom, and the urine starts leaking before you get there. This event was certainly not in the game plan.

Don't be alarmed. This situation is probably only temporary. Bladder surgery and catheterization can temporarily cause bladder instability. Your urgency and frequency of urination and urine loss are probably related to involuntary bladder contractions. As the inflammation from the surgery and catheter subside, so will your symptoms. In the meantime, they can usually be controlled with medications that will relax the bladder musculature. Your problem may last for only several days, although it is more likely to persist for several weeks. After that time it will usually clear up.

The Value of CMG

In chapter 14 we mentioned a test referred to as a cystometrogram (CMG). In this test, a catheter is inserted into the bladder and the bladder is filled with water while monitoring pressure. The test evaluates your bladder function. The circumstances outlined in the previous two questions can sometimes be predicted by a CMG if it is done before surgery. If the CMG indicates incomplete bladder emptying, an atonic bladder (a bladder that doesn't contract well), or a bladder that does not properly sense when it is full, there will be a greater risk of the bladder failing to empty after surgery. Prolonged catheterization of the bladder or intermittent catheterization by the patient may become necessary.

If on the other hand the CMG demonstrates a bladder with a low capacity, heightened sensitivity, or uninhibited contractions upon filling, there will be a greater risk of urgency incontinence after the surgery that may require prolonged use of medication.

Not all physicians feel that CMG testing is necessary prior to surgery in patients who have no evidence of unusual bladder symptoms, but we feel that it is a valuable tool that can inform both the doctor and patient of possible problems that may be faced after surgery.

Why do I have pain in my shoulder after laparoscopic surgery?

"Okay, what did you guys do? Did you wrench my shoulder?" Have no fear. Your shoulder will be fine. Your mind is playing a trick on you. Gas is used to inflate your abdomen during laparoscopy to provide visibility necessary for your surgery. At the end of surgery, most of the gas is evacuated, but some always remains in the abdomen, where it rises and irritates the underside of your diaphragm. Your brain interprets this pain as originating in your shoulder. The body absorbs gas fairly quickly, and the shoulder pain will disappear on its own in a day or two.

Why do I have so many incisions on my abdomen?

Don't be deceived into thinking that laparoscopic surgery involves only one incision for the telescopic instrument. Some procedures, such as tubal ligation or diagnostic laparoscopy, may require only one incision. However, most laparoscopic surgery will involve two to four incisions. As the complexity of the surgery increases, so do the number of incisions. One is used for the laparoscope; the others accommodate surgical instruments. Often, more than one instrument is required simultaneously, so you may have multiple incisions, each one ranging from one-fourth inch to one-half inch in size.

A new technique called single port laparoscopy utilizes one incision that is 2 cm (a little less than 1 inch) in your navel. Because the single incision is larger than usual, it can accommodate multiple instruments, which avoids multiple incision sites on your abdomen. It is too early to tell if this approach is preferable to more standard laparoscopic surgery, but it may become an option as more gynecologists are exposed to it.

Is laparoscopic surgery safer than regular surgery?

This issue is controversial. Doctors who specialize in laparoscopic surgery will often say it is safer than traditional surgery performed through a larger incision. They think the enhanced visibility provided by the laparoscope improves their ability to perform surgery safely. However, many gynecologists are not as facile with laparoscopic surgery as these specialists are. When advanced laparoscopic surgery is attempted by doctors with less experience, the rate of complications may exceed that of the same surgery performed through a traditional approach. Laparoscopic instruments are usually more tedious and cumbersome to use than standard surgical instruments, and in addition, the doctor loses the ability to feel the tissues with his or her hands.

If your doctor has extensive experience in performing a specific laparoscopic operation, he or she can probably perform it safely. Beware of very new laparoscopic procedures. They may sound good, but until all the kinks are worked out, you're probably better off going with a more traditional approach. Although recovery is shorter with laparoscopic surgery, it should not be performed if it might compromise the success of the procedure or increase the possibility of complications.

Can I have laparoscopic surgery as an outpatient?

Most laparoscopic surgery is done in that way. You arrive at the hospital or outpatient surgical facility one to two hours before surgery. After surgery, you spend two to four hours recovering before discharge. If you have excessive pain or nausea and vomiting, your doctor may keep you overnight for observation. Some laparoscopic procedures require a longer postoperative recovery. An operation such as laparoscopic hysterectomy may necessitate one or more days of hospitalization. There is tremendous regional variation in the length of stay after laparoscopic surgery. A woman may be discharged as quickly as eight to twelve hours after this procedure in one region, yet stay two days in another area of the country. Unfortunately, your insurance company often dictates the amount of time that is given for your recovery.

Some doctors perform minor laparoscopic procedures in their office, which provides a more comfortable environment for patients. This setting, however, is usually not equipped to handle major surgical complications. If safety is of paramount importance, you should have your procedure performed at a facility that can expeditiously manage any complication of laparoscopy.

How much pain will I have after laparoscopic surgery?

There is no precise way to gauge how much pain you'll have after surgery. There is usually very little pain after minor laparoscopic procedures such as a tubal ligation. Greater pain will follow advanced laparoscopic surgery that uses multiple incisions. Your pain will be less than the discomfort associated with the same procedure performed through a larger, open incision.

Everybody experiences pain differently. However, most of the time you can obtain adequate relief with oral painkillers. Your doctor should send you home with a prescription for narcotic pain pills. You may be able to get by without them, but keep them on hand just in case.

Can hysteroscopy be done in the office?

Generally, office use of this procedure is confined to diagnostic hysteroscopy. Removal of large polyps and fibroids through the hysteroscope can cause complications that should be managed in a hospital or ambulatory surgery center.

How much pain and bleeding will I have after a hysteroscopy?

Hysteroscopy is usually well tolerated. You can expect to have cramping after the procedure, which can be managed with acetaminophen or other non-narcotic analgesics. If the procedure is particularly long in duration or if it involves removal of a large polyp or fibroid, your pain may be greater and narcotic analgesics may be necessary. Minor bleeding is typical following hysteroscopy. Removal of large fibroids may cause heavier bleeding. Pain after hysteroscopy usually stops after a few days. Bleeding may continue for several weeks, depending on the procedure performed. If you notice progressively worsening pain or bleeding, call your doctor; it may be a sign of a complication.

Epilogue

We hope we haven't confused you. Our goal was to provide answers to most of the questions women ask without getting too technical. You can use this information as a starting point for meaningful discussions with your doctor. He or she can expand on what you have learned and help determine which sections of the book apply to your particular situation.

If you have a problem that is not resolved, it definitely pays to seek another opinion, especially if a specialist deals with the area in question. Keep in mind that not all problems have perfect solutions. Fortunately, medicine is constantly exploring new frontiers and developing new technology. Keep the faith! An answer may be on the horizon.

Finally, make your own healthcare a priority. We see women who continually nurture family and friends while ignoring their own emotional and physical needs. Attending to those who mean a lot to you is admirable, but don't forget yourself.

Glossary

The terms listed here are defined in greater detail throughout the book. To find a fuller explanation, consult the index. Italicized words are defined elsewhere in the glossary.

Abcess—a collection of white blood cells (pus)

Adenomyosis—a condition where the *endometrium* grows into the *myometrium*

Adhesions—scar tissue formed after surgery or from an inflammatory condition

Afterbirth—see *placenta*

AIDS (acquired immunodeficiency syndrome)—a disease caused by the HIV virus that destroys *cells* of the immune system (the body's natural defense against disease)

Amenorrhea—total absence of menstruation

Analgesics—pain relievers

Anesthesia—the induction of a state of diminished sensation; general anesthesia also encompasses a loss of consciousness

Anorexia—short for anorexia nervosa, a disorder manifested by an extreme aversion to food that results in weight loss

Anovulation—the cessation of *ovulation*

Antibody—a protein produced by your immune system to fight anything foreign that invades your body

Anus—the opening of the *rectum*

Areola—the pigmented area surrounding the nipple

Artificial insemination—the placement of sperm (husband's or donor's) at the opening of the uterus or within the uterus to enhance conception

Ascites—excessive free fluid in the abdominal cavity

Aspiration—(1) the withdrawal of fluid from a breast cyst (2) the accidental inhalation of stomach contents during surgery, bringing them into the lungs

Asymptomatic—not causing symptoms

Atrophic vaginitis—thinning of the vaginal *mucosa* secondary to *estrogen* deficiency

Autodonation—the donation of your own blood, typically done in preparation for surgery

Axilla—armpit

Bacterial vaginosis—a condition associated with overgrowth of certain bacteria in the *vagina*, corresponding with a decrease in the number of normal vaginal bacteria

Bartholin's glands—vulvo-vaginal glands located on either side of the opening of the *vagina*, just inside the inner *labia*

Basal body temperature (BBT)—the body's temperature upon awakening; used in natural family planning and infertility evaluation

Benign—not cancerous

Biliary—relating to the bile ducts or gallbladder

Birth control pills—*oral contraceptive* pills containing *estrogen* and/or *progesterone*

Biopsy—sampling a piece of *tissue* for diagnosis

B-HCG(Beta-Human Chorionic Gonadotropin)—the hormone measured in pregnancy tests, which is produced by the *placenta*

Bladder—the pelvic organ that serves as the receptacle for urine prior to voiding

Breast augmentation—a surgical procedure that enlarges the breast

Breast reduction—a surgical procedure that reduces the size of the breast

Bromocryptine—a medication that inhibits the secretion of prolactin, the *pituitary* hormone normally secreted for *lactation*

CA-125—a tumor marker for ovarian cancer that can be measured with a blood test

Candida—a species of yeast that commonly causes vaginal infections

Capsular contracture—the formation of hard scar tissue around a breast implant

Carcinoma-in-situ (CIS)—precancerous changes that immediately precede invasive cancer

Catheter—a flexible tube used for drainage

Cell—the microscopic building block of living matter from which all living plants and animals derive

Cervical polyp—a benign growth derived from glandular cervical tissue

Cervicitis—inflammation of the *cervix*

Cervix—the lower portion of the *uterus* that opens into the *vagina*

Cesarean section—delivery of a baby through an incision made in the wall of the *uterus*

Chemotherapy—substances that are toxic to living cells and used to treat cancer

Chlamydia—a sexually transmitted organism that causes uterine and tubal infection

Chromosome—one of forty-six structures in the nucleus of a cell that bears the genetic blueprint

Clitoris—a sensitive protuberance located just above the vaginal and urethral openings that is important in sexual arousal

Clomiphene citrate—trade names Clomid and Serophene; a substance similar in structure to *estrogen* that is used to stimulate *ovulation*

Colporrhaphy—a surgical procedure that repairs vaginal support of the *bladder* (anterior colporrhaphy) or *rectum* (posterior colporrhaphy)

Colposcope—an instrument that magnifies the *cervix, vagina,* and *vulva* to enhance study of these structures

Conception—successful attainment of pregnancy

Condom—a sheath placed over the penis (male condom) or into the vagina (female condom) prior to intercourse for the prevention of pregnancy and *sexually transmitted infections*

Condylomata—also **condyloma acuminatum**; *genital warts* caused by *Human Papillomavirus*

Condylox—a chemical preparation of *podophylin* used to treat *genital warts*

Conization—excision of a cone of cervical tissue

Contact dermatitis—a rash that results when a substance contacts the skin and induces an allergic reaction

Cornua—the portion of the *uterus* that attaches to the *fallopian tube*

Coronary artery disease—the formation of plaque within the arteries of the heart

Corpus luteum—the *follicular* structure remaining after ovulation, which plays an important role in the secretion of *progesterone*

Cryotherapy—any treatment that uses a freezing technique

CT scan (CAT scan)—computerized tamography scan: a type of radiologic scan used for the detection of certain inflammatory and neoplastic disorders

Cystocele—"dropped bladder"; descent of the *bladder* into the *vagina* from inadequate support

Cystometrogram—a urologic study that evaluates *bladder* function through the measurement of pressures during filling

Cystoplasty—an operation to enlarge the *bladder* (augmentation cystoplasty)

Cystoscopy (cystourethroscopy)—use of a telescopic instrument to look into the *bladder* and *urethra*

Danazol—trade name **Danacrine**; a synthesized steroid used in the medical treatment of *endometriosis*

D&C (dilatation and curettage)—dilation of the *cervix* followed by *endometrial* scraping, which is used to obtain endometrial tissue for diagnosis

D&E (dilatation and evacuation)—dilation of the *cervix* and removal of pregnancy tissue

Deep vein thrombosis (DVT)—blood clot in the deep veins of your legs

Depo-Provera—an intramuscular preparation of Provera, a synthetic *progesterone*

Diaphragm—a dome-shaped flexible device placed into the *vagina* for contraception

Diuretic—"water pill"; any medication or substance that enhances the kidneys' ability to excrete urine

Diverticulitis—inflammation of small outpouchings that extend from the wall of the colon

Diverticulum—an outpouching from an organ

Douche—instilling liquid into the *vagina*

Dysesthesia—disagreeable nerve sensations

Dysmenorrhea—painful *menses*, particularly cramps during the menstrual flow

Dyspareunia—painful intercourse

Dysplasia—atypical cellular changes that are potentially precancerous

Ectopic pregnancy—a pregnancy located outside the intrauterine cavity

Embryo—the earliest stage of life extending from conception to approximately the end of the second month

Endometrial—pertaining to the *endometrium*

Endometrial biopsy—passage of a small catheter into the uterus to obtain a sample of *endometrium*

Endometrial cancer—cancer of the interior glandular lining of the uterus

Endometrial polyp—a benign growth derived from the *endometrium* that projects into the uterine cavity

Endometriosis—a condition where *endometrial* tissue is located outside the *uterus*

Endometrium—the glandular lining inside your *uterus*, which thickens throughout your menstrual cycle and sheds during the menstrual period

Endotracheal tube—a tube inserted into the windpipe during general *anesthesia*

Enterocele—*herniation* between the walls of the *rectum* and *vagina*

Epidural anesthesia—the insertion of a needle or catheter into a space just outside the spinal canal for the administration of anesthetic agents

Estrogen—the fundamental "female" hormone responsible for secondary sexual characteristics; also plays important roles in maintaining bone density and preventing *coronary artery disease*

Excisional biopsy—a breast biopsy with removal of the entire area in question

Fallopian tubes—the two tubes extending from the uterus to the ovaries (one on each side), which allows for the transport of sperm and eggs between the uterus and ovaries

Familial—affecting multiple individuals within a family, usually as a result of genetic inheritance

Fertilization—the impregnation of an egg by a sperm

Fibroadenoma—a noncancerous solid breast tumor

Fibrocystic breasts—the development of cystic glands and fibrotic nodules within breast tissue

Fibroid—a smooth muscle tumor that develops in the muscular wall of the *uterus*

Fimbria—fingerlike projections from the end of the *fallopian tube*, which play an important role in picking up the egg from the ovary after ovulation

Foley—a catheter inserted into the *bladder* through the urethra to drain urine

Follicle—a small fluid-filled structure in your ovary containing an egg, also responsible for the secretion of your female hormones

Follicular—pertaining to the *follicle*

Frozen section—a quick freezing technique used to fix tissue for analysis

Fulguration—destruction of tissue by means of sparks generated with electrical current

Fundus—the upper portion of the uterus, excluding the *cervix*

Galactorrhea—leakage of milk from the breasts that does not occur during pregnancy or nursing

Gamete intrafallopian transfer (GIFT)—transfer of an egg from the ovary to a healthy portion of *fallopian tube*

Gene—a piece of genetic material on a *chromosome* that regulates a specific function

Genitalia—the external organs of the reproductive system

Genital warts—warts located on the external genitals, *vagina*, or *cervix* caused by *human papillomavirus*, also called *condylomata*, and *venereal warts*

Glomerulations—small hemorrhagic areas seen on the inside lining of the bladder in *interstitial cystitis*

GnRH agonists—a group of substances that inhibit the secretion of *gonadotropins* from the *pituitary gland*

Gonadotropins—signals sent to the ovaries from the *pituitary gland* that regulate ovarian function

Gonorrhea—a sexually transmitted bacterium that can cause uterine and tubal infection

G-Spot (Grafenberg Spot)—an area located on the anterior vaginal wall purported to create vaginal orgasm

Hematoma—a collection of extravasated blood

Hepatitis B—one of several hepatitis viruses that may be sexually transmitted and cause liver infection, failure, or cancer

Hepatitis B Immune Globulin—antibodies against *hepatitis B* that can be given shortly after exposure to hepatitis B in order to prevent infection

Hepatitis B Vaccine—a vaccine against *hepatitis B*

Herniation—protrusion through weak support tissue

Herpes Simplex—sexually transmittable virus that causes oral and genital herpes infections

Human immunodeficiency virus (HIV)—a sexually transmitted virus responsible for causing AIDS

Human papillomavirus (HPV)—a sexually transmittable virus that causes *genital warts* and can induce atypical cervical changes

Hydradenitis—infection of the sweat glands

Hyperstimulation syndrome—overstimulation of the ovaries from *ovulation* inducing agents

Hysterectomy—surgical removal of the *uterus*

Hysterosalpingogram (HSG)—an X-ray of the uterus and tubes taken after the injection of radiographic dye into the uterus

Hysteroscopy—looking into the *uterus* with a telescopic instrument placed through the *vagina* and *cervix*

Hymen—a ring of tissue partly occluding the opening of the *vagina*

Incontinence—involuntary loss of urine

Insemination—the placement of semen into the *vagina* or *uterus*

Interferons—naturally occurring proteins that your body uses to fight viruses

Interstitial cystitis—a chronic, inflammatory *bladder* disorder

Intraductal papilloma—a noncancerous growth in a breast duct

Intramural—within the wall of the *uterus*

Intramuscular—within the muscle

Intrauterine—inside the *uterus*

Intravenous (within the vein)—a term used to describe anything administered directly into the bloodstream

Intravenous pyelogram (IVP)—an X-ray of the kidneys, *ureters*, and *bladder* after administering contrast dye

In-Vitro Fertilization (IVF)—a process that includes three steps: (1) removal of eggs from the *ovary* (2) fertilization of the eggs with sperm in a laboratory, and (3) reintroduction of one or more *embryos* into the *uterus*

IUD (intrauterine device)—a device placed into the *uterus* to prevent pregnancy

Kegel exercises—exercises that tighten and strengthen the pelvic muscles

Keloid—an exceedingly thick scar on the skin

Labia—the "lips" or folds of tissue located just outside the opening of the *vagina*

Lactation—the production of breast milk

Lactobacillus—the dominant bacteria in the *vagina*, under normal conditions

Laparoscopy—a means of looking into the abdomen and pelvis through a telescopic instrument (a laparoscope) inserted through a small abdominal incision

Laparotomy—surgery performed through a large abdominal incision

Laser—a high-energy beam

Leiomyoma (fibroid)—a smooth muscle *tumor* that develops within the *myometrium* of the *uterus*

LEEP (loop electrosurgical excision procedure)—a procedure in which a wire loop conducting electrical energy is used to excise cervical tissue

Levator ani—the muscles of the pelvic floor

Libido—sex drive

Lipoma—a noncancerous fatty tumor

Lumpectomy—removal of a cancerous lump, while still preserving the remaining breast tissue

Lymph nodes—oval or round nodules within the lymphatic system, which handles tissue fluids

Malignant—cancerous

Mammogram—an X-ray of the breast

Mastalgia—painful breasts

Mastitis—inflammation of the breast, usually from bacterial infection

Melanoma—a skin cancer derived from pigment-producing cells, usually referred to as malignant melanoma

Menarche—the time of the first menstrual flow or period

Menopause—permanent cessation of the *menses*

Menses—the periodic discharge of blood and *endometrial* tissue from the uterus

Menstrual period—same as *menses*

Menstrual cycle—the monthly cycle of changes in the ovaries and the lining of the *uterus* (*endometrium*)

Microcalcifications—very tiny calcium deposits

Minipill—an *oral contraceptive* that only contains *progesterone*

Mittelschmerz—severe pelvic pain experienced in the middle of the *menstrual cycle*, caused by *ovulation*

Monilia—generic term for a group of fungi that commonly cause vaginal infections

Mucosa—the inside lining of the *vagina*

Multicentric—arising from more than one location

Myolysis—a means of shrinking fibroids by inserting a needle or probe and applying electrical energy or freezing

Myomectomy—removal of a *fibroid* from the *uterus*

Myometrium—the muscular wall of the *uterus*

Nasogastric tube—a tube inserted through the nose into the stomach to drain gastric secretions

Natural family planning—preventing pregnancy without using "artificial" contraception

Neoplasm—a growth of tissue that can be cancerous or noncancerous

Nocturia—getting up to void more than once during the night

Nonpalpable—unable to be felt with the hands

Oligomenorrhea—infrequent menstruation

Omentum—a sheet of fatty tissue that overlays your intestines

Oncologist—a doctor who specializes in treating cancer

Oral contraceptives—pills containing *estrogen* and/or *progesterone* designed to prevent pregnancy

Organ—any part of the body performing a specific function

Orgasm—the climax of sexual response

Osteoporosis—the loss of calcium from bones; thinning of the bones

Ovaries—the two reproductive glands in the female that contain eggs and produce the female hormones

Ovulation—the rupture of a *follicle* in the *ovary* at midcycle, which releases an egg

Paget's disease—a type of skin cancer found on the *vulva*; also, an uncommon cancer that forms in or around the nipple

Palpable—able to be felt with the hands

Pancreatic—relating to the pancreas, an organ that produces enzymes necessary for the digestion of food

Pap smear—a test in which cells from the cervix are submitted for analysis; most commonly used in screening for cervical cancer

Paresthesias—abnormal sensations such as burning, pricking, or numbness

Peau d'orange—French term for a change in skin texture similar to that of an orange peel

Pectoralis muscles—the two large muscles extending across the front of your chest, beneath the breasts

Pelvic inflammatory disease (PID)—bacterial infection of the pelvic organs including the *uterus* and *fallopian tubes*

Pelvic prolapse—general term referring to descent of the pelvic organs (*uterus, bladder, rectum*) due to inadequate support

Perianal—the area around the *anus*

Perineorrhaphy—a surgical procedure that rebuilds the *perineum*

Perineum—the area between the *vagina* and *anus*

Pessary—a device placed into the *vagina* to support pelvic organs

Phytoestrogen—a plant compound with *estrogenic* activity

Pituitary gland—a gland located at the base of the brain that secretes hormonal signals, regulating ovarian function

Placenta—the organ that connects the fetus (by its umbilical cord) to the mother and provides nutrition to the baby from the mother; after delivery, it is expelled as the "afterbirth"

PMS (premenstrual syndrome)—physical and emotional symptoms that occur before the *menstrual period*

Podophylin—a caustic chemical used in the treatment of *genital warts*

Polycystic ovaries—a condition in which the *ovaries* accumulate multiple *follicular cysts*

Polyp—a growth of *tissue* that projects outward from a surface such as the lining of the *uterus, cervix* or *vagina*

Progesterone—the "second female hormone"; made by the *ovary* and *placenta*, it is necessary for supporting pregnancy and plays an important role in balancing the effects of *estrogen* on the *endometrium*

Prolactin—the hormone responsible for inducing *lactation*

Prolapse—an organ falling downward

Prostaglandins—a group of substances that induce contraction of smooth muscle and are released naturally from the *endometrium*

Pubococcygeus—a muscle that stretches from the pubic bone to the sacrum ("tailbone")

Pudendal neuralgia—pain in the pelvic region, caused by disease or injury of the pudendal nerve

Radical hysterectomy—removal of the uterus and its surrounding tissue and lymph nodes

Raloxifene—a *SERM* or an estrogen-like compound that prevents osteoporosis, reduces bone fractures, and lowers the risk of breast cancer

Reanastomosis—reattachment of tubal segments after prior tubal ligation

Rectocele—bulging of the rectum into the vagina from inadequate support

Rectum—the terminal section of large bowel that serves as a receptacle for stool prior to evacuation

Resect—to excise a piece of tissue

RU-486—an anti-progestational agent used to induce early abortion of pregnancy

Sacrospinous vaginal vault suspension—a vaginal operation that suspends the top of the *vagina* to a strong ligament found in the pelvis

Saline—salt water, the foundation of most intravenous solutions

Sebaceous glands—the tiny glands in the skin that secrete an oily substance called sebum

SERM (selective estrogen receptor modulator)—a drug that mimics estrogen in some organs, while blocking it in others

Sexually transmitted infection (STI)—any disease that can be spread through a sexual encounter

Silicone—a plastic based on silicon

Speculum—a device inserted into the vagina that opens to allow inspection of the vagina and cervix

Spermicide—a chemical that kills sperm used in contraceptive creams, gels, and suppositories

Spinal anesthesia—the introduction of a needle or catheter into the spinal canal for the administration of anesthetic agents

Spirometry—the measurement of inspiratory effort

Spontaneous abortion—synonymous with miscarriage, a spontaneous loss of pregnancy before twenty weeks

Squamous intraepithelial lesion (SIL)—atypical cellular changes that are potentially precancerous

Stereotaxis—radiologic technique used for localization

Sterilization—a procedure that permanently renders you incapable of conceiving

Stress incontinence—loss of urine associated with activities that increase abdominal pressure such as coughing, laughing, and sneezing

Submucous—located immediately beneath the *endometrium* or inside lining of the uterus

Subserosal—located immediately beneath the serosa, or outer covering of the uterus

Supracervical hysterectomy—surgical removal of the uterine *fundus* with preservation of the *cervix*

Suprapubic catheter—a tube inserted into the bladder through the abdominal wall immediately above the pubic bone

Tamoxifen—trade name *Nolvadex*; an anti-estrogen used to treat severe *mastalgia* or breast cancer

Teratogenic—anything that induces birth defects

Threatened abortion—bleeding within the first twenty weeks of pregnancy, unassociated with the passage of tissue

Thrombophlebitis—inflammation of veins associated with blood clots

Tissue—a collection of similar cells

Torsion—twisting or being twisted

Tubal pregnancy—a pregnancy located in the *fallopian tube*

Tumor—generic term used to denote a growth or *neoplasm*; can be cancerous or noncancerous

Trichloroacetic acid (TCA)—a chemical used in the treatment of *genital warts*

Trichomonas—a single-cell parasite that causes vaginal infections and is sexually transmitted

Triglycerides—fats that circulate in the bloodstream

Ultrasound—high frequency sound waves used to perform scans

Ureters—the tubes connecting your kidneys with the bladder

Urethra—a tube that extends from your bladder to the outside, allowing you to empty your bladder

Urethral meatus—the opening of the *urethra*; located immediately above the opening of the vagina

Urgency incontinence—loss of urine associated with an urge to empty the bladder

Urinary retention—the excessive retention of urine in the bladder because of an inability of the bladder to empty

Urethral pressure profile—a test that compares bladder pressure to that within the urethra

Uterine descensus—the uterus falling down the vagina from inadequate support

Uterus—also known as your "womb," a muscular organ located in the pelvis in which the fertilized egg develops into a baby; composed of a lower part referred to as the *cervix* (which opens into the vagina) and an upper part referred to as the *fundus*

Vagina—the tubular structure extending from the *uterus* to the *vulva*; also referred to as the birth canal during delivery

Vaginismus—painful spasm of the vagina preventing intercourse

Vaginitis—inflammation of the vagina

Vaporization—destruction of tissue with high-energy laser

Vas defferens—the tubes that carry sperm from the testicles to the penis

Venereal warts—genital warts induced by a sexually transmitted virus

Vestibule—the area at the opening of the vagina between the *labia*

Vestibulitis—an inflammatory condition limited to the *vestibule*

VIN (vulvar intraepithelial neoplasia)—abnormal vulvar skin with potentially precancerous changes

Voiding cystourethrogram—X-rays of the *bladder* and *urethra* (using contrast dye) with the patient standing, bearing down, and voiding

Vulva—the tissue surrounding the opening of the *vagina* that includes the inner and outer "lips" of the *vagina*

Vulvectomy—resection of the *vulva*

Yeast—a form of fungus; may cause vaginal and vulvar infections

Zygote intrafallopian transfer (ZIFT)—transfer of a fertilized egg into a healthy portion of *fallopian* tube

Index

Indexer's note:
Entries for illustrations are in italics, e.g. *137*
Entries for glossary terms are in bold, e.g. **366**
Entries for grey boxes are marked b, e.g. 67b

Numbers

25-OH Vitamin D blood test, 303

A

abdominal biopsy, 224
abdominal cancer, 32
abdominal myomectomy, 182–83
abdominal pain, 31–32, 128, 140, 178
abdominal pregnancy, 161
abdominal surgery, 338–39
abdominal swelling, 223
ablation, 184
abortions, 77–80
abscess, 88, 113, 114, 248, **366**
abstinence, 75b, 131
abuse, 87, 89–90
accelerated partial breast irradiation
    (APBI), 260–61
acetaminophen (Tylenol)
    breast tenderness, 242, 290
    fibroids and, 180, 185
    menstrual pain, 49
    mittel-schmerz, 44
    pain, 35
    in PMS medication, 50
acetic acid, 206
acidic food, 310
acquired immunodeficiency syndrome.
    see AIDS

Actonel (risendronate), 305, 306
acupuncture, 36, 53, 151,
    172, 298
acyclovir (Zovirax), 123, 125
adenomyosis
    defined, **366**
    diagnosing, 189
    explained, 188–89
    heavy flow and, 43
    menstrual pain, 46
    painful, 33
    painful sex and, 89
    treatment, 189–190
adhesions
    defined, **366**
    hysterectomy and, 98
    infertility and, 146
    IUDs and, 73
    miscarriage and, 159
    painful, 33
    painful sex and, 89
    PID and, 113
    tubal, 142
    tubal pregnancy and, 161–62
Administrators in Medicine, 3
adoption, 154
adrenal glands, 97
Advil. *see* ibuprofen
aerobic vaginitis, 112–13
age, 147–49, 278

AID (artificial insemination of donor
    sperm), 147
AIDS (acquired immunodeficiency
    syndrome). *see also* HIV
  death from, 126
  defined, **366**
  in females, 126
  HIV and, 126–27
  treatment, 127
  yeast infections and, 105
AIs. *see* aromatase inhibitors
alcohol
  antibiotics and, 112
  bladder and, 310
  breast cancer and, 249
  headaches and, 53
  IC/PBS and, 324
  infertility and, 145, 149
  insomnia and, 272
  menopause and, 298
  orgasms and, 92–93
  osteoporosis and, 300
  PMS and, 50
  weight and, 25
Aldara (Imiquimod), 119–120, 236, 341
alendronate (Fosamax), 305, 306
Aleve. *see* naproxen sodium
allergies
  IC/PBS and, 323
  latex, 60
  lubricants and, 86, 275
  spermicide, 61
  vaginal itching and, 102–3
  vulvar inflammation and, 86–87
  yeast, 106
Alli (Xenical, Orlistat), 29
almonds, *302*
almotripan (Axert), 52
alpha-lipoic acid, 29
alternative medicine. *see* CAM treatments
amenorrhea, 39, 151, **366**
Amerge (naratripan), 52
American Association of Sex Educators,
    Counselors, and Therapists, 101
American Cancer Society, 247
American College of Obstetrics and
    Gynecology, xxix, xxx, 285
American College of Radiology, 20

American Society for Reproductive
    Medicine, 173
AMH (anti-mullerian hormone), 148
amines, 111
Amitriptyline, 235
ampicillin, 65
anal douche, 100
anal sex, 100–101, 113
analgesics. *see* pain medication, **366**
Anaprox. *see* naproxen sodium
anastrozole (Arimidex), 181, 264
androgens, 97, 170, 275–76
anemia
  chemotherapy and, 228, 263
  continuous oral contraception and,
    67b, 68
  fibroids and, 177, 178
  heavy flow and, 43
  oral contraception and, 62
anesthesia, 35, 346–48, 349–350, **366**
anesthesiologists, 346, 346b, 347
Angie's List, 3
anorexia, 301, **366**
anovulation, 138, 139, **366**
anterior colporrhaphy, 332
antibiotics
  bladder infection, 117, 317, 318
  BV, 112
  cervical infection, 203
  genital cysts, 232
  infertility and, 145
  intravenous, 114
  nipple discharge, 249
  oral contraception and, 65
  penicillin, 117
  PID, 114
  skin infections, 232b–33b
  STIs and, 130
  surgery and, 342
  syphilis, 118
  uterine infections and, 89
  vaginal discharge, 113
  yeast infections and, 105
antibodies, 122b, 123, 128, 160, **366**
anticonvulsants. *see* anti-seizure
    medication
antidepressants
  chronic pain, 35

headaches and, 53
IC/PBS and, 325
libido and, 93, 277
menopause and, 278, 293
PMS and, 50–51
restless leg syndrome, 271
vulvodynia and, 234
weight loss and, 29
antifungal medication, 65, 104, 105,
    107–8, 203
antihistamines, 50, 325
anti-inflammatory medication, 65, 103,
    105, 234, 249, 325
anti-mullerian hormone (AMH), 148
anti-nausea medication, 70, 350
antioxidants, 29, 172
anti-prostaglandins, 46, 53
antipsychotics, 277
antiretroviral therapy (ARV), 127
anti-seizure medication
    chronic pain, 35
    headaches and, 53
    oral contraception and, 65
    osteoporosis and, 301
    restless leg syndrome, 271
    vulvodynia, 234, 235
    weight loss and, 29
antispasmodic medication, 325
antiviral medication, 123, 124, 125, 131
anus
    cancer of, 101, 119
    defined, **366**
    erogenous, 91
    HPV, 119
    picture, *15*
    syphilis, 117
anxiety
    anesthesia and, 347
    cancer, 201b
    libido and, 93
    medication, 271
    menopause, 271, 277
    menstrual cycle and, 39
    ovulation and, 139
    patients and, xxviii, 4–5
    PMS, 46, 51
    sex and, 86, 89–90
    of teens, 8

APBI (accelerated partial breast
    irradiation), 260–61
apnea, 271
apomorphine, 93
appendicitis, 32, 142, 339
appetite changes, 46, 227
appetite suppressants, 28–29, 316
appointment scheduling, 5–7
apps, 26, 76–77
Aredia, 268
areola, 248, **366**
Arimidex (anastrozole), 181, 264
armpit (axilla), 255, 257, 259
Arnica gel, 36
Aromastin (exemestane), 252, 264, 267
aromatase inhibitors (AIs)
    breast cancer, 264
    endometrial cancer, 196
    endometriosis, 171
    fibroids, 181
    metastatic cancer, 267
    osteoporosis and, 301
arousal
    lubrication and, 85–86
    mastectomy and, 259
    menopause and, 275
    orgasm and, 90
    painful sex and, 88b
    testosterone and, 97
    vasectomy and, 83
arthritis, 32, 36, 243, 300
artificial insemination, 146–47, **367**
artificial sweeteners, 310
ARV (antiretroviral) therapy, 127
ascites, 217, 223, **367**
Ashkenazi Jewish, 251
aspiration, 245, 246–47, 346, **367**
aspirin, 160
assumptions, xxix–xxx
asthma, 67, 67b, 347
Astragulus, 150
Astroglide, 275
asymptomatic, **367**
Atelvia (risendronate), 305
atrophic vaginitis, 274–75, **367**
atrophy, vaginal, 264, 274–75, 330
augmentation, breasts, 243–44
augmentation cystoplasty, 326

auras, 63
autodonation, **367**
autoimmune disease, 243–44
autoinoculation, 123
Aveeno, 87, 102
avocados, 51
Axert (almotriptan), 52
axilla (armpit), 255, 257, 259, **367**
AZO, 317

B

bacon, 52
bacteria
  anal sex and, 101
  bladder infections and, 116, 317
  boils and, 232
  BV and, 111
  douching and, 10
  lactobacillus, 108
  MRSA, 232b–33b
  oral sex and, 100
  toxic shock syndrome, 54–55
  yeast infections and, 105
bacterial vaginosis (BV)
  causes, 111
  defined, **367**
  diagnosing, 111–12
  discharge from, 111
  itchy, 102
  IUDs and, 73
  medication, 112
  miscarriage and, 159
  PID and, 111
  probiotics and, 108–9
  spermicide and, 61
Bactroban (mupirocin), 233
bananas, 51
barbiturates, 65
bariatric surgery, 30
barium enema, 34
barrier contraception, 57–60, 77
Bartholin's glands, **367**
basal body temperature (BBT), 137, *137*,
      139, 141, **367**
baths, 145
BBT (basal body temperature), 137, *137*,
      139, 141, **367**

BCMets, 268
Beano, 48
beans, 48, 51, *302*
bed, 272, 298
bee products, 125
Belviq (lorcaserin), 28
benign, **367**
benzocaine, 103
benzodiazepines, 271
berberine, 319
berries, 294
beta human chorionic gonadotropin
      (B-HCG), 32, 156, 164, **367**
beta-blockers, 53
B-HCG (beta human chorionic
      gonadotropin), 32, 156, 164,
      367
bicycle riding, 234, 303
bilateral breast cancer, 251
biliary, 342, **367**
bimanual examination, 14
Binosto (alendronte), 305
biofeedback, 36, 53, 324
bioidentical hormones, 285–86
biopsy
  abdominal, 224
  bladder, 324
  breast, 18, 255
  cervical, 210, 211
  colposcopically directed, 205
  core needle, 256, 257
  defined, **367**
  endometrial. *see* endometrial biopsy
  excisional, **371**
  fine needle, 256
  sentinel node, 259
  skin, 87
  stereotactic core, 256
  vulvar, 236–37, 237
birth control. *see* contraception
birth control pill. *see* oral contraception,
      367
birth defects, 139, 142
bisphosphonates, 268, 305–6
black cohosh, 50, 150, 295, 296
bladder
  biopsy, 324
  changes in, 31

control, 311
cystoscopy, 35
defined, 12, **367**
descended. *see* pelvic prolapse
diverticulum, 318
endometriosis and, 167
enlarging, 326
infections. *see* bladder infections
IVP, 35
neck, 315–16, 333
overactive. *see* overactive bladder
pain in, 32
picture, *13*
radiation and, 196
removal, 326, 359
retraining, 310–11, 324
retrograde ejaculation, 145
spasms, 211
stones, 318
surgery, 360–61
surgery injury, 339
bladder infections
alternative treatments, 318–19
causes, 317, 317–19
cystocele and, 329
diagnosing, 114, 116–17
"honeymoon," 317
overactive bladder and, 310
recurrent, 317–18
sex and, 88
tests, 319–321
bleeding. *see also* menstrual cycle
abnormal, 188, 193, 201b, 210, 223
hormone replacement therapy, 289
blindness, 124
blisters, 118, 122, 131
bloating
clomiphene, 139
Depo-Provera, 72
hormone replacement therapy, 290
Implanon, 71
oral contraception and, 65
ovarian cancer, 223
PMS, 46, 48
blood banks, 126
blood clots
hormone replacement therapy and,
280, 282, 283, 290b, 291–92

menstrual, 43
minipill and, 68
oral contraception and, 62–63, 63b
tamoxifen and, 263
blood donation, 128
blood pregnancy test, 32
blood thinners, 160
blood transfusions, 126, 339
blood vessels, 117
blueberry juice, 318
BMI (Body Mass Index), 28, 30, 72
Board Certified, 3
Body Mass Index (BMI), 28, 30, 72
boils, 231, 232, 233, 233b
bologna, 52
bone cancer, 267
bone density
aromatase inhibitors and, 264
Depo-Provera, 72
GnRH agonists and, 170, 180
testing, 300
testosterone and, 276
bone fracture, 300
bone marrow, 228
bone mineralization, 303
Boniva (ibandronate), 305, 306
boric acid capsules, 107, 109, 112
boswellia, 36
Botox, 53, 312
bowel
cervical cancer and, 211
changes in, 31
chemotherapy and, 227
endometriosis and, 167, 168
fibroids and, 178
ovarian cancer and, 224
radiation and, 196
surgery and, 339, 341–42, 350
bras, 242
BRCA, 23, 220, 221, 251–52
bread, 52
breast cancer
aromatase inhibitors, 181, 264
bilateral, 251
chemotherapy, 262–63
CIS and, 266–67
detection, 254–55
endometrial cancer and, 192

estrogen and, 263
family history, 220, 250–52
fibrocystic breasts and, 242
hormone replacement therapy and,
    280, 282, 288–89, 290b, 291
inflammatory, 245
lifetime risk, 250
lumpectomy, 257b–59b
male, 251
mammograms and, 18, 19–20
mastectomy, 257b–59b
MRI and, 22–23
oral contraception and, 63–64
ovarian cancer and, 221, 251
prevention, 249–250
resources, 269
SERMs and, 298
spreading, 267–68
support groups, 268
symptoms, 254–55
treatment, 257, 257b–59b, 259
"triple negative," 251, 252
breast tenderness
alternative treatments, 49, 241
causes, 241
clomiphene, 139
Depo-Provera, 72
diet and, 241
with fever, 245
hormone replacement therapy, 289
Implanon, 71
medication, 242
oral contraception and, 65
PMS and, 46, 48–49, 241
supplements, 241, 290
breast-feeding
breast cancer and, 249
breast reduction and, 245
dryness and, 86
endometrial cancer and, 193
HIV and, 127
libido and, 93
minipill and, 68
breasts
aspiration, 245, 246–47
augmentation, 243–44, **367**
biopsy, 18, 255
cancer of. *see* breast cancer

cysts, 245, 246–47
erogenous, 91
feeding. *see* breast-feeding
fibrocystic, 18, 21, 241–42, 248
implants, 21, 22, 243–44
infection, 248, 249
large, 244–45
lumps, 245, 254
mammograms. *see* mammograms
MRI, 20, 22–23
prosthetic, 260
reconstruction, 258b, 259–260
reduction, 245, **368**
removal. *see* mastectomy
self-exam, 242, 254, 255
tender. *see* breast tenderness
tumors, 246
ultrasound, 20, 21–22
breathing, 342
broccoli, 48, 250, *302*
bromocriptine (Parlodel), 141, 242, 248,
    368
brushing, teeth, 132
Brussels sprouts, 250
bupropion (Wellbutrin), 29, 93
Burgio, Kathryn L., 311
butt plugs, 101
butter, 303
buttocks, 91, 122
BV. *see* bacterial vaginosis
BVBLUE, 112

C

CA-125 blood test
defined, **368**
endometrial cancer, 202
ovarian cancer and, 221, 222, 228
ovarian cysts and, 217, 219
ovarian tumors and, 220
cabbage, 48, 250
Cabergoline (Dostinex), 248
Cafergot, 52
caffeine, 149
bladder and, 310
breast tenderness and, 241, 290
headaches and, 51, 53
IC/PBS and, 324

insomnia and, 272
in medication, 52
menopause and, 298
miscarriage and, 160
PMS and, 49, 50
restless leg syndrome, 271
calcifications, 18, 256
Calcitonin (Miacalcin, Fortical), 307
calcium, 49, 301, 301–2, *302*
calcium channel blockers, 53
calcium citrate (Citracal), 235, 302
calcium deposits, 18, 256
calendula gel, 341
CAM (complementary and alternative
    medical) treatments
  acupuncture, 36, 53, 151, 172, 298
  bladder infection, 318–19
  breast cancer, 249–250
  breast tenderness, 49, 241
  disclaimer for, xxv–xxvi
  endometriosis, 172–73
  fertility, 149–151
  headaches, 53
  herpes, 125
  hormone replacement therapy, 285–86
  keloids, 341
  menopause, 294–98
  pain, 36
  PMS, 49–50
  sexual dysfunction, 93
  UTIs, 318–19
  vulvodynia, 235
  weight loss, 29
  yeast infections, 108–9
Camrese, 67
cancer
  abdominal, 32
  AIDS and, 126
  anal, 101, 119
  breast. *see* breast cancer
  cervical. *see* cervical cancer
  colon, 192, 220, 280
  colonoscopy, 192
  continuous oral contraception and, 68
  endometrial. *see* endometrial cancer
  family history, 7, 220–21
  fibroids and, 177
  HPV and, 119

interval, 21
liver, 128, 267
lobular, 21
metastasis, 224, 259, 267–68
nipple discharge, 248
oral contraception and, 63–64
ovarian. *see* ovarian cancer
ovarian cysts and, 218–19
Paget's disease, 238, **376**
pancreatic, 251
polyps and, 187
rates, 1–2
rectal, 15
screening, 1–2, 7, 15–16
skin, 238
vaginal, 119, 238–39
vulvar. *see* vulvar cancer
Candida, 107, **368**
Candida vaginitis. *see* yeast infections
candy, 312
caprylic acid, 109
capsaicin cream, 36
capsular contracture, 244, **368**
carbamezapine (Tegretol), 65, 235
carbohydrates, 25, 49
carbonated beverages, 48
carcinoma in situ (CIS), 22, 207, 264–65,
    267, **368**
carcinomas, 191
casual sex, 76b
CAT scan. *see* CT scan
Catapres (clonidine), 294
catheter, 144, 348, 360, 361b, **368**
cauliflower, 250
cautery, 120, 206
CDC (Centers for Disease Control), 61,
    129
Celexa (citalopram), 293, 294
celiac disease, 149
cell, **368**
Centers for Disease Control, 61, 129
centrifuge, 147
Cervarix, 204
cervical biopsy, 210, 211
cervical cancer
  diagnosing, 210–11
  HPV and, 119, 204
  HSIL and, 205

hysterectomy and, 181, 355, 357
oral contraception and, 63
resources, 212
screening, 1–2, 15–16, 17
SIL and, 209
stages of, 211
survival rates, 212
symptoms, 209–10
treatment, 211
cervical caps, 59
cervical conization, 59, 207, **369**
cervical mucus, 57, 139, 144, 146
cervical polyps, 187–88, 190, 232, **368**
cervicitis, 203, **368**
cervix
  biopsy, 210, 211
  cancer of. *see* cervical cancer
  caps, 59
  conization, 59, 207, **369**
  defined, 11
  HPV, 119
  hysterectomy and, 354–55
  "incompetent," 160
  infertility and, 144
  inflammation, 203
  lesions, 43
  mucus, 57, 139, 144, 146
  picture, *13, 38*
  PID and, 113
  polyps, 187–88, 190, 232, **368**
cesarean section, 124, 173, 357, **368**
chancre, 117, 118
Chaste Tree Berry, 150
Chasteberry, 49, 296
cheese, 52, *302*
chemoprevention, 250, 266–67
chemotherapy
  breast cancer, 262–63
  cervical cancer, 211
  defined, **368**
  endometrial cancer, 195, 196
  infertility and, 145
  length of, 228–29, 262
  metastatic cancer, 268
  neoadjuvant, 229, 262
  ovarian cancer, 224–25, 229–230
  side effects, 227–28, 263
  types of, 228–29

vulvar cancer, 238
yeast infections and, 105
chest pain, 63
chewing gum, 312
chicken liver, 51
chickpeas, *302*
childbirth, 89, 106
Children's Oncology Group, 23
chills, 79, 113
Chinese herbal medicine, 172
chlamydia, 113, 114, 115, 130,
    368
chocolate
  bladder and, 310
  breast tenderness and, 241
  headaches and, 51
  IC/PBS and, 324
  insomnia and, 272
  latex and, 132
  PMS and, 49
"chocolate cyst," 214
cholesterol, 214, 276
chromosomes, 158–59, **368**
chronic hepatitis, 128
chronic pain, 31, 35–36
Cialis, 93
CIN 1. *see* LSIL
CIN 2. *see* HSIL
CIN 3. *see* HSIL
CIS (carcinoma in situ), 22, 207,
    264–65, 267, **368**
citalopram (Celexa), 293, 294
Citracal (calcium citrate), 235, 302
citrus fruit, 51, 310, 324
cleaning, 352
Clearblue Easy Fertility Monitor, 57
Cleocin (clindamycin), 113
clindamycin (Cleocin), 112, 113
clitoris
  defined, 12, **368**
  orgasm and, 92, 100
  picture, *13, 15*
  self-exam, 236b
  sexual arousal and, 90–91
  vulvar cancer and, 237
clock, 273
Clomid (clomiphene citrate), 139,
    142, 151–52, **368**

clomiphene citrate (Clomid, Serophene), 139, 142, 151–52, **368**
clonidine (Catapres), 294
clots. *see* blood clots
clumsiness, 46
CMG (cystometrogram), 310, 318, 319–320, 361b, **369**
coconut oil, 109
coffee, 49, 51, 241, 272, 310
cohesive gel, 244
cola. *see* caffeine
cold sores, 122
colitis, 32
collagen, 317
collard greens, 250
colloidal silver, 109
colon cancer, 192, 220, 280
colonoscopy, 35
colporrhaphy, 332, **369**
colposcopy, 205, 205–6, **369**
communication, xxx–xxxi, 133
complementary treatments. *see* CAM treatments
computed tomography. *see* CAT scan
conception, 136, **369**. *see also* infertility
condoms
    anal sex and, 101
    backup, 49, 65
    defined, **369**
    explained, 59–60
    genital warts and, 121
    hepatitis and, 129
    herpes and, 125
    HIV and, 127
    HPV and, 121, 204
    irritation and, 103
    PID and, 115
    spermicide and, 61
    STIs and, 76, 116b, 118, 131, 132
    Vaseline and, 86
condylomata. *see* genital warts, **369**
Condylox (podofilox), 119, **369**
conization, 59, 207, **369**
conjunctivitis, 113
constipation, 31, 312, 329, 331
ConsumerLab.com, xxv
contact dermatitis, 103, 236, **369**

continuous oral contraception. *see* oral contraception, continuous
contraception. *see also* oral contraception
    barrier methods, 57–60, 77
    cervical caps, 59
    choosing, 76–77
    condoms. *see* condoms
    continuous. *see* oral contraception, continuous
    cramps and, 45
    diaphragms, 49, 58–59, 61, 103, **370**
    education, 75b–76b
    emergency, 69–70
    gynecologists and, 2
    implanted, 71–72
    injection, 72–73
    intermenstrual bleeding and, 44
    irritation and, 103
    menstrual cycle and, 40, 62
    menstrual pain and, 44, 46, 62
    natural, 56–57, 76
    NuvaRing, 66, 77
    oral. *see* oral contraception
    patch, 66
    permanent, 77
    pill. *see* oral contraception
    PMS and, 51
    spermicide, 58, 60, 61, 103, **379**
    sterilization, 77, 80–84, **379**
    withdrawal, 60
cooking, 25, 352
copper, 73
CoQ10, 150
core needle biopsy, 256, 257
cornua, 143, **369**
coronary artery disease, **369**
corpus luteum, 37, 141, 142, 163, 213, **369**
cortisone, 105
cottage cheese, *302*
cotton, 103, 298, 318
coughing, 314, 331
counseling, 90, 92, 133, 153, 268
CPAP machine, 271
cramps, 45, 67, 74, 223, 290
cranberries, 318–19
Crinone, 141
cryomyolysis, 184

cryotherapy, 120, 203, 206, 341, **369**
C-section, 124, 173, 357, **368**
CT scan
    bladder infection, 318, 321
    cervical cancer, 210
    chronic pain, 34
    defined, **369**
    endometrial cancer, 202
    ovarian cysts, 213
cultures, 46
curcumin, 36
curettage. *see* D&C
Cycrin (medroxyprogesterone), 171, 272, 280, 284, 286, 288
Cymbalta, 235
cystadenomas, 214
cystdenocarcinomas, 214
cystectomy, 326, 359
cystitis. *see* bladder infections
cystocele, 327, 329, 332, 334, **369**
cystometrogram (CMG), 310, 318, 319–320, 361b, **369**
cystoplasty, **369**
cystoscopy
    bladder infection, 318, 319
    chronic pain, 35
    defined, **370**
    IC/PBS, 324, 325
    overactive bladder, 310, 312
    stress incontinence, 317
cysts
    breast, 245, 246–47
    "complicated," 246–47
    corpus luteal, 213
    dermoid, 214
    genital, 118, 231, 231–32
    labial, 88
    ovarian. *see* ovarian cysts
    vaginal, 88, 231–32
    vestibule, 88
    vulvar, 232
cytokines, 172, 173
cytologists, 15
cytology, 249
cytomegalovirus, 159

D

D&C (dilation and curettage)
    adenomyosis, 189

defined, **370**
    endometrial cancer, 193
    heavy flow, 43
    hospital stays, 345
    intermenstrual bleeding, 44
    polyps, 188
    work leave, 350
D&E (dilation and evacuation), 77, 79, 156–57, **370**
da Vinci surgical system, 353
dairy, 172
Dalkon Shield, 73
damiana leaves, 150
danazol (Danocrine), 170, 172, 242, **370**
dancing, 303, 314
Danocrine, **370**
Danocrine (danazol), 170, 172, 242, **370**
day three levels, 148
DCIS (ductal carcinoma in situ), 22, 267. *see also* CIS
death, 124, 126, 162, 194–95
decongestants, 316
deep vein thrombosis (DVT), 62–63, 66, 291–92, 298, 341, **370**
dehydroepiandrosterone (DHEA), 50
dementia, 310
denosumab (Prolia), 306–7
dental dam, 132
dentists, 128, 306
deodorant, 103
Depo-Provera, 72–73, 171, **370**
depression
    libido and, 93, 97, 276
    menopause and, 271, 277–79
    painful sex and, 89–90
    PMS, 46, 51
dermatitis, 103, 236, 296, 307, **369**
dermatologists, 87, 104
dermoid cysts, 214
desquamative vaginitis, 112–13
detergent, 87, 102
devil's claw, 36
DEXA (dual-energy x-ray absorptiometry), 300
DHEA (dehydroepiandrosterone), 50
diabetes
    estrogen patch and, 283
    gestational, 148
    hepatitis and, 129

hormone replacement therapy and, 290b, 292
medication, 29
miscarriage and, 160
oral contraception and, 63
polycystic ovary syndrome and, 214
testosterone and, 276
yeast infections and, 105
dialators, vaginal, 87, 88, 89
diaphragm (contraceptive), 49, 58–59, 61, 103, **370**
diaphragm (muscle), 162, 328
diaphragm (pelvic floor muscle), 235, 315, 330
diarrhea, 31, 157, 325
diet
    bladder control and, 315
    breast cancer and, 249–250
    breast tenderness and, 241
    cramps and, 45
    endometriosis and, 172
    headaches and, 51–52, 53
    IC/PBS and, 324
    menopause and, 293
    osteoporosis and, 301
    PMS and, 48, 49, 50
    vulvodynia and, 235
    weight and, 25, 28
diethylpropion, 28
Diflucan, 107
digoxin, 307
dihydroergotamine (Migranal), 52
diindolylmethane (DIM), 48, 242, 290
Dilantin (phenytoin), 65
dilation and curettage. *see* D&C
dilation and evacuation. *see* D&E
dilators, 87, 88, 89
DIM (diindolylmethane), 48, 242, 290
disability insurance, 350b
disc disease, 32
discharge
    nipple, 247–49, 255
    penile, 114
    vaginal, 111–13, 113, 263, 331
diuretic, 48, 50, 301, 310, 313, **370**
diverticulitis, 32, 339, **370**
diverticulum, **370**
dizziness, 46, 79, 162
doctors. *see also* gynecologists
    choosing, xxxi, 3–4

family, 9
herbal supplements and, xxv–xxvi
patients, communication with, xxx–xxxi
STI screening, 116b
dong quai, 50, 150, 295
donors, 128, 147, 149
dopamine, 271
dopaminergics, 271
Dostinex (Cabergoline), 248
douche, 10, 100, **370**
Down syndrome, 147, 148
drinking. *see* alcohol
driving, 352
"dropped bladder." *see* pelvic prolapse
drugs. *see* medication
dry mouth, 312
dual-energy x-ray absorptiometry (DEXA), 300
ductal carcinoma in situ (DCIS), 22, 267. *see also* CIS
ductal ectasia, 248, 249
Durex Avanti, 60
DVT (deep vein thrombosis), 62–63, 66, 291–92, 298, 341, **370**
dysesthesia, 340, **370**
dyslipidemia, 214
dysmenorrhea, 34, 44, 45–46, 168, **370**
dyspareunia. *see* painful sex, **370**
dysplasia, **370**
    mild. *see* LSIL
    moderate/severe. *see* HSIL
dysuria, 89, 113, 117, 123

E

ears, 91
eating, 25–26, 272, 346. *see also* diet
echinacea, 125, 150
Ecovag, 108
ectopic pregnancy, 32, 74, 156, 161, 164, **370**
eczema, 307
education, xxx, 75b–76b
Effexor (venlafaxine), 293, 294
Efudex (fluorouracil), 120, 341
egg yolks, 303
eggs, 11, 37–38, 138–39, *143*, 149
ejaculation, 60, 83, 145, 146
electrical stimulation therapy, 324

eletripan (Relpax), 52
eleuthero, 125
Ella (ulipristal acetate), 70, 180
Elmiron (pentosan polysulfate sodium),
    324–25
embedment, 74
embryo, 143, *143*, 156, *161*, **370**
emergency contraception, 69–70
emotional abuse, 89–90
emotional factors
    of hysterectomy, 98–99
    infertility, 153–54
    insomnia and, 273
    mastectomy, 259
    menopause, 277
    miscarriage, 157, 160–61
    painful sex and, 89–90
emotional intimacy, 96, 134, 277
emotional support, 36
endometrial, **371**
endometrial ablation, 184
endometrial cancer
    causes, 192–93
    defined, **371**
    diagnosing, 193
    doctors visits after, 202
    estrogen and, 192, 202, 282
    explained, 191
    family history, 192, 220
    hormone replacement therapy and,
        202, 282, 290b, 291
    hysterectomy and, 181, 263, 357
    infrequent menses and, 39
    oral contraception and, 62, 64, 250
    Pap smears and, 16
    recurrent, 202
    resources, 202
    symptoms, 201b
    tamoxifen and, 263–64
    treatment, 194–96
    types of, 191
endometrial polyps, 187, 188, 190, 263,
    371
endometrioma, 167, 214
endometriosis
    alternative treatments, 172–73
    association, 174, 175
    CA-125 and, 222

causes, 167
classifying, 173–74
continuous oral contraception and,
    67b, 68, 171
defined, **371**
diagnosing, 169
explained, 167
family history, 168
hormone replacement therapy and,
    290b
hysterectomy, 175
IC/PBS and, 323
infertility and, 142, 146, 173–74
intermenstrual bleeding, 43
medication, 170–72
menopause and, 175
menstrual pain, 45–46
ovarian cancer and, 214
painful, 33
painful sex and, 89
picture, *167*
recurrent, 174
support groups, 174
symptoms, 168
treatment, 169–173
tubal pregnancy and, 161–62
Endometriosis Association, 174, 175
endometrium
    ablation, 184
    adenomyosis, 33, 189
    biopsy, 43, 44, 141, 189, 193, **371**
    cancer of. *see* endometrial cancer
    cramps and, 45
    defined, **371**
    endometrioma, 167, 214
    endometriosis. *see* endometriosis
    explained, 11
    hyperplasia, 190–91
    menstrual cycle and, 37, 38
    picture, *38*
    polyps, 187, 188, 190, 263, **371**
    progesterone and, 159
    removal, 354
endoscopy, 35
endotracheal tube, 346, **371**
endrocinologists, 54
enema, 34, 101
enterocele, 328, 333, **371**

epidural anesthesia, **371**
epilepsy, 67, 67b
ER- cancers, 262, 267
ER+ cancers, 262, 263, 264, 267
erections, 83, 93
ergotamine, 52
ergots, 52
erogenous areas, 91
erotic novels, 96
esophagitis, 305
Essure, 80, 83
estradiol, 148, 285
Estratest, 276
estriol, 285
estrogen
    atrophic vaginitis and, 274–75
    bladder and, 310
    bladder infections and, 318
    breast cancer and, 250, 263
    in contraception, 68
    contraceptive patch, 66
    defined, **371**
    dryness and, 86
    emergency contraception, 69
    endometrial cancer and, 192, 202, 282
    fibroids and, 176
    formats, 282–83
    GnRH agonists and, 170
    headaches and, 53
    hot flashes and, 273
    insomnia and, 272
    libido and, 97–98, 276
    menstrual cycle and, 37
    mood changes, 278
    ovaries and, 11
    pelvic prolapse and, 330
    PMS and, 47
    vulvodynia and, 234
    weight gain and, 24
estrogen receptor negative, 262, 267
estrogen receptor positive, 262, 263, 264, 267
Estroven, 295
evacuation. *see* D&E
evening primrose oil, 49, 50, 150, 241, 290
Evista (raloxifene), 250, 252, 267, 298–99, 306, **378**

exams
    bimanual, 14
    family doctors and, 9
    rectal, 15
    rectovaginal, 15
    relaxing during, 14
    self-exam, 236b–37b, 238, 242, 254, 255
    what to expect, 14–15
excision, 120, 325
excisional biopsy, **371**
exemestane (Aromasin), 250, 252, 267
exercise
    after surgery, 352
    breast cancer and, 250
    fertility and, 149
    headaches and, 53
    menopause and, 298
    menstrual cycle and, 39
    osteoporosis and, 301, 303
    PMS and, 50
    weight and, 25, 26–27, 28
expulsion, 74, 75–76
eyes, 113, 122

F

fad diets, 25
faintness. *see* dizziness
fallopian tubes
    defined, 11, **371**
    ectopic pregnancy, 156
    endometrioma, 214
    endometriosis and, 167
    infection, 32
    infertility and, 142–43
    picture, *13, 38, 143, 161*
    PID and, 113
    sterilization, 80
    tubal pregnancy, 161–62
false unicorn root, 150
famciclovir (Famvir), 123
familial, **371**
family doctors, 9
family planning, natural, 2, 56–57, 76.
        see also contraception
Famvir (famciclovir), 123
fast food, 25

fat, 25, 26, 249
fat blockers, 29
fatigue
    chemotherapy and, 227
    hepatitis, 128
    herpes and, 123, 124
    hormone replacement therapy and,
        282
    libido and, 93, 97
    menopause, 277
    misoprostol, 79
    PMS, 46
FBD. *see* fibrocystic breasts
FDA (Food and Drug Administration)
    bladder medication, 312
    breast implants, 243–44
    breast ultrasound and, 21
    emergency contraception, 70
    herbs and supplements regulation, xxv
    HIV testing, 127
    hormone replacement therapy, 285
    IC/PBS medication, 324
    osteoporosis medication, 307
    PMS medication, 51
    SERMs, 298, 299, 306
    testosterone replacement, 276
    weight loss medication, 28, 29
fear
    endometrial cancer, 195, 201b
    of gynecologists, 4–5
    of pregnancy, 97, 99
    of surgery, 343b–45b
feet, 91
felbamate (Felbatol), 65
Felbatol (felbamate), 65
Femal, 50, 297
Femara, 264
Fem-Dophilus, 108
FemiScan, 315
FemSoft, 316
Femstat, 107
femur, 306
ferritin, 149
Fertile-Focus, 57
fertility. *see* infertility
fertility monitors, 57
FertilityBlend, 150
fertilization, 138, 142, 143–44, *143*, **371**

fever, 113, 123, 245
fever blisters, 122
fiber, 48
fibroadenoma, 246, **371**
fibrocystic breasts, 18, 21, 241–42, 248
fibroids
    CA-125 and, 222
    cancer and, 177
    defined, 176, **372**
    estrogen and, 176
    family history, 177
    heavy flow and, 43
    HSG detection, 142
    infertility and, 178
    intermenstrual bleeding, 43
    medication, 179–180
    menstrual pain, 46
    miscarriage and, 159, 178
    painful, 33
    painful sex and, 89
    picture, *177*
    pregnancy and, 178, 179
    problems caused, 177–78
    recurrent, 186–87
    removal, 179, 181–85, 364
    surgery, 181–85
    treatment, 178–79, 185
fibromyalgia, 323
figs, 51, *302*
fimbria, *38*, 143, **372**
fine needle biopsy, 256
fingers, 122
First Response, 57
fish, 303
fish oil, 150
fistula, 340
Flagyl (metronidazole), 112
flaxseed oil, 150
Fleet enema, 101
flossing, 132
fluconazole, 107
fluid retention, PMS, 46, 48
fluorouracil (Efudex), 120, 341
fluoxetine (Prozac), 50, 293
foley, **372**
folic acid, 150, 151
Follicle Stimulating Hormone (FSH), 148
follicles

count, 148
defined, **372**
explained, 11
menstrual cycle and, 37
multiple, 140
ovarian cysts and, 213
ovulation and, 138
picture, *143*
follicular, **372**
follicular phase, 37
Food and Drug Administration. *see* FDA
food cravings, 46
food diary, 310
food intake, 26
foreplay, 85–86, 87–88, 90–91
Forteo (teriparatide), 306, 307
Fortical (Calcitonin), 307
Fosamax (alendronate), 305, 306
fovatripan (Frova), 52
FRAX calculator, 307–8
Frova (fovatripan), 52
frozen section, 218, 223, **372**
fruits, 25, 51, 172, 249
FSH (Follicle Stimulating Hormone), 148
fulguration, 325, **372**
functional pain, 33–34
fundus, *38*, **372**
fungus, 104
furosemide diuretic, 301

G

gabapentin, 35, 235, 294
Gail risk assessment model, 22
galactography, 249
galactorrhea, 247–48, **372**
gallbladder, 32, 283, 290, 290b, 292
gallstones, 292
gamete intrafallopian transfer (GIFT), 143, **372**
garbanzos, *302*
Gardasil, 121, 131, 204
Gardnerella, 111
garlic, 109
gas, 48, 362
gastric banding, 30
gastric bypass, 30
gastritis, 32

gastroenterologists, 32
gastrointestinal problems, 31–32
Gas-X, 48
genetic counseling, 159, 250
genetic technology, 131
genetic testing, 222, 251, **372**
genital warts
defined, **372**
detection, 119
HPV and, 119, 231
itchy, 102
painful sex and, 86
pregnancy and, 119, 120
recurrent, 120–21
sex partners and, 116b, 118
treatment, 119–120
vaccine, 204
vaginal, 231
genitalia. *see* penis; vagina, **372**
germs. *see* bacteria
gestrinone, 172
GIFT (gamete intrafallopian transfer), 143, **372**
ginger, 36
Ginkgo Biloba, 49, 150, 290, 296
Ginseng, 295
girdles, 331
glands
adrenal, 97
Bartholin's glands, **367**
parathyroid, 300
pituitary, 138, 247–48, **377**
salivary, 286
sebaceous, 118, 232, **379**
skin, 232
sweat, 118, 232, 233
glaucoma, 312
Glenville, Marilyn, 149
glomerulations, 324, **372**
glucosamine, 36
gluten, 149, 172
GnRH agonists, 170, 180, 183, 187, **372**
goldenseal, 109
gonadotropins, 138–140, 142, 151–52, **372**
gonorrhea, 113, 114, 115, 130, **373**
Grafenberg spot, 95, 100, **373**
graft insertion, 333

grains, 294
green beans, *302*
green tea extract, 319
griseofulvin, 65
G-spot, 95, 100, **373**
gum disease, 132
gynecologists
    choosing, 3–4
    endometriosis and, 167
    family planning and, 2
    fear of, 4–5
    female, 3, 8
    herbal supplements and, xxvi
    infertility testing, 136
    lifetime risk of breast cancer, 250
    male, 3
    patient's questions and, xxvii–xxviii
    reconstructive surgery and, 334
    regular appointments with, 2–3, 212
    STI screening, 116b
    teens and, 8, 9–10, 54
    urgency incontinence, 310
    vulvar inflammation and, 87
    yeast infections and, 104
Gyne-Lotrimin, 107
Gyne-Moistrin, 86, 275, 293

H

hachimijiogan, 150
hair loss, 227–28, 263, 325
Halsted, William S., 257
hard candy, 312
HCG (human chorionic gonadotropin)
    test, 32. *see also* B-HCG
HE4, 220, 222, 228
headaches
    alternative treatments, 53
    anesthesia and, 347
    clomiphene, 139
    continuous oral contraception and,
        67, 67b
    Depo-Provera, 72
    diet, 51–52, 53
    Elmiron, 325
    estrogen patch and, 283
    fluconazole, 107
    GnRH agonists, 170

gonadotropins, 140
    hormone replacement therapy, 290
    Implanon, 71
    medication, 52–53
    migraines, 51–52, 63b, 67, 67b, 68
    minipill and, 68
    misoprostol, 79
    oral contraception and, 63b, 65
    PMS, 46
health insurance
    disability insurance, 350b
    hormone replacement therapy, 285
    hospital stays and, 345
    HPV vaccine, 121, 204
    IUDs, 73
    MRIs and, 23
heart, 117, 160
heart attacks, 63, 283, 302
heart disease, 280
heartburn, 305
hematoma, 340, **373**
hemorrhage, 42
heparin, 160, 341
hepatitis
    blood transfusions and, 339
    defined, **373**
    explained, 128–29
    hormone replacement therapy and,
        290b, 292
    oral contraception and, 63b
    treatment, 131
hepatotoxicity, 296
HER2, 263
herbs, xxv–xxvi, 150–51, 172, 294–98. *see
    also* supplements
Herceptin (trastuzumab), 263, 267
Hereditary Breast and Ovarian Cancer
    Syndrome, 220
hereditary nonpolyposis colon cancer
    (HNPCC), 192
herniation, 340, 351, **373**
herpes
    alternative treatments, 125
    condoms and, 125
    defined, **373**
    hygiene, 123–24
    itchy, 102
    medication, 122b, 123

miscarriage and, 159
pain and, 32
painful sex and, 86
pregnancy and, 124–25
prevention, 125
recurrent, 124
screening, 131
sex partners and, 116b
sore, 117
symptoms, 122, 123
transmission, 123
types of, 122, 125
herpetic blisters, 118, 122
herring, 51
hesperidin, 297
hidradenitis, 233
high blood pressure. *see* hypertension
high blood sugar. *see* diabetes
high-grade squamous intraepithelial
    lesion. *see* HSIL
Hiprex (methenamine), 318
HIV (human immunodeficiency virus). *see*
    also AIDS
  AIDS and, 126–27
  anal sex and, 101
  blood transfusions and, 339
  defined, **373**
  in females, 126
  hepatitis and, 129
  positive, 127–28
  pregnancy and, 127
  prevention, 127
  spermicide and, 61
  testing, 127, 131
  transmission, 126, 127
  treatment, 131
HNPCC (hereditary nonpolyposis colon
    cancer), 192
hobbies, 268
Holy Redeemer Hospital and Medical
    Center, xxix
homeopathy, 50, 109, 151
"honeymoon cystitis," 317
hormone replacement therapy (HRT)
  bioidentical hormones, 285–86
  bleeding and, 191
  breast cancer and, 250, 288–89
  conditions preventing, 290b, 291–92

dryness and, 86
endometrial cancer and, 202
endometriosis and, 175
formats, 282–83
hysterectomy and, 182
insomnia and, 272
libido and, 93
mammograms and, 18–19
mood changes, 278
myths, 289b
ovarian cancer and, 224
ovarian removal and, 359–360
pelvic prolapse and, 330
risks, 280–82, 288–89
side effects, 289–291
studies on, 280–81
timing, 281, 282, 286–87
types of, 282–84
hormones
  androgens, 97, 170, 275–76
  anti-mullerian, 148
  estradiol, 148, 285
  estriol, 285
  estrogen. *see* estrogen
  Follicle Stimulating Hormone (FSH),
    148
  progesterone. *see* progesterone
  prolactin, 160, 247–48, **378**
  replacement. *see* hormone replacement
    therapy
  testosterone. *see* testosterone
horseback riding, 234
horses, 283
hospital stays, 345, 363–64
hot dogs, 52
hot flashes
  clomiphene, 139
  defined, 273–74
  GnRH agonists and, 170
  hormone replacement therapy and,
    281
  menopause, 270, 271, 277
  tamoxifen, 263
hot tubs, 145
HPV (Human papillomavirus)
  anal sex and, 101
  cervical cancer and, 2, 16, 204, 209
  condoms and, 121, 204

defined, **373**
genital warts and, 119–121, 231
HSIL and, 205
screening, 2, 16, 17, 211b–12b, 212
treatment, 119–120, 131
vaccine, 121, 204
VIN and, 236
HRT. *see* hormone replacement therapy
HSG (hysterosalpingogram), 142, 146,
    159, **373**
HSIL (high-grade squamous
        intraepithelial lesion)
    cervical cancer and, 209
    diagnosing, 205–6
    explained, 205
    recurrent, 208
    treatment, 206–7, 208–9
human chorionic gonadotropin (HCG)
    test, 32. *see also* B-HCG
Human papillomavirus. *see* HPV
hydradenitis, **373**
hydrocortisone, 103
hydrodistention, 324
hydrogen peroxide, 108
hygiene
    anal sex, 100–101
    bladder infections, 318
    dental, 306
    douching, 10
    herpes, 123–24
    oral sex and, 99–100
hymen, *38*, 88, 231, **373**
hypercholesterolemia, 264, 307
hyperparathyroidism, 300
hyperplasia, 22, 190–91, 242
hyperprolactinemia, 141, 160
hyperstimulation syndrome, 140, **373**
hypertension
    bladder medication and, 312
    estrogen patch and, 283
    hormone replacement therapy and,
        290b, 292
    medication, 294
    oral contraception and, 64
    polycystic ovary syndrome and, 214
    pregnancy and, 148
hypertriglyceridemia, 283
hypnosis, 36, 324

hypothyroidism, 24, 97, 141, 247
hysterectomy
    adenomyosis, 190
    cervical cancer, 211, 238
    complete vs. partial, 354–55
    defined, **373**
    endometrial cancer, 194, 238, 263
    endometriosis and, 175
    explained, 357–58
    fibroids and, 181–82, 186–87
    hospital stays, 345
    HSIL and, 207, 208–9
    menopause and, 357–58
    ovarian cancer and, 223–24
    ovaries and, 355–56
    Pap smears and, 16, 358–59
    pelvic prolapse, 332
    restrictions after, 353
    sex and, 98–99
    work leave, 351
hysterosalpingogram (HSG), 142, 146,
    159, **373**
hysteroscopic endometrial ablation, 190
hysteroscopy
    adenomyosis, 189
    defined, **373**
    endometrial cancer, 193
    fibroids and, 184–85
    heavy flow, 43
    hospital stays, 345
    infertility, 142–43
    intermenstrual bleeding, 44
    menstrual pain, 46
    miscarriage and, 159–160
    office visit, 364
    pain from, 364
    polyps, 188
    work leave, 350

I

ibandronate (Boniva), 305, 306
IBS (irritable bowel syndrome), 32, 67,
    67b, 323
ibuprofen (Advil, Motrin)
    adenomyosis, 189
    breast tenderness, 242, 290
    chronic pain, 36

cramps, 45
fibroids and, 180, 185
headaches, 53
menstrual pain, 49
pain, 35
ice cream, *302*
ice packs, 249
IC/PBS (interstitial cystitis/painful
    bladder syndrome)
  causes, 323
  chronic pain, 32
  defined, **374**
  diagnosing, 324
  explained, 323
  other conditions and, 323–24
  resources, 326
  treatment, 324–26
ICSI (Intracytoplasmic Sperm Injection),
    144, 145
Imiquimod (Aldara, Zyclara), 119–120,
    236, 341
Imitrex (sumatripan), 52
immune system, 105, 160
Implanon, 71–72, 77
implanted contraception, 71–72
in vitro fertilization. *see* IVF
incentive spirometer, 342
incisions, 362
incontinence
  cystocele and, 329
  defined, **373**
  resources, 321
  stress incontinence, 314, 314–17,
    333–34, **379**
  urgency incontinence, 309–10, **380**
indegestion, 223
indole-3-carbinol, 250
infertility
  abortion and, 80
  age and, 147–49
  BBT chart, 137, *137*, 139
  cervical problems, 144
  emotional factors, 153–54
  endometriosis and, 67, 168, 173–74
  fertility monitors, 57
  fibroids and, 178
  IUDs and, 73
  IVF, 143–44

luteal phase dysfunction, 140–42
male, 145, 150
medication, 139–140, 141–42,
    151–52
natural methods, 149–151
oral contraception and, 67
ovarian cancer and, 220
ovulatory dysfunction, 138–39
PID and, 113
pregnant, getting, 135
resources, 154
specialists, 136, 140, 144, 174
support groups, 153
testing, 136, 138
timing, 136
tubal problems, 142–43
yeast infections and, 106
inflammatory bowel disease, 323
insemination, 146–47, **373**
insomnia, 271–72, 277
insurance. *see* health insurance
intercourse. *see* sex
interferon, 120, 341, **373**
intermenstrual bleeding, 43–44, 65, 177,
    188
Internet, xxx, 3
interstitial cystitis. *see* IC/PBS
interval cancer, 21
intimacy, 96, 134, 277
InTone, 315
Intracytoplasmic Sperm Injection (ICSI),
    144
intraductal papilloma, 248, 249, 255, **374**
intramural, **374**
intramuscular, **374**
intraperitoneal (IP) chemotherapy,
    228–29
intrauterine, **374**
intrauterine device. *see* IUD
intrauterine insemination (IUI), 146–47
intravenous
  chemotherapy, 228, 229
  defined, **374**
  pyelogram (IVP), 35, 318, 320, **374**
IP (intraperitoneal) chemotherapy,
    228–29
iron deficiency, 62, 97, 149, 271, 277
iron supplements, 43, 189

irritability, 46
irritable bowel syndrome (IBS), 32, 67,
    67b, 323
isoflavones, 294
isolation, 153
IUD (intrauterine device)
    checking, 75–76
    choosing, 77
    defined, **374**
    emergency contraception, 70
    explained, 73
    infertility and, 142
    irritation and, 203
    menstrual cycle and, 74
    Mirena, 73, 74, 171, 180, 189
    risks, 73, 74
    Skyla, 73, 74
IUI (intrauterine insemination), 146–47
IV (intravenous) chemotherapy, 228, 229
IVF (in vitro fertilization)
    after endometriosis, 174
    after tubal pregnancy, 165
    age and, 148
    artificial insemination alternative, 147
    defined, **374**
    infertility, 143–44, 144, 145
    laparoscopy, 146
    sterilization and, 82
IVP (intravenous pyelogram), 35, 318,
    320, **374**

J

jaundice, 128
jaw, 305
joint pain, 264
Jolessa, 67
jumping, 314

K

kale, 250, *302*
kava kava, 50, 295–96
Kegel exercises, 235, 314–15, 330, **374**
keloids, 341, **374**
ketoprofen (Orudis), 45
kidney stones, 32, 302, 307, 318
kidneys, 35, 160, 178

Kohn, Ingrid, 161
K-Y Jelly, 55, 86, 87, 275, 318

L

labia
    arousal and, 91
    cysts, 88
    defined, 12, **374**
    HPV and, 120
    lumpy, 231
    picture, *15, 38*
    self-exam, 236b
    vulvar cancer and, 237
lactation, 245, **374**. *see also* breast-feeding
lactobacillus acidophilus, 108, 111, 112,
    374
laparoscopy
    bariatric, 30
    defined, **374**
    ectopic pregnancy, 164
    endometriosis, 169–170
    explained, 339
    hospital stays, 345, 363–64
    incisions, 362
    infertility, 142, 146
    IUDs and, 76
    menstrual pain, 46
    myomectomy, 179, 183–84
    ovarian cysts, 218
    ovarian torsion, 215
    pain from, 364
    painful sex and, 89
    pelvic prolapse, 333
    restrictions after, 353
    safety, 362–63
    shoulder pain, 362
    single port, 362
    tubal pregnancy, 164
    tubal sterilization, 80–81
    work leave, 350–51
laparotomy, 170, 218, **374**
L-arginine, 93, 150
laryngeal warts, 120
lasers, 120, 203, 207, 236, 238, **374**
latex, 60, 86, 132
laughing, 314
lavender oil, 341

L-carnitine, 150
LCIS (lobular carcinoma in situ), 22, 264.
    see also CIS
LEEP (loop electrosurgical excision
    procedure), 206, **375**
legs, 62–63, 271, 280
legumes, 49
leiomyoma, **374**
leukemia, 105
levator ani (pelvic floor) muscles, 235,
    315, 328, 330, **375**
Levitra, 93
levonorgestrel, 69
levothyroxine, 141
Lexapro, 294
libido, 93, 96–98, 275–77, 282, **375**
lichen planus, 112–13, 236
lichen sclerosis, 103, 236
licorice, 150
lidocaine, 234
Lifestyles SKYN, 60
ligaments, 163, 328
lipase inhibitors, 29
lipoma, **375**
lips, vaginal. *see* labia
liver
    cancer of, 128, 267
    disease, 290b, 292
    hepatitis, 128
    pain, 32
    tumor, 64
    vitamin D, 303
lobular cancer, 21
lobular carcinoma in situ (LCIS), 22, 264.
    see also CIS
loop electrosurgical excision procedure
    (LEEP), 206, **375**
lorcaserin (Belviq), 28
low-grade squamous intraepithelial lesion.
    see LSIL
LSIL (low-grade squamous intraepithelial
    lesion)
    cervical cancer and, 209
    diagnosing, 205–6
    explained, 204, 205
    recurrent, 208
    treatment, 206–7, 208–9
L-Taurine, 150

lubrication
    allergies and, 86, 275
    anal sex, 101
    bladder infections and, 318
    dialators and, 87
    fertility and, 149
    products, 293
    tampons and, 55
    testosterone and, 97
    vaginal, 85–86, 87–88, 91, 275
    vaginal scarring, 89
Lubrin, 275
Lucco, Angelo J., 311
lumpectomy
    DCIS, 267
    defined, **375**
    explained, 257
    lymph nodes and, 259
    vs. mastectomy, 257b–59b
    radiation and, 260–61
lumps, 231–32, 242, 245, 254
lungs, 62, 267, 280, 291, 342
Lupron, 170, 180
lupus erythematosus, 160, 243, 323
luteal phase, 37–38, 140–42, 159
Luvena, 86, 275, 293
Luvox, 294
Lybrel, 45b, 67
lymph nodes
    cervical cancer, 211
    defined, **375**
    endometrial cancer, 194, 195
    hysterectomy and, 357
    mastectomy and, 257, 259
    ovarian cancer and, 224
    ovarian cysts and, 217
    vulvar cancer and, 237–38
lymphedema, 237
Lynch syndrome, 192
Lyrica (pregabalin), 36, 235
lysine, 125
Lysteda (tranexamic acid), 180, 189

M

maca, 150
macromastia, 244–45
magnesium, 45, 49, 302

magnetic resonance imaging. *see* MRI
malignant, **375**
MammaPrint, 262
mammograms
    breast cancer, 251
    defined, **375**
    discomfort and, 18–19
    explained, 18
    fibrocystic breasts and, 242
    frequency of, 20
    implants and, 244
    nipple discharge, 249
    vs. ovarian cancer screening, 221
    reliability, 19–21
    risk, 19
    scheduling, 241
MammoSite, 261
manganese, 150
mannose, 319
manometer, 315
marathons, 149
marijuana, 145
marriage counseling, 90, 133
Marshall test, 321
massage, 50, 101
mastalgia. *see* breast tenderness, **375**
mastectomy
    breast implants and, 243
    DCIS, 267
    emotional factors, 259
    explained, 257
    vs. lumpectomy, 257b–59b
    lymph nodes and, 259
    radiation and, 261–62
    risk reduction, 251–52
mastitis, 245, 248, 249, **375**
masturbation, 97, 136
Mathematica Policy Research, 75b
Maxalt (rizatripan), 52
Mayo Clinic, xxvi
meat, 52, 172
Mederma, 341
media, xxx, 16–17, 96
Medical College of Pennsylvania, xxix
medication
    analgesics. *see* pain medication
    antibacterical, 233
    antibiotics. *see* antibiotics

antidepressants. *see* antidepressants
antifungal, 65, 104, 105, 107–8, 203
antihistamines, 50, 325
anti-inflammatory, 65, 103, 105, 234,
    249, 325
anti-nausea, 70
antinausea, 350
antipsychotics, 277
anti-seizure. *see* anti-seizure medication
antispasmodic, 325
antiviral, 123, 124, 125, 131
aromatase inhibitors. *see* aromatase
    inhibitors
bladder, 312
boils, 233
diabetes, 29
endometriosis, 170–72
ergots, 52
female sexual dysfunction, 93
fertility, 139–140, 141–42, 151–52
fibroids, 179–180
gas, 48
genital warts, 119–120
headaches, 52–53
herpes, 122b, 123
IC/PBS, 324–25
libido and, 97, 277
menopause, 293–94
menstrual cycle and, 39–40
nipple discharge, 247, 248
oral contraception and, 65–66
orgasm and, 92–93
osteoporosis, 304–8
pain. *see* pain medication
PMS, 50–51
restless leg syndrome, 271
sleep disorder, 65
steroids, 113, 234, 300
triptans, 52
tubal pregnancy, 164–65
vulvodynia, 234
weight gain and, 24
weight loss, 28–29
yeast infections, 107–8
meditation, 50, 272, 298
medroxyprogesterone (Provera, Cycrin),
    171, 272, 280, 284, 286, 288
melanoma, 238, 251, **375**

melatonin, 50, 149
menarche, 54, **375**
menopause
    alternative treatments, 294–98
    average age of, 270
    bladder control and, 311
    bleeding during, 190–91
    calcium intake, 301
    defined, **375**
    depression and, 277–79
    diet and, 293
    dryness and, 86, 274–75
    emotional factors, 277, 277–79
    endometriosis and, 175
    fibroids and, 176
    hot flashes, 273–74
    hysterectomy and, 357–58
    libido and, 93, 98, 275–77
    lifestyle changes, 297–98
    mammograms and, 18–19
    non-hormonal treatments, 293–94
    ovarian cancer and, 223
    ovarian cysts and, 217–18
    pelvic prolapse and, 328, 330
    pregnancy and, 84
    sex and, 274–75, 275–77, 278–79
    sleep problems, 271–73
    weight gain, 24, 27
menses. *see* menstrual cycle, **375**
menstrual cycle
    appointment scheduling and, 6
    average length, 37
    bleeding between periods, 43–44, 65,
        177, 188
    blood clots, 43
    breast cancer and, 249
    changes in, 31
    continuous contraception and, 67–68
    cramps, 45–46, 67, 74
    defined, **375**
    endometrial cancer and, 192
    endometriosis and, 168
    headaches, 51–53
    heavy, 42–43
    infrequent, 39–40
    IUDs and, 74
    late, 39
    mammogram scheduling, 18, 241

mittel-schmerz, 44
osteoporosis and, 301
pain, 34, 44, 45–46, 168
phases of, 36–37
progesterone and, 283–84
sterilization and, 82
tamoxifen, 263
uterus and, 11
vaginal discharge and, 111
metastasis, 224, 259, 267–68
metformin, 29
methenamine (Urex, Hiprex), 318
methicillin-resistant Staphylococcus
        Aureus (MRSA), 232b–33b
methotrexate, 164–65
metronidazole (Flagyl), 112
Miacalcin (Calcitonin), 307
microcalcifications, 256, **375**
Midol PMS, 50
"midriff bulge," 24
mifepristone, 78, 172, 180
Migergot, 52
migraines, 51–53, 63b, 67, 67b, 68. *see*
        also headaches
Migranal (dihydroergotamine), 52
milk, 301, *302*, 303
milk production, 68
mind-body techniques, 151
minipill, 68–69, **375**
mirabegron (Mybetriq), 312
Mirena, 73, 74, 171, 180, 189
miscarriage
    age and, 147
    causes, 157, 158–160
    clomiphene and, 139
    D&E, 156–57
    emotional factors, 157, 160–61
    gonadotropins, 140
    infection and, 159
    IUDs and, 74
    pain and, 32, 163–64
    pregnancy after, 158
    progesterone and, 159
    RPL, 158
    successive, 158
    syphilis and, 118
misoprostol, 78, 79, 156–57
mittel-schmerz, 44, **375**

modafinil (Provigil), 65
moles, 231, 237b, 238
monilia, **375**
monilial vaginitis. *see* yeast infections
Monistat, 107
monosodium glutamate (MSG), 52
mood changes
    clomiphene, 139
    Depo-Provera, 72, 171
    GnRH agonists, 170
    hormone replacement therapy, 290
    Implanon, 71
    menopause, 271, 277
    oral contraception and, 65
    PMS, 46
"morning-after" pill, 69–70
Motrin. *see* ibuprofen
mouth, 113, 117, 119, 122
Moyad, Mark, 150
MRI (magnetic resonance imaging)
    breasts, 20, 22–23, 251
    cervical cancer, 210
    defined, 34
    endometrial cancer, 193
    fibroids and, 185
    LCIS, 266
    ovarian cysts, 213
MRSA (methicillin-resistant
        Staphylococcus Aureus),
        232b–33b
MSG (monosodium glutamate), 52
mucosa, 311, 331, **376**
mucous membranes, 117
mucus, cervical, 57, 139, 144, 146
Muira Puama, 296
multicentric, **376**
multiple births, 139, 140
multiple orgasms, 92
multiple sclerosis, 310
multivitamin, 29
mumps, 145
mupirocin (Bactroban), 233
muscular pain, 32
mustard greens, 250
mustard seed oil, 341
MYLICON, 48
Myo-Inositol, 151
myolysis, 184, **376**
myomectomy, 179, 182–83, 187, **376**

myometrium
    adenomyosis, 33
    defined, **376**
    endometrial cancer and, 191
    explained, 11
    picture, *38*
    removal, 354
myPill, 76
Myrbetriq (mirabegron), 312

N

nail clippers, 128, 129
naproxen sodium (Aleve, Anaprox)
    adenomyosis, 189
    chronic pain, 36
    cramps, 45
    fibroids and, 180, 185
    headaches, 52, 53
    pain, 35
naratripan (Amerge), 52
narcotics, 35, 271, 348–49, 349b, 350,
        364
nasogastric tube, 342, **376**
National Campaign to Prevent Teen and
        Unplanned Pregnancy, 75b
National Cancer Institute, 19
National Center for Complementary and
        Alternative Medicine, xxvi, 298
National Headache Foundation, 53
National Institute of Health, xxvi, 298
National Osteoporosis Foundation, 300,
        301, 303b
natural family planning, 56–57, 76, **376**
Naturalamb, 60
nausea
    chemotherapy, 227, 263
    clomiphene, 139
    Depo-Provera, 72
    Elmiron, 325
    emergency contraception and, 70
    with headaches, 51
    hepatitis, 128
    hormone replacement therapy, 290
    Implanon, 71
    misoprostol, 79
    narcotics, 349b
    oral contraception and, 65
    with pain, 31

PID and, 113
PMS, 46
surgery and, 349–350
tamoxifen, 263
neck, 91
neoadjuvant chemotherapy, 229, 262
neoplasms, 219–220, **376**
nerve blocks, 235
nerve entrapment, 341
nerve stimulators, 36, 235, 312, 325
nerves, 340
nervous system, 117, 124, 247–48, 310
Neurontin, 35, 235, 294
neurotransmitters, 47, 271, 277
Neutrogena, 102
New Horizons Menopause Center, xxix
NewGel, 341
Nexplanon, 71. *see also* Implanon
Next Choice, 69
nickel, 103
nicotine. *see* smoking
night sweats, 170, 270, 271, 277, 281
nipple discharge, 247–49, 255
nipples, 91, 244, 245, 248, 255
nocturia, 312–13, **376**
Nolvadex. *see* tamoxifen
Nonoxynol-9, 61
nonpalpable, **376**
non-steroidal anti-inflammatory drugs
    (NSAIDs), 35, 36, 180, 185. *see*
    also ibuprofen; naproxen sodium
Norplant-2, 72, 77
North American Menopause Society, 285
NovaGel, 341
novels, 96
NSAIDs (non-steroidal anti-inflammatory
    drugs), 35, 36, 180, 185. *see also*
    ibuprofen; naproxen sodium
nutrition. *see* diet
nutritionist, 25
nuts, 26, 52
NuvaRing, 66, 77

O

OAB (overactive bladder), 309, 312, 315,
    334
obesity. *see also* weight
    defined, 24

endometrial cancer and, 192
medications, 28
miscarriage and, 160
oral contraception and, 63
surgery, 30
obstructive sleep apnea (OSA), 271
OHSS (ovarian hyperstimulation
    syndrome), 140
oily glands, 118, 232, **379**
oligomenorrhea, 39, 151, **376**
Omega-3 fatty acids, 45, 49, 150, 172
omentum, 224, **376**
oncologists
    chemotherapy and, 228
    defined, **376**
    endometrial cancer and, 196
    lifetime risk of breast cancer, 250
    ovarian cancer and, 224
    ovarian cysts and, 218
    ovarian tumors and, 220
Oncotype DX, 262
oophorectomy, 354, 359
opioids, 271
oral contraception. *see also* contraception
    breast cancer and, 250
    breast tenderness, 242
    breast-feeding and, 68
    cancer and, 63–64
    complications, 62–64
    continuous, 45b, 67–68
    defined, **376**
    DVT and, 62–63
    effectiveness, 61–62
    emergency, 69–70
    endometrial cancer and, 193, 250
    endometriosis and, 171
    fibroids and, 180
    forgotten, 66
    health benefits, 62
    infertility and, 67
    libido and, 98
    medications and, 65–66
    menopause and, 287
    migraines and, 63
    minipill, 68–69
    myths, 64b
    nipple discharge, 247
    ovarian cancer and, 152, 220, 250
    ovarian cysts and, 213

side effects, 64–65
St. John's wort and, 49–50, 66
yeast infections and, 106
oral progestins, 180
oral sex, 99–100, 113, 119, 123, 132
oranges, *302*
OraQuick, 127
oregano oil, 109
organ, **376**
organ donation, 128
orgasms
  anal sex and, 100
  defined, **376**
  lack of, 92–93
  medication, 93
  multiple, 92
  painful sex and, 88b
  stages of, 90–93
  vaginal, 95
orlistat (Xenical, Alli), 29
Ornade (phenylpropanolamine), 316
Ortho Evra, 66
Orudis (ketoprofen), 45
OSA (obstructive sleep apnea), 271
ospemifene (Osphena), 299
Osphena (ospemifene), 299
osteonecrosis, 305, 307
osteopenia, 307
osteoporosis
  aromatase inhibitors and, 264
  bisphosphonates, 268
  calcium and, 301–2
  defined, **376**
  diagnosing, 300
  facts, 303b
  medications, 304–8
  resources, 308
  risk factors, 300–301
  SERMs and, 298–99
  tamoxifen and, 264
  vitamin D and, 303
"ostrich syndrome," 1
ova, 11, 37–38, 138–39, *143*, 149
OVA1, 222
OvaCue Fertility Monitor, 57
ovarian cancer
  breast cancer and, 251
  chemotherapy and, 224–25, 229–230

endometrial cancer and, 192
endometriosis and, 214
family history, 220–21
hysterectomy and, 223–24, 355–56,
  357
infertility medication and, 151–52
MRIs and, 23
oral contraception and, 62, 64, 152,
  250
painful, 33
Pap smears and, 16
pregnancy and, 152
rates, 220–21
recurrent, 229–230
resources, 230
screening, 221–22
symptoms, 222–23
Tensie's story, 226b–27b
ovarian cysts
  cancer and, 218–19
  defined, 213
  diagnosing, 114
  Implanon, 72
  ovarian torsion, 215, 217
  painful, 33, 163, 215
  painful sex and, 89
  removal, 359
  ruptured, 215, 216b
  treatment, 217–18
  types of, 213–15
ovarian hyperstimulation syndrome
  (OHSS), 140
ovarian pregnancy, 161
ovarian torsion, 215, 217
ovarian tumors, 89, 114, 214, 220, 223,
  359
ovaries
  cancer of. *see* ovarian cancer
  cervical cancer, 211
  cysts. *see* ovarian cysts
  defined, 11, **376**
  disorder, 44
  eggs, 11, 37–38, 138–39, *143*, 149
  endometrioma, 167
  endometriosis and, 167
  enlargement, 140
  hysterectomy and, 98, 355–56
  infection, 32

menstrual cycle and, 37
ovulatory dysfunction, 138, 139
painful sex and, 89
picture, *13, 38, 161*
PID and, 113
pregnancy of, 161
removal, 354, 359
testosterone and, 97
torsion, 215, 217
tumors, 89, 114, 214, 220, 223, 359
overactive bladder (OAB), 309, 312, 315,
    334
over-the-counter products, xxx, 10, 103,
    104b
overweight, 24. *see also* weight
ovulation
    BBT and, 137
    dysfunction, 138–39
    family planning and, 56–57, 136
    menstrual cycle and, 37, 39
ovulation predictor kits, 57
oxalates, 235
oxcarbazepine (Trileptal), 65
oxybutynin (Oxytrol), 312
Oxytrol (oxybutynin), 312

P

pads, 103
Paget's disease, 238, **376**
pain
    abdominal, 31–32, 128, 140, 178
    alternative treatments, 36
    back, 178
    breast. *see* breast tenderness
    breasts, large, 244–45
    chest, 63
    chronic, 31, 35–36
    cramps, 45
    functional, 33–34
    headaches, 51–53
    hysteroscopy, 364
    joint, 264
    laparoscopy, 364
    leg, 62–63
    medication. *see* pain medication
    menstrual, 168
    mittel-schmerz, 44

muscular, 32
    ovarian cysts, 214
    pelvic, 32–34, 73, 117, 223
    pregnancy, 163–64
    sex, during. *see* painful sex
    urination, during, 89, 113, 117, 123
    vulvar, 234–35
pain medication
    adenomyosis, 189
    breast tenderness, 242, 290
    chronic pain, 35–36, 36
    cramps, 45
    fibroids and, 180, 185
    headaches, 52, 53
    herpes, 123–24
    menstrual pain, 49, 50
    mittel-schmerz, 44
    pain, 35
    surgery and, 348–49, 364
painful bladder syndrome. *see* IC/PBS
painful sex
    causes, 85–90
    endometriosis and, 168
    fibroids and, 178
    libido and, 97
    menopause and, 274–75
    ovarian cancer and, 223
    ovarian cysts and, 215
    SERMs and, 299
    urgent, 88b
    vulvar vestibulitis, 234
painkillers. *see* pain medication
pajamas, 124
palpable, **376**
palpitations, 312
Pamprin, 50
panax ginseng, 295
pancreas, 32, 251
pancreatic, **377**
pantyhose, 103, 106
Pap smears
    abnormal, 203, 204
    cancer rates and, 1–2
    cervical cancer and, 209
    defined, **377**
    endometrial cancer, 194
    explained, 15–16
    family doctors and, 9

frequency of, 16
HPV and, 204, 211b–12b
HSIL and, 205–6
hysterectomy and, 238, 358–59
intermenstrual bleeding, 44
LSIL and, 205–6
ovarian cancer and, 221
regular, 212
reliability, 16–17
Papanicolaou smear. *see* Pap smears
papayas, 51
papilloma, 248, 249, 255, **374**
ParaGard, 73
parathyroid gland, 300
paresthesias, **377**
Parkinson's disease, 296, 310
Parlodel (bromocriptine), 141, 242, 248, **368**
paroxetine (Paxil), 293
patch, contraceptive, 66
patch, hormonal, 282, 283
pâté, 51
pathologists, 15, 187. *see also* doctors
patient-controlled analgesia (PCA), 348–49
patients
    anxious, xxviii, 4–5
    assumptions of, xxix–xxx
    doctors, communication with,
        xxx–xxxi
    education, xxx
    questions of, xxvii–xxviii, xxx
    self-treatment, xxx
pau d'Arco, 109
Paxil (paroxetine), 293
PCA (patient-controlled analgesia), 348–49
PCT (postcoital test), 144
PDR (*Physicians' Desk Reference*), 93, 247
peanut butter, 52
peanuts, 286
Pearce, K. Lynette, 311
Pearls YB, 108
peau d'orange, 255, **377**
pectoralis, 257, **377**
peeing. *see* urination
pelvic descensus. *see* pelvic prolapse
pelvic floor muscles, 235, 315, 330

pelvic infection, 46
pelvic inflammatory disease (PID). *see* PID
pelvic pain, 32–34, 73
pelvic prolapse
    causes, 328
    danger, 329–330
    defined, **377**
    explained, 327–28
    incontinence and, 329
    lumps from, 232
    management, 330–31
    recurrent, 335
    symptoms, 328–29
    treatment, 331–35
pelvic relaxation. *see* pelvic prolapse
pelvic ultrasound. *see* ultrasound
penicillin, 117
penis, 83, 93, 114
Pensylvania Hospital, xxix
pentosan polysulfate sodium (Elmiron), 324–25
pentoxifylline, 172
pepperoni, 52
perforation, 74, 76
pergabalin, 235
perianal area
    defined, **377**
    massage, 101
    self-exam, 236b
    vulvar cancer and, 237
perineorraphy, 332, **377**
perineum, *15*, 236b, 237, 332, **377**
periods. *see* menstrual cycle
pessaries, 316, 331–32, 334, **377**
PET (positron emission tomography)
    scan, 202, 210, 229
petroleum jelly, 120
PGD (preimplantation genetic diagnosis), 148
pharmacology, 131
Pharmacopeia, xxv
phendimetrazine, 28
phentermine, 28, 29
phentolamine, 93
phenylbutazone, 65
phenylpropanolamine (Ornade), 316
phenytoin (Dilantin), 65
Phisohex, 233

phone apps, 26, 76–77
physical therapy, 36
physicians. *see* doctors
Physicians' Desk Reference (PDR), 93, 247
phytoestrogens, 294, 298, **377**
PID (pelvic inflammatory disease)
   BV and, 111
   CA-125 and, 222
   causes, 113
   defined, **377**
   diagnosing, 114
   infertility and, 142
   IUDs and, 73
   painful, 32
   prevention, 115
   STIs and, 113, 114, 115
   surgery injury and, 339
   symptoms, 113
   tubal pregnancy and, 162
piercings, 103, 132
Pilates, 27, 315
"pill." *see* oral contraception
pimples, 118
Pitocin, 79
pituitary gland, 138, 247–48, **377**
pizza, 52
placenta, 142, 156, **377**
Plan B, 69, 70
plasma, 128
plastic wrap, 132
plums, 51
PMDD (Premenstrual Dysphoric
   Disorder), 46–47, 50–51
PMS (premenstrual syndrome)
   causes, 47
   defined, **377**
   emotional symptoms, 46, 49–51
   lifestyle modifications, 50
   medication, 48–49, 50–51
   physical symptoms, 46, 48–49
   supplements, 49–50
pneumonia, 113, 342
podofilox (Condylox), 119
podophyllin, 119, **377**
pollen, 50, 297
Polycystic Ovarian Syndrome Association,
   214
polycystic ovaries, 192, 214, **377**

polyisoprene, 60
polyps
   bleeding from, 190, 201b
   cancer and, 187
   causes, 187
   cervical, 187–88, 190, 232, **368**
   defined, **378**
   endometrial, 187, 188, 190, 263, **371**
   heavy flow and, 43
   HSG detection, 142
   intermenstrual bleeding, 43
   menstrual pain, 46
   removal, 187–88, 364
   treatment, 232
   uterine, 232
   vaginal, 231, 232
pornography, 96
positron emission tomography (PET)
   scan, 202, 210, 229
postcoital test (PCT), 144
posterior colporrhaphy, 332
potassium chloride, 324
potassium sensitivity test (PST), 324
powders, 102
prayer, 272
Prednisone, 300
pregabalin (Lyrica), 36, 235
Pregitude, 151
pregnancy
   abdominal, 161
   after miscarriage, 158
   age and, 147
   bleeding and, 155–56, 163–64
   BV and, 111
   CA-125 and, 222
   complications, 32
   ectopic, 32, 74, 156, 161, 164, **370**
   endometrial cancer and, 193
   fear of, 97, 99
   fertility. *see* infertility
   fibroids and, 178, 179
   from first-time sex, 56
   genital warts and, 119, 120
   hepatitis and, 128, 129
   herpes and, 124–25
   HIV and, 127
   HPV and, 120
   IUDs and, 74

loss. *see* miscarriage
menopause and, 84
nipple discharge, 247, 248
ovarian, 161
ovarian cancer and, 152
pain, 163–64
syphilis and, 118
tubal. *see* tubal pregnancy
unintended, 2, 76b
preimplantation genetic diagnosis (PGD),
  148
Prelief, 310
Premarin, 280, 283, 288
premature delivery, 74
premature ejaculation, 146
Premenstrual Dysphoric Disorder
  (PMDD), 46–47, 50–51
premenstrual syndrome. *see* PMS
Prempro, 288
Premsyn PMS, 50
probiotics, 108, 112, 319
progesterone
  BBT and, 137
  breast cancer and, 250
  in contraception, 68
  contraceptive patch, 66
  creams, 286, 297
  defined, **378**
  emergency contraception, 69
  endometrial cancer and, 196, 282
  endometriosis and, 171
  endometrium and, 159
  fertility and, 139
  hormone replacement therapy, 283–84
  implant, 71, 72
  injection, 72–73
  insomnia and, 272
  IUD, 73
  luteal phase and, 141–42
  menstrual cycle and, 38
  minipill, 68
  miscarriage and, 159
  natural vs. synthetic, 285–86
  ovaries and, 11
  PMS and, 47, 49
  pregnancy bleeding and, 156
  prescribed, 39, 40, 44
progestins, 180

prolactin, 160, 247–48, **378**
prolapse. *see* pelvic prolapse, **378**
Prolia (denosumab), 306–7
Promensil, 294–95
Prometrium, 171, 272, 284, 285–86
propolis, 125
prostaglandins, 45, 53, 79, 93, **378**
prosthesis, 260
proteolytic enzymes, 36
protein, 26, 49, 149
proton pump inhibitors, 301
Provella, 108
Provera (medroxyprogesterone), 171, 272,
  280, 284, 286, 288
Provigil (modafinil), 65
Prozac (fluoxetine), 50, 293
pseudoephedrine (Sudafed), 316
psoriasis, 104, 236
PST (potassium sensitivity test), 324
psychiatrists, 90, 278
psychologists, 90, 278
pubic hair, 12
pubococcygeus, 314, **378**
pudendal nerve, 235
pudendal neuralgia, **378**
pulmonary embolus, 62, 291
pustules, 232

Q

Qsymia, 29
Q-tip test, 321
Quasense, 67

R

radiation
  breast cancer and, 258b
  cervical cancer, 211
  DCIS, 267
  endometrial cancer, 195–96
  infertility and, 145
  keloids and, 341
  lumpectomy and, 260–61
  mammograms and, 19
  mastectomy and, 261–62
  miscarriage and, 160
  MRIs and, 23

ovarian cancer, 224
vulvar cancer, 238
radical hysterectomy. *see* hysterectomy, **378**
radio, 272
radioisotope, 259
radiologists, 18, 20, 185, 213, 256
raisins, 51, *302*
raloxifene (Evista), 250, 252, 267, 298–99, 306, **378**
rash, 263, 307
razors, 128, 129
reading, 272, 273
reanastomosis, 82, 143, **378**
Reclast (zoledronic acid), 268, 305
rectocele, 327–28, 329, 332, **378**
rectovaginal exam, 15
rectum
    bleeding, 168
    cancer of, 15
    colonoscopy, 35
    defined, **378**
    descended. *see* pelvic prolapse
    examination of, 15
    PID and, 113
    spasms, 178
recurrent pregnancy loss (RPL), 158, 160–61
red clover, 150, 294–95
red plums, 51
red raspberry leaf, 150
reduction mammoplasty, 245
referral service, 3
reflexology, 151
reflux esophagitis, 32
relationships
    hysterectomy and, 98–99
    infertility and, 153
    intimacy and, 96, 134
    mastectomy and, 259
    menopause and, 277, 278–79
    painful sex and, 89–90
    STIs and, 133
relaxation
    in exams, 14
    foreplay and, 87–88, 91
    insomnia and, 272
    menopause and, 298

pain and, 36
    vaginal muscles, 87, 88
Relpax (eltripan), 52
Rely tampons, 55
Remifemin, 295
renal calculi, 302
RepHresh, 86, 108, 112, 275, 293
Replens, 86, 275, 293
resect, **378**
RESOLVE, 153
restless leg syndrome, 271
retraining, bladder, 310–11
retrograde ejaculation, 145, 146
rheumatoid arthritis. *see* arthritis
rifampin, 65
risedronate (Actonel), 306
risedronate (Actonel, Atelvia), 305
rizatripan (Maxalt), 52
robotic surgery, 183, 353–54, 356, 357b
ROMA, 222
romance novels, 96
RPL (recurrent pregnancy loss), 158, 160–61
RU-486, 78, 172, 180, **378**
rubella, 159
running, 314
rutabagas, 250

S

sacral nerve stimulation, 325
sacrospinous vaginal vault suspension, 333, **378**
salad, 26
salami, 52
salicin, 36
saline, 243, 244, **378**
salivary gland, 286
Salix Alba, 36
salpingectomy, 164
salt, 48, 50, 241
salt water, 243, 244
Sarafem, 50
sarcoma, 177, 179, 191–92
saturated fat, 25
saunas, 145
sausage, 52
SavvyCheck, 105

saw palmetto, 150
scallops, *302*
ScarAway, 341
scarring. *see* adhesions
scars, surgical, 341
Schramm, Kathleen, xxix
scintimammography, 20
screening
    breast cancer, 18
    cervical cancer, 1–2, 15–16, 17
    HIV, 127
    HPV, 2, 16, 17
    mammograms. *see* mammograms
    ovarian cancer, 221–22
    Pap smears. *see* Pap smears
    STIs, 116b, 118, 121, 130, 131
scrotum, 145
Seasonale, 67
Seasonique, 45b, 67
sebaceous glands, 118, 232, **379**
sebserosal, **379**
second-look surgery, 229
seeds, 294
selective estrogen receptor modulators
        (SERMs), 298–99, 306, **379**
selective serotonin reuptake inhibitors
        (SSRIs), 50–51, 93, 271, 293–94
selenium, 150
self-exam, 236b–37b, 238, 242, 254, 255
self-treatment, xxx, 104b
semen, 83, 100, 144, 147
SenseRx, 315
sentinel node biopsy, 259
sepsis, 74
Serelys, 50, 297
SERMs (selective estrogen receptor
        modulators), 298–99, 306, **379**
Serophene, 139
serotonin, 47
serotonin–norepinephrine reuptake
        inhibitors (SNRIs), 293
sertraline (Zoloft), 293
sex
    anal, 100–101, 113
    arousal. *see* arousal
    bladder infections and, 318
    casual, 76b
    counseling, 92

dysfunction, 93
education, 75b–76b
extramarital, 133
first time, 56
foreplay, 85–86, 87–88
hysterectomy and, 98–99
insomnia and, 272
intimacy and, 96
libido, 93, 96–98, 275–77, 282, **375**
lubrication, 85–86, 87–88
mastectomy and, 259
menopause and, 274–75, 275–77,
        278–79
oral, 99–100, 113, 119, 123, 132
orgasms, 90–93
painful. *see* painful sex
partners, 116b, 118, 131
surgery, after, 352–53
teens and, 75b–76b
sexual abuse, 87, 89–90
sexual dysfunction, 93
sexually transmitted infections. *see* STIs
shaving, 232
shingles, 247
shock, 162
shoulder pain, 162, 362
shrimp, *302*
SIL (squamous intraepithelial lesion). *see*
        HSIL, LSIL, **379**
sildenafil (Viagra), 93
Silent Sorrow: Pregnancy Loss, 161
silicone, 243, **379**
silicone gel sheets, 341
simethicone, 48
single port laparoscopy, 362
sitz bath, 123, 231–32, 233
skin biopsy, 87
skin cancer, 238
skin glands, 232
Skyla, 73, 74
sleep apnea, 271
sleep disorder medication, 65
sleep problems, 271–73
sleep specialist, 273
smoking
    breast tenderness and, 241
    cervical atypia and, 204
    cervical cancer and, 209

fertility and, 149
infertility and, 145
insomnia and, 272
minipill and, 68
miscarriage and, 160
oral contraception and, 63, 63b
osteoporosis and, 300
pelvic prolapse and, 331
VIN and, 236
snacks, 26, 272
sneezing, 314
snoring, 271
SNRIs (serotonin–norepinephrine
        reuptake inhibitors), 293
soap, 87, 102
soda. *see* caffeine
sonohysterogram, 142
sonohysterosalpingogram, 142
sour cream, 52
sourdough bread, 52
Southampton Psychiatric Associates, xxix
soy, 149, 294
speculum, 14, 44, 141, **379**
sperm, 83, 138, *143*, 144, 147
sperm count, 136, 144, 146, 149
spermicide, 58, 60, 61, 103, **379**
spicy food, 298, 310, 324
spinach, *302*
spinal anesthesia, **379**
spirometry, **379**
sponge, vaginal, 58
spontaneous abortion. *see* miscarriage, **379**
sports, 27, 352
sprays, 102
sprouts, 294
squamous cell hyperplasia, 103, 236
squamous intraepithelial lesion (SIL). *see*
        HSIL, LSIL, **379**
Sreophene (clomiphene citrate), 139, 142,
        151–52, **368**
SSRIs (selective serotonin reuptake
        inhibitors), 50–51, 93, 271,
        293–94
St. John's wort, 49–50, 66, 150, 296
Staphylococcus aureus, 55
*Staying Dry: A Practical Guide to Bladder
        Control*, 311
STDs. *see* STIs

stent, 143
step climbing, 303
stereotactic core biopsy, 256
stereotaxis, **379**
sterilization, 77, 80–84, **379**
steroids, 113, 234, 300
stillbirth, 118
STIs (sexually transmitted infections)
    anal sex, 101
    chlamydia, 113, 114, 115, 130,
        368
    chronic, 130–31
    condoms and, 60, 76, 116b, 118, 121
    defined, **379**
    education, 76b
    emotional impact, 132–34
    genital warts. *see* genital warts
    gonorrhea, 113, 114, 115, 130, **373**
    hepatitis, 128–29
    herpes. *see* herpes
    HPV. *see* HPV
    infertility and, 145
    IUDs and, 73
    multiple, 130
    oral sex and, 99, 123
    painful sex and, 86
    pelvic pain, 32
    PID and, 113, 114, 115
    prevention, 131–32
    quiz on, 109b–10b
    relationships and, 133
    screening, 116b, 118, 121, 130
    stigma, 132–33
    support groups, 134
    syphilis, 86, 117–18
    treatment, 130–31
stomach, 32
stress
    headaches and, 53
    herpes and, 124
    IC/PBS and, 324
    insomnia and, 272
    menopause and, 298
    menstrual cycle and, 39
    midlife and, 277–78
    ovulation and, 139
    PMS and, 50
    sex and, 90–91, 91

stress incontinence, 314, 314–17, 333–34, **379**
strokes
    bladder and, 310
    calcium supplements and, 302
    hormone replacement therapy and, 280, 283
    oral contraception and, 63
    SERMs and, 298
submucous, **379**
Sudafed (pseudoephedrine), 316
sugar, 49, 50, 106, 172
sumatripan (Imitrex), 52
superficial phlebitis, 245
supplements. *see also* herbs
    breast cancer and, 249, 250
    breast tenderness, 49, 241, 290
    calcium, 301–2
    cramps, 45
    disclaimer, xxv–xxvi
    estrogen, 53
    fertility and, 150
    heavy flow, 43
    menopause, 294–98
    pain, 36
    PMS, 49
    weight loss, 29
support, emotional, 36
support groups, 128, 134, 174, 268
supracervical hysterectomy, 354–55, **379**
suprapubic catheter, **380**
surgeons, 32
surgery
    abdominal, 338–39
    anesthesia, 346–48
    complications, 338–342
    fear of, 343b–45b
    hospital stays, 345
    infertility, 142
    laparoscopic. *see* laparoscopy
    nausea, 349–350
    pain medication, 348–49
    reconstructive, 334–35
    restrictions after, 352–53
    robotic, 353–54
    safety, 362–63
    tubal pregnancy, 164–65
    USI, 316

weight loss, 30
work leave, 350–51
sweat glands, 118, 232, 233
sweats. *see* night sweats
swelling, 48
Synarel, 170, 180
syphilis, 86, 117–18
Syracuse Medical Devices, 87

T

talcs, 102
tamoxifen
    vs. aromastase inhibitors, 264
    breast cancer and, 250, 252, 263
    breast tenderness, 242
    defined, **380**
    endometrial cancer and, 193
    LCIS and, 267
    metastatic cancer, 267
    SSRIs and, 293–94
tampons, 54–55
    bladder control and, 316
    irritation and, 103, 203
TCA (trichloroacetic acid), 119, **380**
tea, 49, 51, 241, 272, 310
technicians, 15, 18
teens
    calcium intake, 301
    gynecologists and, 8
    sex and, 56
    sex education, 75b–76b
    sexual development, 54
Tegretol (carbamazepine), 65, 235
television, 16–17, 27, 272
tenderness, breast. *see* breast tenderness
TENS (transcutaneous electrical nerve stimulation), 36, 325
Tensie's story, 226b–27b
teratogenic, **380**
Terazol, 107
teriparatide (Forteo), 306, 307
testes, 83
testosterone
    infertility and, 145
    libido and, 97–98, 275–76, 282
    mood changes, 278, 282
    vulvodynia and, 234

tetracycline, 65
therapists, 36, 128, 268, 277
thermography, 20
thighs, 91
Thiosinaminum 5C, 341
Thornton, R. Scott, xxix
threatened abortion, **380**
throat, 119
thrombophlebitis, 263, **380**
thyroid disease, 40, 145, 149, 160
thyroid replacement, 301
tibolone, 299–300
Tindamax (tinidazole), 112
tinidazole (Tindamax), 112
tiredness. *see* fatigue
tissue, **380**
tobacco. *see* smoking
tofu, 294
toilet paper, 87, 102
tomatoes, 310, 324
tomosynthesis, 21
toothbrushes, 128, 129
tooth brushing, 132
Topamax (topiramate), 29, 65
topiramate (Topamax), 29, 65
torsion, 215, 217, **380**
TOT sling procdure, 316, 317
toxic shock syndrome (TSS), 54–55
toxoplasmosis, 159
tranexamic acid (Lysteda), 180, 189
trans fat, 25
transcutaneous electrical nerve stimulation
    (TENS), 36, 325
transdermal. *see* patches
transobturator procdure, 316
transvaginal procdure, 316
trastuzumab (Herceptin), 263, 267
Treximet, 52
triathlons, 149
Tribulus, 150
trichloroacetic acid (TCA), 119, **380**
trichomonas, **380**
trichomoniasis, 112
triglycerides, 214, 283, **380**
Trileptal (oxcarbazepine), 65
Trimo-San, 331
"triple negative" breast cancers, 251, 252
triptans, 52

tryptophan, 50
TSS (toxic shock syndrome), 54–55
tubal ligation, 220
tubal pregnancy
    defined, **380**
    explained, 161–62
    infertility and, 142
    medication, 164–65
    pain and, 163–64
    picture, *161*
    PID and, 113
    pregnancy after, 165
    surgery, 164–65
tubal reanastomosis, 82, 143
tubal sterilization, 77, 80–81, 82–83,
        351, 353
tumors
    "boderline," 225
    breast, 246
    defined, 219–220, **380**
    Depo-Provera, 72
    ER-, 262
    ER+, 262
    genital, 231, 232
    ovarian, 89, 114, 214, 220, 223, 359
    pituitary, 248
turnip greens, *302*
turnips, 250
TVT sling procedure, 316, 317
twins, 139, 140
Tylenol. *see* acetaminophen

U

ulcerations, 103, 113, 118, 131, 237b
ulcers, 32
ulipristal acetate (Ella), 70, 180
ultrasound
    adenomyosis, 189
    bladder infection, 321
    breast, 20, 21–22, 245
    cervical cancer, 210
    chronic pain, 34
    defined, **380**
    endometrial cancer, 193
    fibroids, 179, 185
    heavy flow, 43
    infertility, 142

intermenstrual bleeding, 44
IUDs and, 75
luteal development, 141
menstrual pain, 46
nipple discharge, 249
ovarian cancer and, 221–22
ovarian cysts, 213, 218, 219
ovulatory dysfunction, 139
pain, 34
painful sex, 89
polyps, 188
teens and, 8
tubal pregnancy, 164
underwear
boils and, 233
infertility and, 145
irritation and, 87, 102, 103
yeast infections and, 106
United States Pharmacopeia, xxv
Univeristy of Michigan, 150
University of Pennsylvania School of
        Medicine, xxix
Urelle, 325
ureters, 35, 178, 179, **380**
urethra
defined, 12, **380**
diverticulum, 318
fibroids and, 178
infection, 88
picture, *15*
PID and, 113
self-exam, 236b
sphincter, 316–17
urethral meatus, 14, *15*, **380**
urethral pressure profile, 320–21, **381**
urethritis, 88
Urex (methenamine), 318
urgency incontinence, 309–10, **380**
Uribel, 325
urinalysis, 117
urinary diversion, 326
urinary retention, 342, **380**
urinary stress incontinence (USI), 314,
        314–17, 333–34, **379**
urinary tract infection (UTIs). *see also*
        bladder infection
alternative treatments, 319
IC/PBS and, 324

painful sex and, 88–89
spermicide and, 61
surgery and, 342
urination
bladder surgery and, 360–61
coughing and, 314
difficult, 210
frequent, 89, 117, 168, 178, 211, 323
laughing and, 314
overactive bladder
overnight, 312–13
painful, 89, 113, 117, 123
stress incontinence, 314, 314–17,
        333–34, **379**
urgency incontinence, 309–10, **380**
urgent, 89, 117, 168, 178, 211, 323
urine, 12, 117, 168. *see also* urination
urine culture, 117, 317
Uristat, 317
urogynecologists, 335
urologists
bladder infections, 117
bladder infections and, 318
male infertility, 145
STI screening, 116b, 121, 131
urgency incontinence, 310
USI (urinary stress incontinence), 314,
        314–17, 333–34, **379**
USP (United States Pharmacopeia), xxv
uterine artery embolization, 185, 190
uterine descensus, 328, **381**
uterus
adenomyosis, 189
arousal and, 91
defined, 11, **381**
descended. *see* pelvic prolapse
endometriosis and, 167
fibroids. *see* fibroids
heavy flow and, 43
infection, 32, 43–44, 74, 89
orgasm and, 92
picture, *13, 38, 161*
PID and, 113
polyps, 43, 46, 142, 187–88, 232
removal. *see* hysterectomy
shape, unusual, 142, 159
UTIs (urinary tract infection). *see also*
        bladder infection

alternative treatments, 319
    IC/PBS and, 324
    painful sex and, 88–89
    spermicide and, 61
    surgery and, 342
uva ursi, 319

V

vaccines, 121, 128, 129
vagina
    arousal and, 91
    atrophy, 264, 274–75, 330
    bacteria, 108
    cancer of, 119, 238–39
    cones, 315
    cysts, 88, 231–32
    defined, 12, **381**
    dilators, 87, 88, 89
    discharge, 111–13, 113, 331
    dryness, 86, 98, 170, 274–75, 281,
        293
    erogenous, 91
    G-spot, 95, 100, **373**
    HPV, 119
    hysterectomy and, 98
    infections, 102
    inflammation, 86, 113
    itchy, 102–4
    lesions, 43
    "lips." *see* labia
    lubrication, 85–86, 91, 97, 275
    lumps, 231–32
    orgasm and, 92
    pain in, 32
    picture, *13, 15, 38*
    polyps, 231, 232
    scarring, 89
    self-exam, 236b
    spasms, 87
    sponge, 58
    syphilis, 117
    ulcerations, 103, 113
    vault suspension, 333, **378**
    vestibule. *see* vestibule
    warts, 231
vaginal atrophy, 264, 274–75, 330
vaginal dilators, 87, 88, 89

vaginal discharge, 111–13, 113, 331
vaginal polyps, 231, 232
vaginal sponge, 58
vaginal vault suspension, 333, **378**
vaginismus, 87, **381**
vaginitis, 32, 86, **381**
Vagisil Intimate Moisturizer, 275
Vagistat-1, 107
valacyclovir (Valtrex), 122b, 123, 125, 131
Valtrex (valacyclovir), 122b, 123, 125, 131
vaporization. *see* lasers, **381**
varicose veins, 145
vas deferens, 83, **381**
vascular disease, 63b
vasectomy, 77, 83–84
Vaseline, 86
VD (venereal disease). *see* STIs
vegetables, 25, 49, 172, 249–250, 294
vegetarian diet, 45
veneral disease. *see* STIs
veneral warts. *see* genital warts, **381**
venlafaxine (Effexor), 293, 294
vestibule
    cysts, 88
    defined, 14, **381**
    inflammation, 88
    painful, 234
    picture, *15, 38*
    vulvar cancer and, 237
vestibulitis. *see* vulvar vestibulitis
Viagra (sildenafil), 93
vibrators, 101
VIN (vulvar inrapithelial neoplasia),
    236–37, **381**
vinegar, 206
virgins, 55
vitamin A, 150, 172
vitamin B1, 45
vitamin B6, 45, 49, 150
vitamin B12, 150
vitamin C, 150, 172, 297, 319
vitamin D, 45, 249, 302, 303
vitamin E
    breast tenderness, 49, 241, 290
    cramps, 45
    endometriosis, 172
    fertility and, 150
    menopause, 296–97

surgical scars, 341
Vitex, 150
Vivag, 108
voiding cystourethrogram, 320, **381**
vomiting
    chemotherapy, 263
    emergency contraception and, 70
    with headaches, 51
    misoprostol, 79
    with pain, 31
    PID and, 113
    tamoxifen, 263
vulva
    biopsy, 236–37, 237
    cancer of. *see* vulvar cancer
    cysts, 232
    defined, 12, **381**
    dystrophy, 103
    HPV and, 119, 120
    infections, 102, 236
    inflammation, 86–87
    pain, 234–35
    pain in, 32
    picture, *13*, *15*
    removal, 237, 238
    vestibulitis, 88, 234
    VIN, 236–37, **381**
    vulvodynia, 234–35
vulvar biopsy, 236–37, 237
vulvar cancer
    HPV and, 119
    lumps and, 231
    Pap smears and, 16
    resources, 239
    treatment, 237–38
    VIN and, 237
    yeast infections and, 104
vulvar dystrophy, 103
vulvar inrapithelial neoplasia (VIN),
    236–37, **381**
Vulvar Pain Foundation, 235
vulvar vestibulitis, 88, 234, **381**
vulvectomy, 237, 238, **381**
vulvitis, 86–87
vulvodynia, 234–35, 323

W

walking, 27, 303

warts
    genital. *see* genital warts
    laryngeal, 120
    self-exam, 237b
    sexual partners, 131
    vaginal, 231
water, 26, 43, 324
"water pill" (diuretic), 48, 50, 301, 310,
    313, **370**
weight
    breast cancer and, 249
    breast tenderness and, 242
    Depo-Provera, 72, 171
    diet and excersize, 24–27
    fertility and, 149
    hormone replacement therapy and, 291
    medications for, 28–29
    menopause and, 293
    menstrual cycle and, 39
    miscarriage and, 160
    oral contraception and, 65
    OSA and, 271
    ovulation and, 139
    pelvic prolapse and, 331
    surgery, 30
weightlifting, 303
Weil, Andrew, xxvi
Wellbutrin (bupropion), 29, 93
wheat, 149, 172
WHI (Women's Health Initiative), 280–
    81, 287, 288
whipped cream, 132
white willow bark, 36
WHO (World Health Organization), 61
whole grains, 49
withdrawal, 60
Wobenzym, 36
Women's Health Initiative (WHI), 280–
    81, 287, 288
Women's Health Seminars, xxix
Wong, Cathy, xxvi
work leave, 350–51
working, 268
World Health Organization (WHO), 61

X

Xenical (orlistat, Alli), 29
x-rays, 18, 34, 142, 202, 308

Y

yams, 50, 150, 297
Yaz, 51
yeast, **381**
yeast infections
    atypical, 107
    causes, 105–6
    danger, 106
    diagnosing, 104–5
    discharge from, 111
    itchy, 102
    medication, 107–8
    misdiagnosed, 234
    natural treatments, 108–9
    painful sex and, 86
    preventing, 106
    probiotics and, 108
    self-treatment, 104b
    spermicide and, 61
    testing, 107–8
    yogurt and, 108
yoga
    bladder control and, 315
    insomnia and, 272

menopause and, 298
PMS and, 50
weight and, 27
yogurt, 108, *302*
yohimbine, 93
youth oriented, 278

Z

ZIFT (zygote intrafallopian transfer), 143,
    381
zinc, 125, 150
Zoladex, 170
zoledronic acid (Reclast), 268, 305
zolmitriptan (Zomig), 52
Zoloft (sertraline), 293
Zometa, 268
Zomig (zolmitripan), 52
zonisamide, 29
Zovirax (acyclovir), 123, 125
Zyclara (Imiquimod), 119–120, 236, 341
zygote intrafallopian transfer (ZIFT), 143,
    381